D1760196

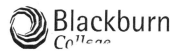

Nutrition and Football

The benefits of good nutrition to the health and performance of players and officials at all levels of the game of soccer are widely recognised, and optimal nutrition is now a key strategy in the preparation of top teams. Covering the significant advances made in soccer-specific research and practice in recent years, this book presents the first formal scientific consensus on nutrition for the game. It includes:

- Analysis of the physical and metabolic demands of training and match-play
- Nutrition for training, competition and recovery, and for coping with different conditions
- Strategies to counter the effects on the immune system of intensive training and competition
- Water and electrolyte needs
- Dietary supplements
- The effects of alcohol on performance and recovery
- The role of the brain in fatigue, and nutritional interventions to combat late-game fatigue
- Nutrition for female and youth players, and for officials.

Written by leading international researchers and practitioners, and covering all key aspects of nutrition for soccer, this book provides scientists and professionals with an accessible guide to a rapidly developing field.

Ron Maughan is Professor of Sport and Exercise Nutrition at Loughborough University and Chair of the Nutrition Working Group of the International Olympic Committee.

Nutrition and Football

The FIFA/FMARC Consensus on Sports Nutrition

Edited by R.J. Maughan

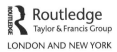

Routledge
Taylor & Francis Group

LONDON AND NEW YORK

First published 2007
by Routledge
2 Park Square, Milton Park, Abingdon, Oxon OX14 4RN

Simultaneously published in the USA and Canada
by Routledge
270 Madison Ave, New York, NY 10016

Routledge is an imprint of the Taylor & Francis Group, an informa business

© 2007 Ron Maughan for editorial material and selection.
Individual chapters the contributors

Typeset in Goudy by BC Typesetting Ltd, Bristol

British Library Cataloguing in Publication Data
A catalogue record for this book is available from the British Library

Library of Congress Cataloging in Publication Data
Nutrition and football : the FIFA/FMARC consensus on sports nutrition/
    edited by Ron Maughan. – 1st ed.
    p.   cm.
    Includes bibliographical references and index.
    ISBN-13: 978-0-415-41229-2 (hardback)
    ISBN-10: 0-415-41229-3 (hardback)
    1. Soccer players–Nutrition. I. Maughan, Ron J., 1951–
    TX361.S58N88 2006
    613.202'4796334–dc22
    2006019597

ISBN 10: 0-415-41229-3 (hbk)
ISBN 10: 0-203-96743-7 (ebk)
ISBN 13: 978-0-415-41229-2 (hbk)
ISBN 13: 978-0-203-96743-0 (ebk)

Contents

List of contributors

Lawrence Armstrong, Human Performance Laboratory, Departments of Kinesiology and Nutritional Sciences, University of Connecticut, Storrs, CT, USA

Jens Bangsbo, Institute of Exercise and Sport Sciences, University of Copenhagen, Copenhagen Muscle Research Centre, Copenhagen, Denmark

Nicolette Bishop, School of Sport and Exercise Sciences, Loughborough University, Loughborough, UK

Nick Broad, Birmingham City Football Club, Birmingham and Blackburn Rovers Football Club, Blackburn, UK

Louise Burke, Department of Sports Nutrition, Australian Institute of Sport, Canberra, ACT, Australia, and School of Nutrition and Exercise Sciences, Deakin University, Melbourne, VIC, Australia

Jiri Dvorak, Department of Neurology and FIFA Medical Assessment and Research Centre (F-MARC), Schulthess Clinic, Zurich, Switzerland

Bjorn Ekblom, Department of Physiology and Pharmacology, Karolinska Institute, Stockholm, Sweden

Paul Greenhaff, Centre for Integrated Systems Biology and Medicine, School of Biomedical Sciences, University of Nottingham Medical School, Queen's Medical Centre, Nottingham, UK

Warren Gregson, Research Institute for Sport and Exercise Sciences, Liverpool John Moores University, Liverpool, UK

John Hawley, School of Medical Sciences, RMIT University, Bundoora, VIC, Australia

Peter Hespel, Exercise and Health Laboratory, Faculty of Kinesiology and Rehabilitation Sciences, Katholieke Universiteit Leuven, Leuven, Belgium

Peter Krustrup, Institute of Exercise and Sport Sciences, University of Copenhagen, Copenhagen Muscle Research Centre, Copenhagen, Denmark

Anne Loucks, Department of Biological Sciences, Ohio University, Athens, OH, USA

Ron Maughan, School of Sport and Exercise Sciences, Loughborough University, Loughborough, UK

Romain Meeusen, Department of Human Physiology and Sports Medicine, Faculty of Physical Education and Physiotherapy, Vrije Universiteit Brussel, Brussels, Belgium

Mindy Millard-Stafford, Exercise Physiology Laboratory, School of Applied Physiology, Georgia Institute of Technology, Atlanta, GA, USA

Magni Mohr, Institute of Exercise and Sport Sciences, University of Copenhagen, Copenhagen Muscle Research Centre, Copenhagen, Denmark

David Nieman, Department of Health and Exercise Science, Appalachian State University, Boone, NC, USA

Tom Reilly, Research Institute for Sport and Exercise Sciences, Liverpool John Moores University, Liverpool, UK

Chris Rosenbloom, College of Health and Human Sciences, Georgia State University, Atlanta, GA, USA

Mike Sawka, Thermal and Mountain Medicine Division, US Army Research Institute of Environmental Medicine, Natick, MA, USA

Luis Serratosa, Department of Sports Medicine, Real Madrid Football Club, Madrid, Spain

Susan Shirreffs, School of Sport and Exercise Sciences, Loughborough University, Loughborough, UK

Mike Stone, Manchester United Football Club, Manchester, UK

Kevin Tipton, School of Sport and Exercise Sciences, University of Birmingham, Birmingham, UK

Phil Watson, School of Sport and Exercise Sciences, Loughborough University, Loughborough, UK

Clyde Williams, School of Sport and Exercise Sciences, Loughborough University, Loughborough, UK

Introduction

In 1993, a small group of experts gathered at FIFA house in Zurich, Switzerland, to discuss the role of nutrition in the performance of soccer players. Their discussions, under the guidance of Professors Clyde Williams and Bjorn Ekblom, represented the state of knowledge in the field at that time, and their recommendations were widely applied throughout the game. Indeed, the suggestion that players would benefit from better access to fluids during matches led to a change in the rules relating to the provision of drinks during games. One recurring theme throughout those discussions was the limited information specific to the game of soccer – in many cases, extrapolation had to be made from laboratory studies of cycling or running, usually involving exercise at constant power output. The inadequacies of this information were clearly recognized. Nonetheless, the information generated at this meeting was widely disseminated and was used by many players, clubs and national teams as the basis of their nutritional strategies.

Since that meeting, a lot of new information has emerged, much of it using exercise models that are more representative of the game of soccer. Intermittent shuttle running tests of various descriptions have been used to simulate activity patterns of players in competition, and soccer-specific skills tests have been used to evaluate performance after various nutritional interventions. New techniques, such as remote monitoring of heart rate and body temperature, have allowed the assessment of physiological strain with much better time resolution than before, while computerized motion analysis systems and the use of GPS technology have refined the study of movement patterns of individual players.

Completely new areas of study have emerged, including the application of molecular biology to assess the role of diet in modulating and promoting the adaptations taking place in muscle in response to training. There has been a growing recognition that the stress of frequent competition, especially in the top players, where games for club and country impose special demands, can lead to a greater risk of illness and under-performance. Again, the foods that a player chooses will influence their ability to cope with these demands. It is also increasingly recognized that the brain plays a vital role in the fatigue process, and strategies that target this central fatigue can help sustain performance, especially in the later stages of the game when deterioration in function can affect the match outcome and also the risk of injury.

Recognizing these new developments, another Consensus Conference was convened at FIFA House at the end of August 2005. With the support of FIFA and F-MARC (the FIFA Medical Assessment and Research Centre), a group of international experts spent three days reviewing the evidence relating to nutrition and soccer. Their discussions resulted in the preparation of a short Consensus Statement. The evidence on which that statement is based is presented here as a series of scientific papers, each subjected to the scrutiny of the assembled experts.

From the information presented, it was clear that the nutritional goals of soccer players at every level of the game can be achieved by using normal foods. It was also very clear that the foods that a player chooses will influence the effectiveness of the training programme, and can also decide the outcome of matches. A varied diet, eaten in amounts sufficient to meet the energy needs, should supply the whole range of essential nutrients in adequate amounts. In a few exceptional situations, the targeted use of a few supplements may be necessary, as, for example, in the case of iron-deficiency anaemia where iron supplements may meet the short-term need while an appropriate dietary solution is identified and implemented. The conference also recognized that there are special needs of the female player and of the young player, and recognized too that more information on these special populations is urgently needed. The needs of the referees were not forgotten, and the importance of the decisions made by the referee, especially late in the game when some fatigue is inevitable, was highlighted.

RON MAUGHAN, *Loughborough University*
MICHEL D'HOOGHE, *Chairman, FIFA Sports Medical Committee*
JIRI DVORAK, *Chairman, F-MARC*

Consensus Statement

Nutrition for football:
The FIFA/F-MARC Consensus Conference

Soccer players can remain healthy, avoid injury and achieve their performance goals by adopting good dietary habits. Players should choose foods that support consistent, intensive training and optimize match performance. What a player eats and drinks in the days and hours before a game, as well as during the game itself, can influence the result by reducing the effects of fatigue and allowing players to make the most of their physical and tactical skills. Food and fluid consumed soon after a game and training can optimize recovery. All players should have a nutrition plan that takes account of individual needs.

The energetic and metabolic demands of soccer training and match-play vary across the season, with the standard of competition and with individual characteristics. The typical energy costs of training or match-play in elite players are about 6 MJ (1500 kcal) per day for men and about 4 MJ (1000 kcal) per day for women. Soccer players should eat a wide variety of foods that provide sufficient carbohydrate to fuel the training and competition programme, meet all nutrient requirements, and allow manipulation of energy or nutrient balance to achieve changes in lean body mass, body fat or growth. Low energy availability causes disturbances to hormonal, metabolic and immune function, as well as bone health. An adequate carbohydrate intake is the primary strategy to maintain optimum function. Players may require 5–7 g of carbohydrate per kilogram of body mass during periods of moderate training, rising to about $10 \, \mathrm{g \cdot kg^{-1}}$ during intense training or match-play.

Nutritional interventions that modify the acute responses to endurance, sprint and resistance training have the potential to influence chronic training adaptations. The everyday diet should promote strategic intake of carbohydrate and protein before and after key training sessions to optimize adaptation and enhance recovery. The consumption of solid or liquid carbohydrate should begin during the first hour after training or match-play to speed recovery of glycogen. Consuming food or drinks that contain protein at this time could promote recovery processes.

Match-day nutrition needs are influenced by the time since the last training session or game. Players should try to ensure good hydration status before kick-off and take opportunities to consume carbohydrate and fluids before and after the game according to their nutrition plan. Fatigue impairs both physical and mental performance, but the intake of carbohydrate and other nutrients can reduce the negative effects of fatigue. Training for and playing soccer lead to sweat loss even in cool environments. Failure to replace water and electrolyte losses can lead to fatigue and the impaired performance of skilled tasks. Breaks in play currently provide opportunities for carbohydrate and fluid intake, and may not be adequate in some conditions. Soccer is a team sport, but the variability in players' seating responses dictates that monitoring to determine individual requirements should be an essential part of a player's hydration and nutrition strategy.

There is no evidence to support the current widespread use of dietary supplements in soccer, and so the indiscriminate use of such supplements is strongly discouraged. Supplements should only be taken based on the advice of a qualified sports nutrition professional.

Female players should ensure that they eat foods rich in calcium and iron within their energy budget. Young players have specific energy and nutrient requirements to promote growth and development, as well as fuelling the energy needs of their sport. Many female and youth players need to increase their carbohydrate intake and develop dietary habits that will sustain the demands of training and competition.

Players may be at increased risk of illness during periods of heavy training and stress. For several hours after heavy exertion, the components of both the innate and adaptive immune system exhibit suppressed function. Carbohydrate supplementation during heavy exercise has emerged as a partial countermeasure.

Heat, cold, high altitude and travel across time zones act as stressors that alter normal physiological function, homeostasis, metabolism and whole-body nutrient balance. Rather than accepting performance decrements as inevitable, well-informed coaches and athletes should plan strategies for training and competition that offset environmental challenges.

Alcohol is not an essential part of the human diet. Recovery and all aspects of performance could be impaired for some time after the consumption of alcohol. Binge drinking should be avoided at all times.

The needs of the referee and assistant referee are often overlooked, but high standards of fitness and decision making are expected of all officials. At every standard of competition, training regimens and nutritional strategies, including fluid intake during the game, should be similar to those followed by players.

Talent and dedication to training are no longer enough to ensure success in soccer. Good nutrition has much to offer players and match officials, including improved performance, better health and enjoyment of a wide range of foods.

Zurich, 2 September 2005

1 Physical and metabolic demands of training and match-play in the elite football player

JENS BANGSBO, MAGNI MOHR AND
PETER KRUSTRUP

In soccer, the players perform intermittent work. Despite the players performing low-intensity activities for more than 70% of the game, heart rate and body temperature measurements suggest that the average oxygen uptake for elite soccer players is around 70% of maximum ($\dot{V}O_{2max}$). This may be partly explained by the 150–250 brief intense actions a top-class player performs during a game, which also indicates that the rates of creatine phosphate (CP) utilization and glycolysis are frequently high during a game. Muscle glycogen is probably the most important substrate for energy production, and fatigue towards the end of a game may be related to depletion of glycogen in some muscle fibres. Blood free-fatty acids (FFAs) increase progressively during a game, partly compensating for the progressive lowering of muscle glycogen. Fatigue also occurs temporarily during matches, but it is still unclear what causes the reduced ability to perform maximally. There are major individual differences in the physical demands of players during a game related to physical capacity and tactical role in the team. These differences should be taken into account when planning the training and nutritional strategies of top-class players, who require a significant energy intake during a week.

Keywords: Match-play activity pattern, substrate utilization, muscle metabolites, fatigue, recovery after matches, training intensity

Introduction

Since the last FIFA conference on nutrition in soccer in 1994, soccer at the elite level has developed and much research regarding match performance and training has been conducted. It is also clear that science has been incorporated to a greater extent in the planning and execution of training. Earlier scientific studies focused on the overall physiological demands of the game, for example by performing physiological measurements before and after the game or at half-time. As a supplement to such information, some recent studies have examined changes in both performance and physiological responses throughout the game with a special focus on the most demanding activities and periods. New technology has made it possible to study changes in match performance with a high time resolution. Another aspect to have received attention in practical training is information regarding individual differences in the physical demands to which players are exposed in games and training. These differences are not only related to the training status of the players and their playing position, but also to their specific tactical roles. Thus, some top-class clubs have integrated the tactical and physical demands of the players into their fitness training.

This review addresses information on the demands of the game at a top-class level and provides insights into training at the elite level. Thus, it should form the basis for deciding nutritional strategies for these players. The review deals mainly with male players, but at relevant points information about female players is provided.

Match activities

Many time–motion analyses of competitive games have been performed since the first analysis of activities in the 1960s (Bangsbo, 1994; Bangsbo, Nørregaard, & Thorsøe, 1991; Krustrup, Mohr, Ellingsgaard, & Bangsbo, 2005; Mayhew & Wenger, 1985; Mohr, Krustrup, & Bangsbo, 2003; Reilly & Thomas, 1979; Rienzi, Drust, Reilly, Carter, & Martin, 1998; Van Gool, Van Gerven, & Boutmans, 1988). The typical distance covered by a top-class outfield player during a match is 10–13 km, with midfield players covering greater distances than other outfield players. However, most of this distance is covered by walking and low-intensity running, which require a limited energy turnover. In terms of energy production, the high-intensity exercise periods are important. Thus, it is clear that the amount of high-intensity exercise separates top-class players from players of a lower standard. In one study, computerized time–motion analysis demonstrated that international players performed 28% more ($P < 0.05$) high-intensity running (2.43 vs. 1.90 km) and 58% more sprinting (650 vs. 410 m) than professional players of a lower standard (Mohr *et al.*, 2003). It should be emphasized that the recordings of high-intensity running do not include a number of energy-demanding activities such as short accelerations, tackling, and jumping. The number of tackles and jumps depends on the individual playing style and position in the team, and at the highest level has been shown to vary between 3 and 27 and between 1 and 36, respectively (Mohr *et al.*, 2003). Most studies have used video analysis followed by manual computer analysis to examine individual performance during a match. New developments in technology have allowed the study of all 22 players during each one-sixth of a second throughout a match, and the systems are used by many top teams in Europe. There are reasons to believe that in the future such systems will provide significant additional information and will soon find their way into scientific research. For example, using a high time resolution, Bangsbo and Mohr (2005) recently examined fluctuations in high-intensity exercise, running speeds, and recovery time from sprints during several top-class soccer matches. They found that sprinting speed in games reached peak values of around $32 \, \text{km} \cdot \text{h}^{-1}$ and that sprints over more than 30 m demanded markedly longer recovery than the average sprints (10–15 m) during a game.

There are major individual differences in the physical demands of players, in part related to his position in the team. A number of studies have compared playing positions (Bangsbo, 1994; Bangsbo *et al.*, 1991; Ekblom, 1986; Reilly & Thomas, 1979). In a study of top-class players, Mohr *et al.* (2003) found that the central defenders covered less overall distance and performed less high-intensity running than players in the other positions, which probably is closely linked to the tactical roles of the central defenders and their lower physical capacity (Bangsbo, 1994; Mohr *et al.*, 2003). The full-backs covered a considerable distance at a high-intensity and by sprinting, whereas they performed fewer headers and tackles than players in the other playing positions. The attackers covered a distance at a high intensity equal to the full-backs and midfield players, but sprinted more than the midfield players and defenders. Furthermore, Mohr *et al.* (2003) showed that the attackers had a more marked decline in sprinting distance than the defenders and midfield players. In addition, the performance of the attackers on the Yo-Yo intermittent recovery test was not as good as that of the full-backs and midfield players. Thus, it would appear that the modern top-class attacker needs to be able to perform high-intensity actions repeatedly throughout a game.

The midfield players performed as many tackles and headers as defenders and attackers. They covered a total distance and distance at a high-intensity similar to the full-backs and attackers, but sprinted less. Previous studies have shown that midfield players cover a greater distance during a game than full-backs and attackers (Bangsbo, 1994; Bangsbo *et al.*, 1991; Ekblom, 1986; Reilly & Thomas, 1979). These differences may be explained by the development of the physical demands of full-backs and attackers, since, in contrast to earlier studies (Bangsbo, 1994), Mohr *et al.* (2003) observed that players in all team positions experienced a significant decline in high-intensity running towards the end of the match. This indicates that almost all elite soccer players utilize their physical capacity during a game. Individual differences are not only related to position in the team. Thus, in the study by Mohr *et al.* (2003), within each playing position there was a significant variation in the physical demands depending on the tactical role and the physical capacity of the players. For example, in the same game, one midfield player covered a total distance of 12.3 km, with 3.5 km being covered at a high intensity, while another midfielder covered a total distance of 10.8, of which 2.0 km was at a high intensity. The individual differences in playing style and physical performance should be taken into account when planning the training and nutritional strategy.

Aerobic energy production in soccer

Soccer is an intermittent sport in which the aerobic energy system is highly taxed, with mean and peak heart rates of around 85 and 98% of maximal values, respectively (Ali & Farrally, 1991; Bangsbo, 1994; Ekblom, 1986; Krustrup *et al.*, 2005; Reilly & Thomas, 1979). These values can be "converted" to oxygen uptake using the relationship between heart rate and oxygen uptake obtained during treadmill running (Bangsbo, 1994; Esposito *et al.*, 2004; Krustrup & Bangsbo, 2001). This appears to be a valid method, since in studies in which heart rate and oxygen uptake (by the so-called K_4 apparatus) have been measured during soccer drills, similar heart rates have been observed for a given oxygen uptake as found during treadmill running (Castagna *et al.*, 2005; Esposito *et al.*, 2004). However, it is likely that the heart rates measured during a match lead to an overestimation of the oxygen uptake, since such factors as dehydration, hyperthermia, and mental stress elevate the heart rate without affecting oxygen uptake. Nevertheless, with these factors taken into account, the heart rate measurements during a game seem to suggest that the average oxygen uptake is around 70% $\dot{V}O_{2max}$. This suggestion is supported by measurements of core temperature during a soccer game. Core temperature is another indirect measurement of energy production during exercise, since a linear relationship has been reported between rectal temperature and relative work intensity (Saltin & Hermansen, 1966). During continuous cycling exercise at 70% $\dot{V}O_{2max}$ with an ambient temperature of 20°C, the rectal temperature was 38.7°C. In soccer, the core temperature increases relatively more compared with the average intensity due to the intermittent nature of the game. Hence, it has been observed that at a relative work rate corresponding to 60% of $\dot{V}O_{2max}$, the core temperature was 0.3°C higher during intermittent than continuous exercise (Ekblom *et al.*, 1971). Nevertheless, core temperatures of 39–40°C during a game suggest that the average aerobic loading during a game is around 70% $\dot{V}O_{2max}$ (Ekblom, 1986; Mohr *et al.*, 2004b; Smodlaka, 1978).

More important for performance than the average oxygen uptake during a game, may be the rate of rise in oxygen uptake during the many short intense actions. A player's heart rate during a game is rarely below 65% of maximum, suggesting that blood flow to the exercising leg muscle is continuously higher than at rest, which means that oxygen delivery is high. However, the oxygen kinetics during the changes from low- to high-intensity exercise during the game appear to be limited by local factors and depend, among other things, on the oxidative capacity of the contracting muscles (Bangsbo *et al.*, 2002; Krustrup, Hellsten, & Bangsbo, 2004a). The rate of rise of oxygen uptake can be changed by intense interval training (Krustrup *et al.*, 2004a).

Anaerobic energy production in soccer

That elite soccer players perform 150–250 brief intense actions during a game (Mohr *et al.*, 2003) indicates that the rate of anaerobic energy turnover is high at certain times. Even though not studied directly, the intense exercise during a game leads to a high rate of creatine phosphate breakdown, which to some extent is resynthesized in the following low-intensity exercise periods (Bangsbo, 1994). On the other hand, creatine phosphate may decline (i.e. below 30% of resting values) during parts of a game if a number of intense bouts are performed with only short recovery periods. Analysis of creatine phosphate in muscle biopsies obtained after intense exercise periods during a game have provided values above 70% of those at rest, but this is likely to be due to the delay in obtaining the biopsy (Krustrup *et al.*, 2006).

Mean blood lactate concentrations of 2–10 mmol·l^{-1} have been observed during soccer games, with individual values above 12 mmol·l^{-1} (Agnevik, 1970; Bangsbo, 1994; Ekblom, 1986; Krustrup *et al.*, 2006). These findings indicate that the rate of muscle lactate production is high during match-play, but muscle lactate has been measured in only a single study. In a friendly game between non-professional teams, it was observed that muscle lactate rose four-fold (to around 15 mmol·kg dry weight^{-1}) compared with resting values after intense periods in both halves, with the highest value being 35 mmol·kg dry weight^{-1} (Krustrup *et al.*, 2006). Such values are less than one-third of the concentrations observed during short-term intermittent exhaustive exercise (Krustrup *et al.*, 2003). An interesting finding in that study was that muscle lactate was not correlated with blood lactate (Figure 1). A scattered relationship with a low correlation coefficient has also been observed between muscle lactate and blood lactate when participants performed repeated intense exercise using the Yo-Yo intermittent recovery test (Krustrup *et al.*, 2003) (Figure 1). This is in contrast to continuous exercise where the blood lactate concentrations are lower but reflect well the muscle lactate concentrations during exercise (Figure 1). These differences between intermittent and continuous exercise are probably due to different turnover rates of muscle lactate and blood lactate during the two type of exercise, with the rate of lactate clearance being significantly higher in muscle than in blood (Bangsbo, Johansen, Graham, & Saltin, 1993). This means that during intermittent exercise in soccer, the blood lactate concentration can be high even though the muscle lactate concentration is

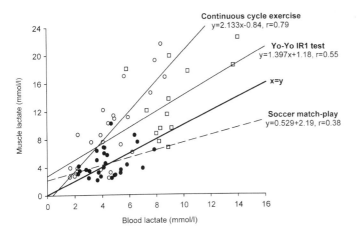

Figure 1. Individual relationships between muscle lactate (expressed in mmol per litre of cell water) and blood lactate during a soccer match (solid circles; data from the present study), at exhaustion in the Yo-Yo intermittent level 1 recovery test (solid squares; data from Krustrup *et al.*, 2003), and after 20 min of continuous cycle exercise at 80% $\dot{V}O_{2max}$ (open circles; data from Krustrup *et al.*, 2004b).

relatively low. The relationship between muscle lactate and blood lactate also appears to be influenced by the activities immediately before sampling (Bangsbo et al., 1991; Krustrup & Bangsbo, 2001). Thus, the rather high blood lactate concentration often seen in soccer (Bangsbo, 1994; Ekblom, 1986; Krustrup et al., 2006) may not represent a high lactate production in a single action during the game, but rather an accumulated/balanced response to a number of high-intensity activities. This is important to take into account when interpreting blood lactate concentration as a measure of muscle lactate concentration. Nevertheless, based on several studies using short-term maximal exercise performed in the laboratory (Gaitanos et al., 1993; Nevill et al., 1989), and the finding of high blood lactate and moderate muscle lactate concentrations during match-play, it is suggested that the rate of glycolysis is high for short periods of time during a game.

Substrate utilization during a soccer match

To provide nutritional strategies for a soccer player it is important to understand the energy demands and which substrates are utilized during a game. Muscle glycogen is an important substrate for the soccer player. Saltin (1973) observed that muscle glycogen stores were almost depleted at half-time when the pre-match values were low ($\sim$200 mmol $\cdot$ kg dry weight^{-1}). In that study, some players also started the game with normal muscle glycogen concentrations ($\sim$400 mmol $\cdot$ kg dry weight^{-1}), with the values still rather high at half-time but below 50 mmol $\cdot$ kg dry weight^{-1} at the end of the game. Others have reported concentrations of $\sim$200 mmol $\cdot$ kg dry weight^{-1} after a match (Jacobs, Westlin, Karlsson, Rasmusson & Houghton, 1982; Krustrup et al., 2006; Smaros 1980), indicating that muscle glycogen stores are not always depleted in a soccer game. However, analyses of single muscle fibres after a game have revealed that a significant number of fibres are depleted or partly depleted at the end of a game (Krustrup et al., 2006; see below).

It has been observed that the concentration of free fatty acids (FFA) in the blood increases during a game, most markedly so during the second half (Bangsbo, 1994; Krustrup et al., 2006). The frequent periods of rest and low-intensity exercise in a game allow for a significant blood flow to adipose tissue, which promotes the release of free fatty acids. This effect is also illustrated by the finding of high FFA concentrations at half-time and after the game. A high rate of lipolysis during a game is supported by elevated glycerol concentrations, even though the increases are smaller than during continuous exercise, which probably reflects a high turnover of glycerol (e.g. as a gluconeogenic precursor in the liver; Bangsbo, 1994). Hormonal changes may play a major role in the progressive increase in the concentrations of free fatty acids. The insulin concentrations are lowered and catecholamine concentrations are progressively elevated during a match (Bangsbo, 1994), stimulating a high rate of lipolysis and thus the release of free fatty acids into the blood (Galbo, 1983). The effect is reinforced by lowered lactate concentrations towards the end of a game, leading to less suppression of mobilization of free fatty acids from the adipose tissue (Bangsbo, 1994; Bülow & Madsen, 1981; Galbo, 1983; Krustrup *et al.*, 2006). The changes in free fatty acids during a match may cause a higher uptake and oxidation of such acids by the contracting muscles, especially during the recovery periods in a game (Turcotte, Kiens, & Richter, 1991). In addition, a higher utilization of muscle triglycerides might occur in the second half due to elevated catecholamine concentrations (Galbo, 1992). Both processes may be compensatory mechanisms for the progressive lowering of muscle glycogen and are favourable in maintaining a high blood glucose concentration.

Fatigue during a soccer game

A relevant question when planning training is when fatigue occurs during a soccer game and what the cause of that fatigue is. Several studies have provided evidence that players' ability to perform high-intensity exercise is reduced towards the end of games in both elite and sub-elite soccer (Krustrup *et al.*, 2006; Mohr *et al.*, 2003, 2004; Mohr, Krustrup, & Bangsbo, 2005; Reilly & Thomas, 1979). Thus, it has been demonstrated that the amount of sprinting, high-intensity running, and distance covered are lower in the second half than in the first half of a game (Bangsbo *et al.*, 1991; Bangsbo, 1994; Mohr *et al.*, 2003; Reilly & Thomas, 1979). Furthermore, it has been observed that the amount of high-intensity running is reduced in the final 15 min of a top-class soccer game (Mohr *et al.*, 2003) and that jumping, sprinting, and intermittent exercise performance is lowered after versus before a soccer game (Mohr *et al.*, 2004b, 2005; Rebelo, 1999) (Figure 2). However, the underlying mechanism behind a reduced exercise performance at the end of a soccer game is unclear. One candidate is depletion of glycogen stores, since development of fatigue during prolonged intermittent exercise has been associated with a lack of muscle glycogen. Moreover, it has been demonstrated that elevating muscle glycogen before prolonged intermittent exercise using a carbohydrate diet elevates performance during such exercise (Balsom, Gaitanos, Söderlund, & Ekblom, 1999; Bangsbo, Nørregaard & Thorsøe, 1992a). Some (Saltin, 1973) but not all (Jacobs *et al.*, 1982; Krustrup *et al.*, 2006; Smaros, 1980) authors have observed that muscle glycogen during a game decreases to values below that required to maintain maximal glycolytic rate ($\sim$200 mmol · kg dry weight^{-1}; Bangsbo *et al.*, 1992b). In a study by Krustrup *et al.* (2006), the muscle glycogen concentration at the end of the game was reduced to 150–350 mmol · kg dry weight^{-1}. Thus, there was still glycogen available. However, histochemical analysis revealed that about half of the individual muscle fibres of both types were almost depleted or depleted of glycogen. This reduction was associated with a decrease in sprint performance immediately after the game. Therefore, it is possible that such a depletion of glycogen in some fibres does not allow for a maximal effort in single and repeated sprints. Nevertheless, it is unclear what the mechanisms are behind the possible causal relationship between muscle glycogen concentration and fatigue during prolonged intermittent exercise.

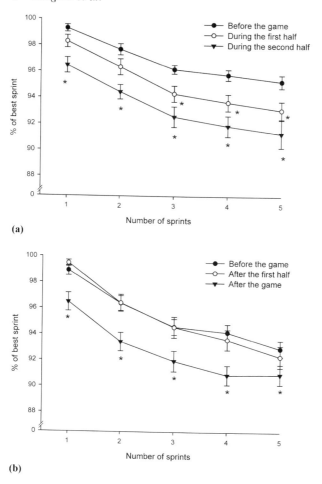

Figure 2. Sprint time (% of the best sprint) of five 30 m sprints separated by a 25 s period of recovery. (a) Before the game (solid circles) and after the first (open circles) and second (solid triangles) half. (b) Before the game (solid circles) and after an intense period in the first (open circles) and second half (solid triangles). Data are means ± standard errors of the mean.

Factors such as dehydration and hyperthermia may also contribute to the development of fatigue in the later stages of a soccer game (Magal *et al.*, 2003; Reilly, 1997). Soccer players have been reported to lose up to 3 litres of fluid during games in temperate thermal environments and as much as 4–5 lires in a hot and humid environment (Bangsbo, 1994; Reilly, 1997), and it has been observed that 5 and 10 m sprint times are slowed by hypohydration amounting to 2.7% of body mass (Magal *et al.*, 2003). However, in the study by Krustrup *et al.* (2006) a significant reduction in sprint performance was observed, although the fluid loss of the players was only about 1% of body mass, and no effect on core or muscle temperature was observed in a study with a similar loss of fluid (Mohr *et al.*, 2004). Thus, it would appear that fluid loss is not always an important component in the impaired performance seen towards the end of a game.

Temporary fatigue during a soccer match

Recent research using computerized time–motion analysis of top-class professional male soccer players has indicated that players become fatigued during a game (Mohr *et al.*, 2003). Thus, in the 5 min following the most intense period of the match, the amount of high-intensity exercise was reduced to levels below the game average. This phenomenon has also been observed in elite women's soccer (unpublished observations). These findings suggest that performance was reduced after a period of intense exercise, which could have been a result of the natural variation in the intensity in a game due to tactical or psychological factors. However, in another study players performed a repeated sprint test immediately after intense match-play and also at the end of each half (Krustrup *et al.*, 2006). It was shown that after intense periods in the first half, the players' sprint performance was significantly reduced, whereas at the end of the first half the ability to perform repeated sprints had recovered (Figure 2). Together, these results suggest that soccer players experience fatigue temporarily during the game.

An interesting question is what causes fatigue during a game of soccer. Fatigue during match-play is a complex phenomenon with a number of contributing factors. One of these may be cerebral in nature, especially during hot conditions (see Meeusen, Watson, & Dvorak, 2006; Nybo & Secher, 2004). However, it has been shown that for well-motivated individuals the cause of fatigue is muscular in nature (Bigland-Ritchie, Furbush, & Woods, 1986). In the study by Krustrup *et al.* (2006), the decrement in performance during the game was related to muscle lactate. However, the relationship was weak and the changes in muscle lactate were moderate. Furthermore, several studies have shown that accumulation of lactate does not cause fatigue (Bangsbo *et al.*, 1992; Krustrup *et al.*, 2003; Mohr *et al.*, 2004a). Another candidate for muscle fatigue during intense exercise is a low muscle pH (Sahlin, 1992). However, muscle pH is only moderately reduced (to about 6.8) during a game and no relationship with lowered performance has been observed (Krustrup *et al.*, 2006). Thus, it is unlikely that elevated muscle lactate and lowered muscle pH cause fatigue during a soccer game. It may be due to low muscle creatine phosphate concentrations, since performance in intense intermittent exercise has been demonstrated to be elevated after a period of creatine supplementation (Balsom, Seger, Sjödin, & Ekblom, 1995; Greenhaff, Bodin, Söderlund, & Hultman, 1994). After intense periods in a soccer game, muscle creatine phosphate has been observed to be lowered by only 25% (Krustrup *et al.*, 2006). This was due in part to the fast recovery of creatine phosphate and the 15–30 s delay in collecting the muscle biopsy in that study. Creatine phosphate may have been significantly lower in individual muscle fibres, since creatine phosphate stores have been reported to be almost completely depleted in individual fibres at the point of fatigue after intense exercise (Søderlund & Hultman, 1991). However, during the Yo-Yo intermittent recovery test where the speed is progressively increased to the point of exhaustion, no changes were observed in muscle creatine phosphate in the final phase of exercise (Krustrup et al., 2003). This fact argues against creatine phosphate having an inhibitory effect on performance during intense intermittent exercise. During the matches studied by Krustrup et al. (2006), muscle inosine monophosphate (IMP) concentrations were higher than before the game and elevated blood NH_3 levels also indicate that the adenosine monophosphate (AMP) deaminase reaction was significantly stimulated. On the other hand, the muscle IMP concentrations were considerably lower than observed during exhaustive exercise (Hellsten, Richter, Kiens, & Bangsbo, 1999) and ATP was only moderately reduced. Thus, it is unlikely that fatigue occurred as a result of a low energy status of the contracting muscles. Together, these findings suggest that temporary fatigue in soccer is not causally linked to high muscle lactate, high muscle acidosis, low muscle creatine phosphate, or low muscle ATP.

One has to look for other explanations of the fatigue that occurs after periods of intense exercise in soccer. It has been suggested that the development of fatigue during high-intensity exercise is related to an accumulation of potassium in the muscle interstitium and the concomitant electrical disturbances in the muscle cell (Bangsbo et al., 1996; Sejersted & Sjøgaard, 2000). This hypothesis is supported by the observation of muscle interstitial potassium concentrations of more than $11 \, \text{mmol} \cdot l^{-1}$ during exhaustive exercise (Mohr et al., 2004a; Nielsen et al., 2004; Nordsborg et al., 2003), which according to *in vitro* studies is high enough to depolarize the muscle membrane potential and reduce force development markedly (Cairns & Dulhunty, 1995). In addition, it has been observed that the maximal activity of the Na^+/K^+ pump is reduced with different types of exercise (Fraser et al., 2002), which could lead to greater transient accumulation of potassium during a match. Mean arm venous plasma potassium concentration during a soccer game has been observed to be $5 \, \text{mmol} \cdot l^{-1}$, with individual values above $5.5 \, \text{mmol} \cdot l^{-1}$, which is only slightly lower than values observed after exhaustive incremental intermittent exercise (Krustrup et al., 2003). However, these plasma values do not provide a clear picture of the concentrations around the contracting muscle fibres in soccer. Further research is needed to reveal what causes fatigue during soccer matches.

Training of a top-class player

Based on the analysis of the game it is clear that the training of elite players should focus on improving their ability to perform intense exercise and to recover rapidly from periods of high-intensity exercise. This is done by performing aerobic and anaerobic training on a regular basis (Bangsbo, 2005).

In a typical week for a professional soccer team with one match to play, the players have six training sessions in 5 days (i.e. one day with two sessions), with the day after the match free. If there is a second match in midweek the team often trains once a day on the other days. However, there are marked variations depending on the experience of the coach. Table I presents examples of programmes for an international top-class team during the season.

To obtain information about the loading of the players, heart rate monitoring can be used. It should, however, be emphasized that such measurements do not provide a clear picture about the anaerobic energy production during training. Figure 3 shows an example of the heart rate response for two top-class players during high-intensity aerobic training (drill "Pendulum"; Bangsbo, 2005) consisting of eight 2 min exercise periods separated by 1 min recovery periods. The length of time the heart rate was 80–90, 90–95, and 95–100% of maximum was 8.3, 10.9, and 4.7 min respectively for one player, and 4.8, 11.1, and 5.3 min

Table 1. An in-season weekly programme for a professional soccer team when playing one or two matches a week

Day	*One match a week*	*Two matches a week*
Sunday	Match	Match
Monday	Free	Low-/moderate-intensity aerobic training, 30 min Strength training, 30 min
Tuesday	Warm-up, 15 min Technical/tactical, 30 min High-intensity aerobic training, 23 min Play, 15 min	Warm-up, 15 min Technical/tactical, 30 min High-intensity aerobic training, 10 min Play, 15 min
Wednesday	*Morning* Strength training, 60 min *Afternoon* Warm-up, 15 min Technical/tactical, 30 min Speed endurance training, 20 min	Match
Thursday	Warm-up, 15 min Technical/tactical, 30 min Play, 30 min	Low-/moderate-intensity aerobic training, 40 min Strength training, 30 min
Friday	Warm-up/technical, 25 min Speed training (long), 20 min High-intensity aerobic training, 18 min	Warm-up/technical, 25 min Speed training (long), 10 min High-intensity aerobic training, 20 min
Saturday	Warm-up/technical, 25 min Speed training (short), 20 min Play, 30 min	Warm-up/technical, 25 min Speed training (short), 20 min Play, 30 min
Sunday	Match	Match

Note: For a definition of "training", see Bangsbo (2005).

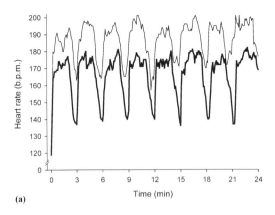

(a)

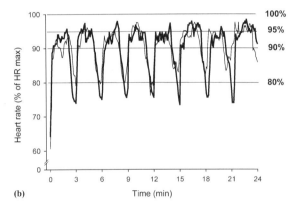

(b)

Figure 3. (a) Absolute (beats · min^{-1}) and (b) relative (percent of maximal) heart rate for two players during a high-intensity aerobic exercise drill called "Pendulum". The maximal heart rate of the players was 206 and 185 beats · min^{-1} respectively.

respectively for the other player. To understand the total demand on a player during a period, it is also important to perform measurements in the training sessions that are not specifically aimed at improving the fitness of the players. Table 2 shows the heart rates of three players during all training sessions over a 2 week preparation period for the World Cup in 2002, with the exception of two strength training sessions. The midfield player had a mean heart rate of 146 and 143 beats · min^{-1} respectively during the training sessions in week 1 and 2, corresponding to 78 and 76% of maximal heart rate, with heart rates of 90–95 and 95–100% of maximum for 144 and 11.5 min in week 1 and 135 and 8.5 min in week 2 respectively. The estimated mean energy expenditure was 7.6 and 7.5 MJ · day^{-1} in week 1 and 2 respectively. In comparison, the attacker had a lower relative mean heart rate (~70% maximum) and an estimated mean energy expenditure of 5.6 and 6.3 MJ · day^{-1} in week 1 and 2 respectively. Note the marked individual differences in heart rate distribution

Table 2. Training frequency, duration, heart rate response, and estimated energy expenditure during 2 weeks of training for a defender, a midfield player, and an attacker in the Danish National team in the first part of the preparation period for the 2002 World Cup

		Number of training sessions (n)	Time per session (min)	Total training time (min)	Mean heart rate (b.p.m^{-1})	Mean heart rate (% of max)	Heart rate zone*			Energy expenditure per week (MJ)	Energy expenditure per day (MJ)
							80–90% max (min)	90–95% max (min)	95–100% max (min)		
Defender	Week1	9	83.5	751	143.1	71.9	76.9	31.3	10.1	42.9	6.1
	Week 2	11	82.3	905	142.5	71.6	67.4	53.7	3.9	51.3	7.3
Midfielder	Week1	10	85.3	853	146.4	77.5	156.3	143.5	11.5	53.4	7.6
	Week 2	11	79.0	869	143.1	75.7	133.7	135.5	8.5	52.6	7.5
Attacker	Week1	8	85.9	687	129.8	68.3	63.3	52.1	16.2	39.0	5.6
	Week 2	9	80.9	728	136.0	71.6	104.4	60.1	21.9	44.4	6.3

* Expressed as a percentage of maximal heart rate.

and energy demand among the players (Table II). Such differences should be taken into account when planning training and nutritional strategies for individual players.

Muscle glycogen concentrations and adaptations to training

A study with the elite players of the Swedish team Malmø FF in the 1970s not only showed that muscle glycogen was lowered after a game, as discussed above, but also that muscle glycogen concentration was only 50% of the pre-match value 2 days after the match (Jacobs *et al.*, 1982). In a recent study, in addition to confirming these earlier findings, we observed that even though the players received a high carbohydrate diet after the game, they only had slightly higher muscle glycogen (Figure 4). Thus, muscle glycogen may be low before a training session 2 days after a game, which is often associated with the players' feelings of tiredness. This has obviously a negative effect on the intensity of the training session. However, one important aspect in relation to the lower muscle glycogen prior to the training should be discussed. Several studies have focused on the effect of nutrition intake and muscle glycogen concentration on the adaptations that occur with training. Pilegaard *et al.* (2002) found that reducing muscle glycogen before exercise elevated the transcriptional activation of some metabolic genes in response to exercise. Similarly, glucose supplementation has been shown to attenuate the increase in muscle mRNA for several enzymes and transporters, such as PDK-4, UCP-3, and GLUT-4, following exercise (Cluberton, McGee, Murphy, & Hargeaves, 2005; Kuo *et al.*, 1999). However, it is unclear what the effect is at the protein level. A recent study compared training twice a day every second day with one training session a day (Hansen

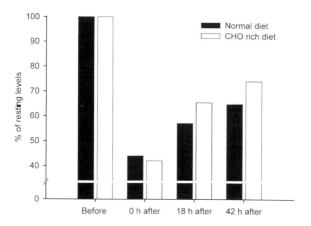

Figure 4. Muscle glycogen concentration (expressed as a percentage of resting values) after a competitive soccer match. Biopsies were obtained from the vastus lateralis muscle 0, 18, and 42 h after a game on two occasions, with a normal diet (solid bars) and a diet high in carbohydrates (open bars).

et al., 2005). The increase in citrate synthase was significantly greater in the group that trained twice a day, whereas no differences were observed for the increase in 3-hydroxyacyl-CoA dehydrogenase (HAD). It was proposed that the difference was caused by the group training twice a day performing a number of training sessions (in the afternoon) with lowered muscle glycogen. However, the true differences in citrate synthase were small, and it is unclear whether such an effect also applies to well-trained athletes. Furthermore, the quality of training should also be taken into consideration. The amount of high-intensity work performed during a soccer training session is likely to be higher if the players have high glycogen stores before the training. For a further discussion of these issues, see the article by Hawley, Tipton and Millard-Stafford (2006).

Acknowledgement

The original studies by the authors of this review were supported by Team Danmark and The Sports Research Council, Ministry of Culture, Denmark.

References

Ali, A., & Farrally, M. (1991). Recording soccer players' heart rate during matches. *Journal of Sports Sciences, 9*, 183–189.

Agnevik, G. (1970). Fotboll. Rapport Idrottsfysiologi, Trygg-Hansa, Stockholm.

Balsom, P. D., Seger, J. Y., Sjödin, B., & Ekblom, B. (1995). Skeletal muscle metabolism during short duration high-intensity exercise: influence of creatine supplementation. *Acta Physiologica Scandinavica, 154* (3), 303–310.

Balsom, P. D., Gaitanos, G. C., Söderlund, K., & Ekblom, K. (1999). High-intensity exercise and muscle glycogen availability in humans. *Acta Physiologica Scandinavica, 165*, 337–345.

Bangsbo, J. (1994). The physiology of soccer – with special reference to intense intermittent exercise. *Acta Physiologica Scandinavica, 151* (suppl. 619), 1–155.

Bangsbo, J. (2005). Aerobic and anaerobic training in soccer – with special emphasis on training of youth players. In *Fitness training in soccer I* (pp. 1–225). Bagsvaerd, Denmark: HO + Storm.

Bangsbo, J., Gibala, M., Krustrup, P., González-Alonso, J., & Saltin, B. (2002). Enhanced pyruvate dehydrogenase activity does not affect muscle O_2 uptake at onset of intense exercise in humans. *American Journal of Physiology, 282*, R273–R280.

Bangsbo, J., Graham, T. E., Kiens, B., & Saltin, B. (1992). Elevated muscle glycogen and anaerobic energy production during exhaustive exercise in man. *Journal of Physiology, 451*, 205–227.

Bangsbo, J., Johansen, L., Graham, T., & Saltin, B. (1993). Lactate and H^+ effluxes from human skeletal muscles during intense dynamic exercise. *Journal of Physiology, 462*, 115–133.

Bangsbo, J., Madsen, K., Kiens, B., & Richter, E. A. (1996). Effect of muscle acidity on muscle metabolism and fatigue during intense exercise in man. *Journal of Physiology (Lond), 495*, 587–596.

Bangsbo, J., & Mohr, M. (2005). Variations in running speed and recovery time after a sprint during top-class soccer matches. *Medicine and Science in Sports and Exercise*, 37, 87.

Bangsbo, J., Nørregaard, L., & Thorsøe, F. (1992a). The effect of carbohydrate diet on intermittent exercise performance. *International Journal of Sports Medicine*, 13, 152–157.

Bangsbo, J., Nørregaard, L., & Thorsøe, F. (1991). Activity profile of competition soccer. *Canadian Journal of Sports Sciences*, 16, 110–116.

Bigland-Ritchie, B., Furbush, F., & Woods, J. J. (1986). Fatigue of intermittent submaximal voluntary contractions: Central and peripheral factors. *Journal of Applied Physiology*, 61, 421–429.

Bulow, J., & Madsen, J. (1981). Influence of blood flow on fatty acid mobilization forms lipolytically active adipose tissue. *Pflügers Archive*, 390, 169–174.

Cairns, S. P., & Dulhunty, A. F. (1995). High-frequency fatigue in rat skeletal muscle: role of extracellulary ion concentrations. *Muscle and Nerve*, 18, 890–898.

Castagna, C., Belardinelli, R., & Abt, G. (2005). The VO_2 and HR response to training with the ball in youth soccer players. In T. Reilly, J. Cabri, & D. Araújo (Eds.), *Science and Football V* (pp. 462–464). London/New York: Routledge, Taylor & Francis Group.

Cluberton, L. J., McGee, S. L., Murphy, R. M., & Hargreaves, M. (2005). Effect of carbohydrate ingestion on exercise-induced alterations in metabolic gene expression. *Journal of Applied Physiology*, 99, 1359–1363.

Ekblom, B. (1986). Applied physiology of soccer. *Sports Medicine*, 3, 50–60.

Ekblom, B., Greenleaf, C. J., Greenleaf, J. E., & Hermansen, L. (1971) Temperature regulation during continuous and intermittent exercise in man. *Acta Physiologica Scandinaviaca*, 81, 1–10.

Esposito, F., Impellizzeri, F. M., Margonato, V., Vanni, R., Pizzine, G., & Veicsteinas, A. (2004). Validity of heart rate as an indicator of aerobic demand during soccer activities in amateur soccer players. *European Journal of Applied Physiology*, 93, 167–172.

Fraser, S. F., Li, J. L., Carey, M. F., Wang, X. N., Sangkabutra, T., Sostaric, S. *et al.* (2002). Fatigue depresses maximal *in vitro* skeletal muscle Na(+)-K(+)-ATPase activity in untrained and trained individuals. *Journal of Applied Physiology*, 93, 1650–1659.

Gaitanos, G. C., Williams, C., Boobis, L. H., & Brooke, S. (1993). Human muscle metabolism during intermittent maximal exercise. *Journal of Applied Physiology*, 75(2): 712–719.

Galbo, H. (1983). *Hormonal and metabolic adaptations to exercise* (pp. 1 144). New York: Thime-Stratton.

Galbo, H. (1992). Exercise physiology: Humoral function. *Sport Science Reviews*, 1, 65–93.

Greenhaff, P. L., Bodin, K., Söderlund, K., & Hultman, E. (1994). The effect of oral creatine supplementation on skeletal muscle phosphocreatine resynthesis. *American Journal of Physiology*, 266, E725–E730.

Hansen, A. K., Fischer, C. P., Plomgaard, P., Andersen, J. L., Saltin, B., & Pedersen, B. K. (2005). Skeletal muscle adaptation: Training twice every second day vs. training once daily. *Journal of Applied Physiology*, 98, 93–99.

Hawley, J. A., Tipton, K. D., & Millard-Stafford, M. L. (2006). Promoting training adaptations through nutritional interventions. *Journal of Sports Sciences*, 24, 709–721.

Hellsten, Y., Richter, E. A., Kiens, B., & Bangsbo, J. (1999). AMP deamination and purine exchange in human skeletal muscle during and after intense exercise. *Journal of Physiology*, *529*, 909–920.

Jacobs, I., Westlin, N., Karlsson, J., Rasmusson, J., & Houghton, B. (1982). Muscle glycogen and diet in elite soccer players. *European Journal of Applied Physiology*, *48*, 297–302.

Krustrup, P., & Bangsbo, J. (2001). Physiological demands of top-class soccer refereeing in relation to physical capacity: Effect of intense intermittent exercise training. *Journal of Sports Sciences*, *19*, 881–891.

Krustrup, P., Hellsten, Y., & Bangsbo, J. (2004a). Intense interval training enhances human skeletal muscle oxygen uptake in the initial phase of dynamic exercise at high but not at low intensities. *Journal of Physiology*, *559*(1), 335–345.

Krustrup, P., Mohr, M., Amstrup, T., Rysgaard, T., Johansen, J., Steensberg, A. *et al.* (2003). The Yo-Yo intermittent recovery test: Physiological response, reliability and validity. *Medicine and Science in Sports and Exercise*, *35*, 695–705.

Krustrup, P., Mohr, M., Ellingsgaard, H., & Bangsbo, J. (2005). Physical demands during an elite female soccer game: Importance of training status. *Medicine and Science in Sports and Exercise*, *37*, 1242–1248.

Krustrup, P., Mohr, M., Steensburg, A., Bencke, A., Kjær, M., & Bangsbo, J. (2006). Muscle and blood metabolites during a soccer game: Implications for sprint performance. *Medicine and Science in Sports and Exercise*, *38*(6), 1–10.

Krustrup, P., Soderlund, K., Mohr, M., & Bangsbo, J. (2004b). The slow component of oxygen uptake during intense sub-maximal exercise in man is associated with additional fibre recruitment. *Pflügers Archive*, *44*, 855–866.

Kuo, C. H., Hunt, D. G., Ding, Z., & Ivy, J. L. (1999). Effect of carbohydrate supplementation on postexercise GLUT-4 protein expression in skeletal muscle. *Journal of Applied Physiology*, *87*, 2290–2295.

Magal, M., Webster, M. J., Sistrunk, L. E., Whitehead, M. T., Evans, R. K., & Boyd, J. C. (2003). Comparison of glycerol and water hydration regimens on tennis-related performance. *Medicine and Science in Sports and Exercise*, *35*, 150–156.

Mayhew, S. R., & Wenger, H. A. (1985). Time-motion analysis of professional soccer. *Journal of Human Movement Studies*, *11*, 49–52.

Meeusen, R., Watson, P., & Dvoraak, J. (2006). The brain and fatigue: New opportunities for nutritional interventions? *Journal of Sports Sciences*, *24*, 773–782.

Mohr, M., Krustrup, P., & Bangsbo, J. (2003). Match performance of high-standard soccer players with special reference to development of fatigue. *Journal of Sports Sciences*, *21*, 439–449.

Mohr, M., Krustrup, P., & Bangsbo, J. (2005). Fatigue in soccer: A brief review. *Journal of Sports Sciences*, *23*, 593–599.

Mohr, M., Krustrup, P., Nybo, L., Nielsen, J. J., & J. Bangsbo, J. (2004b). Muscle temperature and sprint performance during soccer matches – beneficial effects of re-warm-up at half time. *Scandinavian Journal of Medicine and Science in Sports*, *14*, 156–162.

Mohr, M., Nordsborg, N., Nielsen, J. J., Pedersen, L. D., Fischer, C., Krustrup, P. *et al.* (2004a). Potassium kinetics in human interstitium during repeated intense exercise in relation to fatigue. *Pflügers Archive*, *448*, 452–456.

Nevill, M. E., Boobis, L. H., Brooks, S., & Williams, C. (1989). Effect of training on muscle metabolism during treadmill sprinting. *Journal of Applied Physiology*, *67*(6), 2376–2382.

Nielsen, J. J., Mohr, M., Klarksov, C., Kristensen, M., Krustrup, P., Juel, C. *et al.* (2004). Effects of high-intensity intermittent training on potassium kinetics and performance in human skeletal muscle. *Journal of Physiology*, 554, 857–870.

Nordsborg, N., Mohr, M., Pedersen, L. D., Nielsen, J. J., & Bangsbo, J. (2003). Muscle interstitial potassium kinetics during intense exhaustive exercise – effect of previous arm exercise. *American Journal of Physiology*, 285, 143–148.

Nybo, L., & Secher, N. (2004). Cerebral perturbations provoked by prolonged exercise. *Progress in Neurobiology*, 72, 223–261.

Pilegaard, H., Keller, C., Steensberg, A., Helge, J. W., Pedersen, B. K., Saltin, B. *et al.* (2002). Influence of pre-exercise muscle glycogen content on exercise-induced transcriptional regulation of metabolic genes. *Journal of Physiology*, 541, 261–271.

Rebelo, A. N. C. (1999). *Studies of fatigue in soccer.* PhD thesis, University of Porto, Porto, Portugal.

Reilly, T. (1997). Energetics of high-intensity exercise (soccer) with particular reference to fatigue. *Journal of Sports Sciences*, 15, 257–263.

Reilly, T., & Thomas, V. (1979). Estimated energy expenditures of professional association footballers. *Ergonomics*, 22, 541–548.

Rienzi, E., Drust, B., Reilly, T., Carter, J. E., & Martin, A. (1998). Investigation of anthropometric and work-rate profiles of elite South American international soccer players. *Journal of Sports Medicine and Physical Fitness*, 40, 162–169.

Sahlin, K. (1992). Metabolic factors in fatigue. *Sports Medicine*, 13(2), 99–107.

Saltin, B. (1973). Metabolic fundamentals in exercise. *Medicine and Science in Sports and Exercise*, 5, 137–146.

Saltin, B., & Hermansen, L. (1966). Esophageal, rectal and muscle temperature during exercise. *Journal of Applied Physiology*, 21, 1757–1762.

Sejersted, O. M., & Sjogaard, G. (2000). Dynamics and consequences of potassium shifts in skeletal muscle and heart during exercise. *Physiological Reviews*, 80(4), 1411–1481.

Smaros, G. (1980). Energy usage during a football match. In L. Vecchiet (Ed.), *Proceedings of the First International Congress on Sports Medicine Applied to Football* (pp. 795–801). Rome, Italy: D. Guanello.

Smodlaka, V. J. (1978). Cardiovascular aspects of soccer. *Physiology and Sportsmedicine*, 18, 66–70.

Søderlund, K., & Hultman, E. (1991). ATP and phosphocreatine changes in single human muscle fibers after intense electrical stimulation. *American Journal of Physiology*, 162, E737–E741.

Turcotte, L. P., Kiens, B., & Richter, E. A. (1991). Saturation kinetics of palmitate uptake in perfused skeletal muscle. *Federation of European Biochemical Societies*, 279, 327–329.

Van Gool, D., Van Gerven, D., & Boutmans, J. (1988). The physiological load imposed on soccer players during real matchplay. In T. Reilly, A. Lees, K. Davids, & W. J. Murphy (Eds.), *Science and Football* (pp. 51–59). London/New York: E. & F.N. Spon.

2 Energy and carbohydrate for training and recovery

LOUISE M. BURKE, ANNE B. LOUCKS AND
NICK BROAD

Soccer players should achieve an energy intake that provides sufficient carbohydrate to fuel the training and competition programme, supplies all nutrient requirements, and allows manipulation of energy or nutrient balance to achieve changes in lean body mass, body fat or growth. Although the traditional culture of soccer has focused on carbohydrate intake for immediate match preparation, top players should adapt their carbohydrate intake on a daily basis to ensure adequate fuel for training and recovery between matches. For players with a mobile playing style, there is sound evidence that dietary programmes that restore and even super-compensate muscle glycogen levels can enhance activity patterns during matches. This will presumably also benefit intensive training, such as twice daily practices. As well as achieving a total intake of carbohydrate commensurate with fuel needs, the everyday diet should promote strategic intake of carbohydrate and protein before and after key training sessions to optimize the adaptations and enhance recovery. The achievement of the ideal physique for soccer is a long-term goal that should be undertaken over successive years, and particularly during the off-season and pre-season. An increase in lean body mass or a decrease in body fat is the product of a targeted training and eating programme. Consultation with a sports nutrition expert can assist soccer players to manipulate energy and nutrient intake to meet such goals. Players should be warned against the accidental or deliberate mismatch of energy intake and energy expenditure, such that energy availability (intake minus the cost of exercise) falls below 125 kJ (30 kcal) per kilogram of fat-free mass per day. Such low energy availability causes disturbances to hormonal, metabolic, and immune function.

Keywords: Glycogen, refuelling, low energy availability, female athlete triad

Introduction

During a typical training week, a soccer player undertakes individual and team-based sessions encompassing endurance, speed and strength conditioning, skills practice, tactical drills, and match-play (Bangsbo, Mohr, & Krustrup, 2006). The nature, volume, and intensity of the training programme vary according to the time of the season, the calibre of player, and the player's position and individual goals. For professional players, pre-season camps may involve a schedule of twice daily practices. During the competitive season, the week may also include one or two matches. This review will cover the players' needs for energy and carbohydrate to fuel, recover, and optimize the adaptations from these sessions. Ideas for future research in which the timing and macronutrient composition of energy intake might be manipulated to further enhance training adaptations are covered by Hawley, Tipton and Millard-Stafford (2006). The present review is limited to strategies for which there is good support for positive outcomes, and warns against strategies for which there is clear evidence of detrimental outcomes. It will also focus on research undertaken over the last decade, and thus on the enhancements in our knowledge since the 1994 Consensus on Food, Nutrition and Soccer Performance.

Energy needs

The total energy expenditure and requirements of each soccer player are unique, arising from the contribution of basal metabolic rate, thermic effect of food, thermic effect of activity, and in some cases growth (Manore & Thompson, 2006). For many athletes, and in particular professional players undertaking multiple training sessions in a day or more than one match in a week, the energy cost of training and games is substantial. The importance of adequate energy intake in underpinning the nutritional goals of training is emphasized in other sections of this review. In the scientific literature there are several reports of the energy expenditure of particular groups of soccer players, derived from techniques such as doubly labelled water (Ebine *et al.*, 2002) and indirect calorimetry (Fogelholm *et al.*, 1995). However, the expense and complex technology involved in these techniques confine them to the realms of research.

In the field, an accessible and practical way to assess the daily energy expenditure of an athlete is to use prediction equations based on assessments of resting metabolic rate and the energy cost of daily activities (Manore & Thompson, 2006). Once resting metabolic rate is estimated from one of the available prediction equations, it is then multiplied by various activity factors to determine the daily total energy expenditure. Most simply, a general activity factor is applied to the whole day to represent the athlete's typical exercise level. More complex, an athlete might complete an intricate activity diary, with the predicted or measured energy cost of each activity undertaken over the day being summed to predict total daily energy expenditure. While this "factorial method" can provide a general estimation of a soccer player's energy requirements, there is considerable potential for error.

An alternative field method is the "energy availability model" (Loucks, 2004) in which the amount of energy available to the body to undertake its physiological processes is considered. Energy availability is calculated as total energy intake minus the energy cost of the daily exercise programme. Typically, energy balance in normal, healthy adults is achieved at a mean energy availability of $\sim$45 kcal per kilogram of fat-free mass (FFM) (189 kJ $\cdot$ kg FFM^{-1}). Since information about the energy expended in exercise can be provided by various commercial heart rate monitors, calculations of energy availability may be simple to undertake and interpret. The Appendix to this review compares the concepts of energy balance and energy availability, demonstrating the utility of the energy availability model.

Whether it is assessed in absolute terms or in comparison to estimates of energy requirement, the energy intake of a soccer player is of interest for several reasons (Burke, 2001):

1. It sets the potential for achieving the player's requirements for energy-containing macronutrients such as protein and carbohydrate, and the food needed to provide vitamins, minerals, and other non-energy-containing dietary compounds required for optimal function and health.
2. It assists the manipulation of muscle mass and body fat to achieve the specific physique that is ideal for training and match performance.
3. It affects the function of the hormonal and immune systems.
4. It challenges the practical limits to food intake set by issues such as food availability and gastrointestinal comfort.

The available information on intakes of energy and macronutrients in the everyday diets of adult soccer players, ranging from collegiate to elite/professional players, is summarized in Table 1. These data were collected by self-reported prospective techniques that are limited by errors of accuracy and reliability (how well they represent usual intake) (for a review, see Burke *et al.*, 2001). In addition, only three of the studies attempted to measure energy balance (intake vs. expenditure) in their groups. One study of Japanese male professional soccer players found that mean reported energy intake accounted for only 88% of energy expenditure, estimated from doubly labelled water techniques (Ebine *et al.*, 2002). The authors concluded that this discrepancy was due to under-reporting; this is the usual error in self-reported dietary intake. Another study that used daily activity records to assess energy expenditure found closer agreement with estimates of energy intake and expenditure of a group of players from the Olympic team of Puerto Rico (Rico-Sanz *et al.*, 1998).

Although the spread of time periods of data collection makes it difficult to make firm conclusions about the dietary practices of contemporary soccer players, it appears that the reported energy intake of the typical male player is about $13–16 \, \text{MJ} \cdot \text{day}^{-1}$, equivalent to approximately $160–200 \, \text{kJ} \cdot \text{kg}^{-1} \cdot \text{day}^{-1}$. This would appear to reflect high levels of activity during game play and the conditioning required to achieve or maintain fitness, especially among professional players (Bangsbo, Norregaard, & Thorsoe, 1992; Jacobs, Westlin, Karlsson, Rasmusson, & Houghton, 1982; Rico-Sanz *et al.*, 1998). Data for female soccer players are scarce, but tend to show the usual phenomenon of a lower energy intake relative to body mass in female players than in their male counterparts. Of course, the training demands of female players are likely to be substantially less than those of male players, since the opportunities for elite competition are fewer. The one study to investigate energy balance in female soccer players

Table 1. Reported dietary intakes of male soccer players during training (mean daily intake ± s) (adapted from Burke, 2006)

Reference	Team population	Survey method	Age (years)	BM (kg)	Energy MJ	Energy kJ·kg⁻¹	CHO g	CHO g·kg⁻¹	CHO % Energy	Protein g	Protein g·kg⁻¹	Protein % Energy	Fat g	Fat % Energy
Jacobs et al. (1982)	Swedish professional players (n = 15)	7-day food diary (household measures)	24	74	20.7 ± 4.7	282	596 ± 127	8.1	47 ± 3	170 ± 27	2.3	13.5 ± 1.5	217 ± 36	29 ± 8
Short and Short (1983)	US collegiate players (n = 8)	3-day food diary (household measures)			12.4		320		43	113		16	135	41
Hickson et al. (1987)	US collegiate players – conditioning on campus (n = 17)	3-day food diary (household measures)	20	72	18.7	260	596	8.3	52			14		34
	– season on campus (n = 8)				15.99 ± 2.7	221	487 ± 107	6.8	52 ± 11			16		32 ± 9
	– season off campus (n = 9)				12.8 ± 4.9	178	306 ± 118	4.2	42 ± 15			16		42 ± 18
Van Erp-Baart et al. (1989)	Dutch international players (n = 20)	4-7 day food diary (household measures)	20	74	14.3	192	420	5.6	47	111	1.5	13	134	35
Caldarone et al. (1990)	Italian professional players (n = 33)	7 day dietary recall (household measures)	26	76	12.8 ± 2.4	169	449	5.9	56					
Bangsbo et al. (1992)	Danish professional players (n = 7)	10 day food diary (household measures)	23	77	15.7	204	426	5.5	46	144	1.9	16	152	38
Schena et al. (1995)	Italian national players (n = 16)	7 cay food diary (household measures)	25	74	13.4 ± 1.5	180	454 ± 32	6.1	57	86 ± 16	1.2	19	90 ± 14	24
Zuliani et al. (1996)	Italian professional players (n = 25)	4 cay food diary (household measures)	25	71	15.3 ± 1.8	213	532	7.4	56					
Maughan (1997)	Scottish professional players from two clubs (n = 51)	7-day weighed food diary	23	80	11.0 ± 2.6	137	354 ± 95	4.4	51 ± 8	103 ± 26	1.3	16 ± 2	93 ± 33	31 ± 5
Rico-Sanz et al. (1998)	Puerto Rican Olympic team players (n = 8)	12 day food diary (household measures)	26	75	12.8 ± 2.2	171	397 ± 94	5.3	48 ± 4	108 ± 20	1.4	14 ± 2	118 ± 24	35 ± 4
			17	63	16.5 ± 4.5	260 ± 50	526 ± 62	8.3	53 ± 6	143 ± 23	2.3	14 ± 2	142 ± 17	32 ± 4
Ebine et al. (2002)	Japanese professional players (n = 7)	7 day food diary (household measures)	22	70	13.0 ± 2.4	186	–	–	–	–	–	–	–	–
Reeves and Collins (2003)	English professional players (n = 21)	7 day food diary (household measures)	20	74	12.8 ± 0.8	173	437 ± 40	5.9	57 ± 4	115 ± 2	1.6	15 ± 2	94 ± 1	27 ± 3
Ruiz et al. (2005)	Basque club players (n = 24)	3 day weighed food diary	21	73	12.7 ± 2.9	173 ± 43	334 ± 78	4.7 ± 1.0	45	133 ± 31	1.8 ± 0.5	18	128 ± 49	38

Abbreviations: BM = body mass. CHO = carbohydrate.

during the post-season (Fogelholm *et al.*, 1995) found reasonable agreement between reported energy intake and energy expenditure (using indirect calorimetry to estimate resting metabolic rate). However, energy expenditure was not different from that of sedentary controls, raising some doubts about the appropriateness of the techniques or the timing of the investigation. Alternatively, resting metabolism may have been suppressed by chronic energy deficiency in the soccer players.

Manipulating energy balance and body composition

Energy balance is not the objective for many athletes, at least for some portions of the season or their athletic career. Instead, the athlete may wish to manipulate body composition (lean body mass or body fat) and fuel stores (glycogen stores), and these changes might require temporary periods of energy deficit or surplus, or manipulation of multiple components of these body compartments in apparently conflicting directions (for a review, see Loucks, 2004). The optimal physique for a soccer player in terms of lean body mass and body fat varies according to the position and playing style of the individual. However, there is at least anecdotal evidence that elite modern players are leaner and stronger than players from previous times or those who compete at a lower standard (Reilly, 2005). Mean body fat values in high-level adult male soccer players using a variety of methods (dual-energy X-ray absorptiometry; skinfold thicknesses) and prediction equations have been reported to range from 8.2 to 13.0% (Kraemer *et al.*, 2004; Maughan, 1997; Reilly & Gregson, 2006; Wittich, Oliveri, Rotemberg, & Mautalen, 2001). Data for top-class female players are limited. Using hydrostatic weighing, Clark, Reed, Crouse and Armstrong (2003) reported percent body fat to be approximately 16% in US collegiate division 1 players (see Table 2).

The best time to undertake conditioning programmes aimed at increasing lean body mass and/or reducing body fat is during the off-season or pre-season. At lower levels of competition, achievement of the desired body composition for the playing season may also require a dedicated effort to reduce the loss of conditioning caused by a long off-season that is often marked by inactivity, poor eating, and excessive intake of alcohol. The off-season for elite players is usually brief (about 6 weeks) and generally involves a player- or club-determined conditioning programme. However, breaks required for the treatment and rehabilitation of injuries in elite players also present a risk for deconditioning.

Optimizing lean body mass and body fat requires manipulation of both training and dietary strategies. Adequate energy intake, including perhaps an increase in energy intake, appears to be important in promoting the gains from a resistance training programme (Gater, Gater, Uribe, & Bunt, 1992), although information pinpointing the optimal intake of energy and the macronutrient contribution to this intake is lacking. There is emerging evidence that resistance training may be assisted by strategic intake of protein and carbohydrate before, during,

Table 2. Reported dietary intakes of female soccer players during training (mean daily intake ± s) (adapted from Burke, 2006)

Reference	Team population	Survey method	Age (years)	BM (kg)	Energy MJ	Energy kJ · kg⁻¹	CHO g	CHO g · kg⁻¹	CHO % Energy	Protein g	Protein g · kg⁻¹	Protein % Energy	Fat g	Fat % Energy
Fogelholm et al. (1995)	Finnish national players (n = 12)	7-day food diary (household measures)	18	61	9.0 ± 1.7	147								
Clark et al. (2003)	US collegiate players (n = 13)	3-day food diary (household measures)	20	62										
		– season			9.6 ± 1.3	155	320 ± 70	5.2 ± 1.1	55 ± 8	87 ± 19	1.4 ± 0.3	15 ± 3	75 ± 13	29 ± 6
		– post-season			7.8 ± 2.2	126	263 ± 71	4.3 ± 1.2	57 ± 7	59 ± 17	1.0 ± 0.3	13 ± 2	66 ± 29	31 ± 7
Gropper et al. (2003)	US collegiate players (n = 15)	3-day food diary (household measures)	19	59	8.5 ± 2.5	143				71 ± 29	1.3	14		

Abbreviations: BM = body mass, CHO = carbohydrate.

and after the session (Hawley *et al.*, 2006). Guidelines to assist players to increase their energy intake to meet high energy requirements or to provide nutritional support at strategic times in relation to training or a match are summarized in Table 3. These strategies may be useful to support an increase in lean body mass during the pre-season or a growth spurt in adolescent players, or to meet high energy requirements during a demanding schedule of training or matches.

A reduction in body fat is achieved by manipulation of diet and training to create a negative fat balance and negative energy balance over the total day or for substantial portions of the day. Guidelines to achieve this outcome with minimal interference with other goals of training or performance are outlined in Table 3. There is considerable evidence that a low availability of energy, previously defined as total energy intake minus the energy cost of the athlete's exercise programme, has serious consequences on the hormonal, immunological, and health status of the athlete (see Loucks, 2004). This is best demonstrated in female athletes and the characterisation of the female athlete triad in which low energy availability, impaired menstrual status, and poor bone health are interrelated (Loucks & Nattiv, 2005; Otis, Drinkwater, Johnson, Loucks, & Wilmore, 1997). Many female athletes develop metabolic, reproductive, and bone disruptions because they over-restrict their energy intake to achieve loss of body fat. Incremental changes in energy availability (Loucks & Thuma, 2003) lead to a dose-dependent relationship between energy restriction and metabolic and hormonal function; the threshold for maintenance of normal menstrual function in females is an energy availability of above 30 kcal (125 kJ) per kilogram of fat free mass. The Appendix to this paper illustrates the concepts of low and normal energy availability.

Although team sport athletes, and soccer players in particular, are generally not identified in the literature as being at high risk of over-zealous dieting or the pursuit of inappropriate thinness, practitioners who work with soccer teams will be familiar with individual players to whom this does apply. The prevalence of this concern may increase as an outcome of the general increase in the leanness achieved by elite soccer players. Anecdotally, we have noted that the imposition of lycra "body suit" uniforms on female competitors in some team sports has increased the concerns related to body image and body fatness in these populations. Indeed, the wearing of a figure-hugging or revealing uniform has been identified as a risk factor for the development of disordered eating among athletes (Otis *et al.*, 1997). The suggestion that women's soccer should follow this fashion statement in an attempt to increase the television interest and popularity of the sport must be balanced by consideration of the possible harmful outcomes from such a change (Burke, 2006).

It is likely that male athletes who expose themselves to periods of low energy availability will also suffer from metabolic and reproductive disturbances (Friedl *et al.*, 2000). Of course, not all cases of low energy availability in males, or females, are due to deliberate restriction of energy to reduce body mass and body fat. It can be due to the practical challenges faced by the soccer player

Table 3. Guidelines for adjusting energy intake according to goals of training or physique

Recommendations for

- Soccer players should adjust their energy intake according to their activity level and goals for growth, increased lean body mass, or loss of body fat. These goals are specific to the individual player and will vary over the season and over the player's career. An energy surplus will occur if energy intake is not reduced when a player who normally undertakes a heavy training programme becomes suddenly inactive, such as during the off-season or when injured.
- The ideal physique for match performance is individual to each player and should be achieved gradually as the player matures in age and training history.
  The achievement of the ideal physique should not compromise health, long-term performance, sound eating practices, or the enjoyment of food. Major programmes to manipulate muscle mass and body fat should be confined to the pre-season or off-season.
- Soccer players should not monitor body mass as a measure of physique. Rather, they should monitor changes in objective measures of body fat (e.g. skinfold thickness) or functional capacity (e.g. strength), taking into account the reliability and relevance of these measures.
- An increase in lean body mass is the product of appropriate resistance training and a diet providing adequate energy and nutrients. Strategic intake of protein and carbohydrate before and after a workout may enhance the adaptations achieved by the session, as well as increasing total energy intake to meet higher energy requirements
- Other strategies that may assist the soccer player to meet high energy needs include:
  ○ Planning food intake with appropriate supplies organized for consumption at key times
  ○ Consuming small, frequent meals and snacks throughout the day
  ○ Avoiding excessive intake of low energy-dense and fibre-rich foods when these foods would reduce appetite or impair total food intake
  ○ Making use of energy- and nutrient-dense fluids such as fortified milk drinks and liquid meal supplements
- Loss of body fat is achieved by careful planning of training and food intake to achieve a negative fat balance and a negative energy balance. A strategic spread and choice of foods over the day and in relation to training should achieve these goals while maintaining adequate intake of fuel and nutrients and avoiding hunger.
  ○ Fat intake should be moderated, especially saturated fats
  ○ Foods that are energy-dense but low in nutrient density should be avoided
  ○ Priority should be given to foods that are high in nutrient density so that nutrient needs are met from a lower intake of energy
  ○ Foods that are low in energy density or high in satiety value (e.g. low glycaemic index or protein-containing) should be chosen to manage hunger
- Soccer players should consult a sports nutrition expert for an individualised eating plan to assist with goals of fat loss or increased muscle mass. Players who are seen to be following unsound nutritional practices, especially those related to weight loss, should be referred to appropriate specialists for early intervention.

continued on facing page

Recommendations against

- Soccer players should not undertake a diet and exercise programme that allows or specifically promotes a substantial energy deficit. In particular, daily energy availability (total energy intake minus the cost of exercise) should not be less than about 125 kJ (30 kcal) per kilogram of fat-free mass daily. This may happen unintentionally when food intake is not sufficiently increased to compensate for a sudden increase in training. More often, however, this situation is the outcome of restricted energy intake to achieve fat loss goals.
- A low-carbohydrate diet is not a suitable weight-loss programme for an active soccer player. Low carbohydrate availability may underpin some of the metabolic disturbances seen in instances of low energy availability.

---

with high energy requirements, an over-committed daily timetable and travel schedule, and poor nutrition knowledge. The guidelines in Table 3 address the needs of these players.

Carbohydrate needs for training and recovery between games

The "training" diet of a soccer player must include strategies to refuel effectively between matches undertaken every 4–7 days during the competition season, as well as the conditioning sessions undertaken between matches or during pre-season preparation. The fuel needs of training and matches, including the effects of inadequate fuel stores on performance, are reviewed by Bangsbo *et al.* (2006). We now consider the effect of dietary interventions that manipulate muscle glycogen content on the outcomes of actual or simulated soccer match-play. While some strategies to promote fuel availability for match-play and prolonged training sessions are achieved by nutritional practices on the day (Williams & Serratosa, 2006), tactics to restore or even super-compensate muscle glycogen content must commence in the 24–48 h before a game. As such, they form a cycle of recovery between activities in the training week.

The value of "fuelling up" before a match has been demonstrated in laboratory studies. In the study of Balsom, Gaitanos, Soderlund and Ekblom (1999a), participants followed 48 h of either a high- or low-carbohydrate diet before short-term (< 10 min) and prolonged (> 30 min) protocols of intermittent exercise (6 s bouts at 30 s intervals). Muscle glycogen concentrations were reduced by at least 50% in the low-carbohydrate trial compared to the high-carbohydrate trial, and were associated with a dramatic reduction in the work performed in both exercise protocols. In another study (Bangsbo *et al.*, 1992), professional soccer players completed an intermittent high-intensity protocol of field and treadmill running lasting approximately 90 min, after 48 h on a high-carbohydrate ($\sim 8 \text{ g} \cdot \text{kg}^{-1} \cdot \text{day}^{-1}$) or control ($\sim 4.5 \text{ g} \cdot \text{kg}^{-1} \cdot \text{day}^{-1}$) diet. Intermittent running to fatigue at the end of the protocol was increased by about 1 km by the high-carbohydrate diet ($P < 0.05$), although the performance enhancement was more marked in some participants than others. These studies show that higher pre-exercise glycogen stores enhance the capacity to undertake repeated bouts of exercise, even when these are as short as 6 s in duration.

Other studies using applied or real-life protocols in prolonged team sports have confirmed these findings. Balsom, Wood, Olsson and Ekblom (1999b) undertook movement analysis of a four-a-side indoor game lasting 90 min, following 48 h of high ($\sim$8 g·kg^{-1}·day^{-1}) or moderate ($\sim$3 g·kg^{-1}·day^{-1}) carbohydrate intake. Compared with the control trial, the high-carbohydrate diet increased muscle glycogen content by 38% and allowed the soccer players to complete approximately 33% more high-intensity work during the game. In another investigation, Akermark, Jacobs, Rasmusson and Karlsson (1996) found that elite ice hockey players who "carbohydrate-loaded" (8.4 g·kg^{-1}·day^{-1}) during the 3 day recovery between two games were able to skate for longer distances and at higher intensities than when their normal dietary preparation (6.2 g·kg^{-1}·day^{-1}) was followed. Muscle glycogen concentrations were reduced after the first game for all players (43 mmol·kg wet weight^{-1}), but restoration levels were 45% higher in the carbohydrate-loaded players before the next game (99 vs. 81 mmol·kg wet weight^{-1}; $P < 0.05$). Distance skated, number of shifts skated, amount of time skated within shifts, and skating speed were all increased in the carbohydrate-loaded players compared with the control group, with the differences being most marked in the third period. Individual differences in performance were thought to be related to muscle glycogen metabolism (Akermark *et al.*, 1996).

Twenty-four hour recovery was studied in team sport players who undertook a 60 min treadmill test involving multiple sprints, and were then randomized into groups of low (12% of energy), normal (47% of energy), and high (79% of energy) carbohydrate intake (Nevill, Williams, Roper, Slater, & Nevill, 1993). Power outputs during 6 s sprints interspersed over the 60 min declined over the duration of the test on day 1, and were even lower when repeated on day 2. Performance on day 2 was not different between dietary groups for the total 60 min; performance declined by 5%, 0.5%, and 0.2% compared with day 1 for the low, normal, and high carbohydrate trials respectively, but this was not statistically significant. However, over the first 20 min of the test on day 2, the high-carbohydrate group did perform better than the low-carbohydrate group. This study shows the difficulty of repeating performance of high-intensity exercise on successive days, but suggests that better restoration of muscle carbohydrate stores can enhance recovery.

Whether enhanced muscle fuel status will prevent the apparent deterioration of skills towards the end of a soccer game is hard to determine. Abt, Zhou and Weatherby (1998) attempted to address this question by having recreational soccer players consume different carbohydrate intakes (8 vs. 4 g·kg^{-1}·day^{-1}) in the 48 h before a simulated match. Shooting and dribbling tasks were undertaken before and after a 60 min intermittent treadmill run. There was no deterioration in the performance of these drills over time in the control trial. It is not surprising, therefore, that the high-carbohydrate treatment did not change the outcome. The authors concluded that either their treadmill protocol failed to achieve sufficient glycogen degradation to impair the execution of skills, or that factors other than fuel depletion are responsible for the decline that occurs during real match-play (Abt *et al.*, 1998). However, the ability of the test protocol to provide a reliable and valid measure of match skills in these players must also be questioned.

Overall, the literature supports the value of restoring glycogen between matches, and of providing adequate fuel for training sessions requiring high-intensity intermittent exercise. However, there has been little systematic study of the amounts of dietary carbohydrate needed to achieve optimal refuelling of soccer players. Early studies suggested that professional players were unable to replete muscle glycogen during the 48 h after a match, despite minimal training and a mean daily carbohydrate intake of $8 \, g \cdot kg^{-1}$ (Jacobs *et al.*, 1982). Muscle glycogen concentrations determined from biopsy samples increased from ~46 to ~69 mmol $\cdot$ kg wet weight^{-1} during the first 24 h of sedentary recovery, with restoration correlated to the extent of depletion at the end of the game. However, no further refuelling appeared to take place during the second 24 h recovery period that included light training; muscle glycogen concentrations were 73 mmol $\cdot$ kg wet weight^{-1} at the end of this period. It should be noted that the reported values for glycogen content in this study are low in comparison to other values in the literature for well-trained and rested athletes, and are in contrast to more recent studies that suggest that the well-trained muscle can normalize or even super-compensate glycogen stores within 24–36 h of the last exercise bout (Bussau, Fairchild, Rao, Steele, & Fournier, 2002). This may reflect an artifact of the study or a specific impairment of glycogen resynthesis in team sport players – for example, as a result of muscle damage from high-intensity running or contact injuries.

In contrast, a study using magnetic resonance spectroscopy monitored muscle glycogen utilization during a simulated soccer match and its repletion over 24 h of recovery while players consumed their habitual diet (Zehnder, Rico-Sanz, Kuhne, & Boutellier, 2001). Mean muscle glycogen content decreased from 134 to 80 mmol $\cdot$ kg wet weight^{-1} over the exercise protocol, but was almost restored to pre-"match" values (122 mmol $\cdot$ kg wet weight^{-1}) after 24 h. Players reported an intake of 327 g carbohydrate (4.8 g $\cdot$ kg body mass^{-1}) during this period. Whether this is a suitable simulation of the true fuel demands of match-play, and whether players would benefit from a higher carbohydrate intake to ensure full glycogen repletion, was not addressed by this study.

Carbohydrate intake guidelines for daily training and preparation for games

Further study is needed before clear guidelines for daily carbohydrate intake can be provided to soccer players. In addition, the variability in the fuel needs of different players, even in the same team, causes additional complexity in formulating and implementing such guidelines. However, in at least some circumstances it is prudent to undertake strategies that optimize muscle glycogen storage – these factors were addressed by the 2003 International Olympic Committee Consensus on Nutrition for Athletes (Burke, Kiens, & Ivy, 2004). The outcomes of this consensus regarding daily fuel needs have been translated into guidelines appropriate for soccer players (see Table 4).

The major dietary factor involved in post-exercise refuelling is the amount of carbohydrate consumed. As long as total energy intake is adequate (Tarnopolsky et al., 2001), increasing amounts of dietary carbohydrate promote increased muscle glycogen storage until the upper limit for glycogen synthesis is reached at intakes of about $10 \, \text{g} \cdot \text{kg}^{-1} \cdot \text{day}^{-1}$ (see Burke et al., 2004). Each player needs to match daily carbohydrate intake to the fuel needs of the schedule of training and the competition programme, including the weekly and seasonal variations that occur. A reasonable target range for carbohydrate intake by high-level players in less mobile roles, or teams or individuals with a less demanding training and competition schedule, is $5–7 \, \text{g} \cdot \text{kg}^{-1} \cdot \text{day}^{-1}$. For mobile players who want to maximize muscle glycogen refuelling, in preparation for matches or for recovery during an intensive training schedule, a target of $7–10 \, \text{g} \cdot \text{kg}^{-1} \cdot \text{day}^{-1}$ may be required (see Table 4). Historically, many team sport players have considered carbohydrate intake as a priority for the night before the game or for the pre-game meal only. It may take a change in culture for some modern players to eat adequate carbohydrate to keep pace with the daily fuel demands of training and match-play. The limited range of dietary surveys of serious soccer players (Table 1) shows that only a few groups of players (Rico-Sanz et al., 1998; Zuliani et al., 1996), and perhaps some individuals within groups, report daily carbohydrate intakes that fall within these higher target ranges.

Manipulation of the timing of intake and type of carbohydrate may provide some practical or metabolic advantages for refuelling. Carbohydrate-rich foods with a moderate or high glycaemic index (GI) appear to have some advantages over low-GI choices in promoting glycogen synthesis (Burke, Collier, & Hargreaves, 1993), but the form of the carbohydrate – fluids or solids – does not appear to affect glycogen synthesis (Keizer, Kuipers, Van Kranenburg, & Guerten, 1986). The highest rates of muscle glycogen storage occur during the first hour after exercise, due to enhancement of glucose delivery and enzyme activity within the muscle. While carbohydrate intake immediately after exercise appears to take advantage of these effects (Ivy, Katz, Cutler, Sherman, & Coyle, 1988), failure to consume carbohydrate in the immediate phase of post-exercise recovery leads to very low rates of glycogen restoration until feeding occurs. Early intake of carbohydrate following strenuous exercise is valuable because it provides an immediate source of substrate to the muscle cell to start effective recovery. This may be important when there is only 4–8 h between exercise sessions (Ivy et al., 1988), such as when training twice a day, but may have less impact over a longer recovery period (Parkin, Carey, Martin, Stojanovska, & Febbraio, 1997).

The pattern of food intake does not appear to affect glycogen storage in overall daily recovery as long as total carbohydrate needs are met (Burke et al., 1996;

Table 4. Guidelines for the intake of carbohydrate in the everyday or training diets of soccer players (based on Burke *et al.*, 2004).

Recommendations for

- Soccer players should aim to achieve a carbohydrate intake that meets the fuel requirements of their training programme and optimizes restoration of muscle glycogen stores between training sessions and before matches. General recommendations can be provided, but these should be fine-tuned with individual consideration of total energy needs, specific training needs, and feedback from training/match performance.
  - o Moderate daily recovery and match preparation (e.g. less mobile players, moderate training programme, periods of energy restriction for fat loss) = $5\text{--}7 \text{ g} \cdot \text{kg}^{-1} \cdot \text{day}^{-1}$
  - o Enhanced daily recovery and match preparation (e.g. heavy training such as twice daily practices, or fuelling up for matches, in mobile players) = $7\text{--}12 \text{ g} \cdot \text{kg}^{-1} \cdot \text{day}^{-1}$
- Players should recognize that their fuel requirements will vary over the week, over the season, and over their career. They should be prepared to adjust their carbohydrate intake accordingly. Many soccer clubs provide opportunities for players to eat together (e.g. pre-match meals, post-match or post-training recovery eating, catering during camps or travel). Menus and food choices on these occasions should be sufficiently flexible to provide for the range of energy and carbohydrate needs of various players.
- Soccer players should give priority to nutrient-rich carbohydrate foods and may need to add other foods to recovery meals and snacks to provide a good source of protein and other nutrients. These nutrients may assist in other recovery processes. The soccer club should invest in resources, such as the services of a sports nutrition expert, to help young players to develop nutrition knowledge and the practical skills required to eat well.
- When the period between exercise sessions is less than about 8 h, players should consume carbohydrate as soon as practical after the first workout to maximize the effective recovery time between sessions. There may be some advantages in meeting carbohydrate intake targets as a series of snacks during the early recovery phase.
  - o Carbohydrate intake target for immediate recovery after a match or training session (0–4 h) = $1.0\text{--}1.2 \text{ g} \cdot \text{kg}^{-1} \cdot \text{h}^{-1}$ consumed at frequent intervals
- During longer recovery periods (24 h), soccer players should organize the pattern and timing of carbohydrate-rich meals and snacks according to what is practical and comfortable for them individually. There is no difference in refuelling when liquid or solid forms of carbohydrate are consumed.
- Carbohydrate-rich foods with a moderate to high glycaemic index provide a readily available source of carbohydrate for muscle glycogen synthesis, and should be the major carbohydrate choices in recovery meals.
- Adequate energy intake is also important for optimal glycogen recovery; the restrained eating practices of some players, particularly females, make it difficult to meet carbohydrate intake targets and to optimize glycogen storage from this intake.

continued on next page

Recommendations against

- Guidelines for carbohydrate (or other macronutrients) should not be provided in terms of percentage contributions to total dietary energy intake. Such recommendations are neither user-friendly nor strongly related to the muscle's absolute needs for fuel.
- Soccer players should not consume excessive amounts of alcohol after training or matches, since this is likely to interfere with their ability or interest to follow guidelines for post-exercise eating. Players should follow sensible drinking practices at all times, but particularly in the period after exercise.

Costill *et al.*, 1981). However, rapid refuelling during the first hours of recovery may be achieved by a total carbohydrate intake of approximately $1.0-1.2 \, g \cdot h^{-1}$, perhaps as a series of small snacks every 15–30 min (see Jentjens & Jeukendrup, 2003). The effect of the co-ingestion of protein with carbohydrate on refuelling has been debated (see Burke *et al.*, 2004), but any enhancement of glycogen storage appears to be limited to the first hour of recovery (Ivy *et al.*, 2002) or to when the total amount of carbohydrate or pattern of intake is below the threshold for maximal glycogen synthesis and when the protein is consumed as an additional energy source. There may be some merit in investigating further the effects of consuming large amounts of carbohydrate with or without protein during the half-time interval of a soccer match. In general, the intake of protein within carbohydrate-rich recovery meals is encouraged and may allow the players to meet other nutritional goals, including the enhancement of net protein balance after exercise. Excessive alcohol intake during the post-game period is likely to interfere with refuelling goals, particularly by its indirect effects on behaviour and commitment to optimal nutrition strategies (Burke *et al.*, 2003; Maughan, 2006).

References

Abt, G., Zhou, S., & Weatherby, R. (1998). The effect of a high-carbohydrate diet on the skill performance of midfield soccer players after intermittent treadmill exercise. *Journal of Science and Medicine in Sport*, 1, 203–212.

Akermark, C., Jacobs, I., Rasmusson, M., & Karlsson, J. (1996). Diet and muscle glycogen concentration in relation to physical performance in Swedish elite ice hockey players. *International Journal of Sport Nutrition*, 6, 272–284.

Balsom, P. D., Gaitanos, G. C., Soderlund, K., & Ekblom, B. (1999a). High-intensity exercise and muscle glycogen availability in humans. *Acta Physiologica Scandinavica*, 165, 337–345.

Balsom, P. D., Wood, K., Olsson, P., & Ekblom, B. (1999b). Carbohydrate intake and multiple sprint sports: With special reference to football (soccer). *International Journal of Sports Medicine*, 20, 48–52.

Bangsbo, J., Mohr, M., & Krustrup, P. (2006) Physical and metabolic demands of training and match-play in the elite footballer. *Journal of Sports Sciences*, 24, 665–674.

Bangsbo, J., Norregaard, L., & Thorsoe, F. (1992). The effect of carbohydrate diet on intermittent exercise performance. *International Journal of Sports Medicine, 13*, 152–157.

Burke, L. M. (2001). Energy needs of athletes. *Canadian Journal of Applied Physiology, 26* (suppl.), S202–S219.

Burke, L. M. (2006). *Applied sports nutrition.* Champaign, IL: Human Kinetics.

Burke, L. M., Collier, G. R., Broad, E. M., Davis, P. G., Martin, D. T., Sanigorski, A. J. and Hargreaves, M. (2003). Effect of alcohol intake on muscle glycogen storage after prolonged exercise. *Journal of Applied Physiology, 95*, 983–990.

Burke, L. M., Collier, G. R., Davis, P. G., Fricker, P. A., Sanigorski, A. J., & Hargreaves, M. (1996). Muscle glycogen storage after prolonged exercise: Effect of the frequency of carbohydrate feedings. *American Journal of Clinical Nutrition, 64*, 115–119.

Burke, L. M., Collier, G. R., & Hargreaves, M. (1993). Muscle glycogen storage after prolonged exercise: The effect of the glycemic index of carbohydrate feedings. *Journal of Applied Physiology, 75*, 1019–1023.

Burke, L. M., Cox, G. R., Cummings, N. K., & Desbrow, B. (2001). Guidelines for daily CHO intake: Do athletes achieve them? *Sports Medicine, 31*, 267–299.

Burke, L. M., Kiens, B., & Ivy, J. L. (2004). Carbohydrates and fat for training and recovery. *Journal of Sports Sciences, 22*, 15–30.

Bussau, V. A., Fairchild, T. J., Rao, A., Steele, P., & Fournier, P. A. (2002). Carbohydrate loading in human muscle: An improved 1 day protocol. *European Journal of Applied Physiology, 87*, 290–295.

Caldarone, G., Tranquilli, C., & Giampietro, M. (1990). Assessment of the nutritional state of top level football playes. In G. Santilli (Ed.), *Sports medicine applied to football* (pp. 133–141). Rome: Instituto dietian Scienza della Sport del Coni.

Clark, M., Reed, D. B., Crouse, S. F., & Armstrong, R. B. (2003). Pre- and post-season dietary intake, body composition, and performance indices of NCAA Division I female soccer players. *International Journal of Sport Nutrition and Exercise Metabolism, 13*, 303–319.

Costill, D. L., Sherman, W. M., Fink, W. J., Maresh, C., Witten, M., & Miller, J. M. (1981). The role of dietary carbohydrates in muscle glycogen resynthesis after strenuous running. *American Journal of Clinical Nutrition, 34*, 1831–1836.

Ebine, N., Rafamantanantsoa, H. H., Nayuki, Y., Yamanaka, K., Tashima, K., Ono, T. et al. (2002). Measurement of total energy expenditure by the doubly labelled water method in professional soccer players. *Journal of Sports Sciences, 20*, 391–397.

Fogelholm, G. M., Kukkonen-Harjula, T. K., Taipale, S. A., Sievanen, H. T., Oja, P., & Vuori, I. M. (1995). Resting metabolic rate and energy intake in female gymnasts, figure-skaters and soccer players. *International Journal of Sports Medicine, 16*, 551–556.

Friedl, K. E., Moore, R. J., Hoyt, R. W., Marchitelli, L. J., Martinez-Lopez, L. E., & Askew, E. W. (2000). Endocrine markers of semistarvation in healthy lean men in a multistressor environment. *Journal of Applied Physiology, 88*, 1820–1830.

Gater, D. R., Gater, D. A., Uribe, J. M., & Bunt, J. C. (1992). Impact of nutritional supplements and resistance training on body composition, strength and insulin-like growth factor-1. *Journal of Applied Sport Science Research, 6*, 66–76.

Gropper, S. S., Sorrels, L. M., & Blessing, D. (2003). Copper status of collegiate female athletes involved in different sports. *International Journal of Sport Nutrition and Exercise Metabolism, 13*, 343–357.

Hawley, J. A., Tipton, K. D., & Millard-Stafford, M. L. (2006). Promoting training adaptations through nutritional interventions. *Journal of Sports Sciences, 24*, 709–721.

Hickson, J. F., Johnson, C. W., Schrader, J. W., & Stockton, J. E. (1987). Promotion of athletes' nutritional intake by a university food service facility. *Journal of the American Dietetic Association, 87*, 926–927.

Ivy, J. L., Goforth, H. W., Damon, B. D., McCauley, T. R., Parsons, E. C., & Price, T. B. (2002). Early post-exercise muscle glycogen recovery is enhanced with a carbohydrate-protein supplement. *Journal of Applied Physiology, 93*, 1337–1344.

Ivy, J. L., Katz, A. L., Cutler, C. L., Sherman, W. M., & Coyle, E. F. (1988). Muscle glycogen synthesis after exercise: Effect of time of carbohydrate ingestion. *Journal of Applied Physiology, 64*, 1480–1485.

Jacobs, I., Westlin, N., Karlsson, J., Rasmusson, M., & Houghton, B. (1982). Muscle glycogen and diet in elite soccer players. *European Journal of Applied Physiology, 48*, 297–302.

Jentjens, R., & Jeukendrup, A. E. (2003). Determinants of post-exercise glycogen synthesis during short-term recovery. *Sports Medicine, 33*, 117–144.

Keizer, H. A., Kuipers, H., Van Kranenburg, G., & Guerten, P. (1986). Influence of liquid and solid meals on muscle glycogen resynthesis, plasma fuel hormone response, and maximal physical working capacity. *International Journal of Sports Medicine, 8*, 99–104.

Kraemer, W. J., French, D. N., Paxton, N. J., Hakkinen, K., Volek, J. S., Sebastianelli, W. J. et al. (2004). Changes in exercise performance and hormonal concentrations over a big ten soccer season in starters and non-starters. *Journal of Strength and Conditioning Research, 18*, 121–128.

Loucks, A. B. (2004). Energy balance and body composition in sports and exercise. *Journal of Sports Sciences, 22*, 1–14.

Loucks, A. B., & Nattiv, A. (2005). The female athlete triad. *The Lancet, 366*, S49–S50.

Loucks, A. B., & Thuma, J. R. (2003). Luteinizing hormone pulsatility is disrupted at a threshold of energy availability in regularly menstruating women. *Journal of Clinical Endocrinology and Metabolism, 88*, 297–311.

Manore, M., & Thompson, J. (2006). Energy requirements of the athlete: Assessment and evidence of energy efficiency. In L. Burke & V. Deakin (Eds.), *Clinical sports nutrition* (3rd edn., pp. 113–134). Sydney, NSW: McGraw-Hill.

Maughan, R. J. (1997). Energy and macronutrient intake of professional football (soccer) players. *British Journal of Sports Medicine, 31*, 45–47.

Maughan, R. J. (2006) Alcohol and football. *Journal of Sports Sciences, 24*, 741–748.

Myerson, M., Gutin, B., Warren, M. P., May, M. T., Contento, I., Lee, M. et al. (1991). Resting metabolic rate and energy balance in amenorrheic and eumenorrheic runners. *Medicine and Science in Sports and Exercise, 23*, 15–22.

Nevill, M. E., Williams, C., Roper, D., Slater, C., & Nevill, A. M. (1993). Effect of diet on performance during recovery from intermittent sprint exercise. *Journal of Sports Sciences, 11*, 119–126.

Otis, C. L., Drinkwater, B., Johnson, M., Loucks, A., & Wilmore, J. (1997). American College of Sports Medicine position stand: The female athlete triad. *Medicine and Science in Sports and Exercise, 29*, i–ix.

Parkin, J. A. M., Carey, M. F., Martin, I. K., Stojanovska, L., & Febbraio, M. A. (1997). Muscle glycogen storage following prolonged exercise: Effect of timing of ingestion of high glycemic index food. *Medicine and Science in Sports and Exercise*, *29*, 220–224.

Reeves, S., & Collins, K. (2003). The nutritional and anthropometric status of Gaelic football players. *International Journal of Sport Nutrition and Exercise Metabolism, 13*, 539–548.

Reilly, T. (2005). Science and football: A history and an update. In T. Reilly, J. Cabri, & D. Araújo (Eds.), *Science and football V* (pp. 3–12). London: Routledge.

Reilly, T., & Gregson, W. (2006). Special populations: The referee. *Journal of Sports Sciences, 24*, 795–801.

Rico-Sanz, J., Frontera, W. R., Mole, P. A., Rivera, M. A., Rivera-Brown, A., & Meredith, C. N. (1998). Dietary and performance assessment of elite soccer players during a period of intense training. *International Journal of Sport Nutrition, 8*, 230–240.

Ruiz, F., Irazusta, A., Gil, S., Irazusta, J., Casis, L., & Gil, J. (2005). Nutritional intake in soccer players of different ages. *Journal of Sports Sciences, 23*, 235–242.

Schena, F., Pattini, A., & Mantovanelli, S. (1995). Iron status in athletes involved in endurance and prevalently anaerobic sports. In C. V. Kies & J. A. Driskell (Eds.), *Sports nutrition: Minerals and electrolytes* (pp. 65–79). Boca Raton, FL: CRC Press.

Short, S. H., & Short, W. R. (1983). Four-year study of university athletes' dietary intake. *Journal of the American Dietetic Association, 82*, 632–645.

Tarnopolsky, M. A., Zawada, C., Richmond, L. B., Carter, S., Shearer, J., Graham, T. *et al.* (2001). Gender differences in carbohydrate loading are related to energy intake. *Journal of Applied Physiology, 91*, 225–230.

Van Erp-Baart, A. M. J., Saris, W. H. M., Binkhorst, R. A., Vos, J. A., & Elvers, J. W. H. (1989). Nationwide survey on nutritional habits in elite athletes. Part I: Energy, carbohydrate, protein, and fat intake. *International Journal of Sports Medicine, 10* (suppl.1), S3–S10.

Williams, C., & Serratosa, L. (2006) Nutrition on match day. *Journal of Sports Sciences, 24*, 687–697.

Wittich, A., Oliveri, M. B., Rotemberg, E., & Mautalen, C. (2001). Body composition of professional football (soccer) players determined by dual x-ray absorptiometry. *Journal of Clinical Densitometry, 4*, 51–55.

Zehnder, M., Rico-Sanz, J., Kuhne, G., & Boutellier, U. (2001). Resynthesis of muscle glycogen after soccer specific performance examined by 13C-magnetic resonance spectroscopy in elite players. *European Journal of Applied Physiology and Occupational Physiology, 84*, 443–447.

Zuliani, G., Baldo-Enzi, G., Palmieri, E., Volpato, S., Vitale, E., Magnanini, P. *et al.* (1996). Lipoprotein profile, diet and body composition in athletes practicing mixed and anaerobic activities. *Journal of Sports Medicine and Physical Fitness, 36*, 211–216.

Appendix

Energy considerations using energy balance

Consider a healthy, adult athlete with an energy intake (EI) sufficient to maintain all the body's physiological processes and an exercise energy expenditure

(EEE) of $15 \, \text{kcal} \cdot \text{kg FFM}^{-1} \cdot \text{day}^{-1}$. The athlete's energy balance (EB) is calculated in terms of resting metabolic rate (RMR), the thermic effect of food (TEF), and non-exercise activity thermogenesis (NEAT) as:

$$EB = EI - (RMR + TEF + NEAT) - EEE$$

$$= 60 - (30 + 6 + 9) - 15 \, \text{kcal} \cdot \text{kg FFM}^{-1} \cdot \text{day}^{-1}$$

$$= 0 \, \text{kcal} \cdot \text{kg FFM}^{-1} \cdot \text{day}^{-1}$$

The athlete's energy availability (EA) is:

$$EA = EI - EEE$$

$$= 60 - 15 \, \text{kcal} \cdot \text{kg FFM}^{-1} \cdot \text{day}^{-1}$$

$$= 45 \, \text{kcal} \cdot \text{kg FFM}^{-1} \cdot \text{day}^{-1}$$

Thus, at an energy availability of $45 \, \text{kcal} \cdot \text{kg FFM}^{-1} \cdot \text{day}^{-1}$, the athlete is in energy balance.

Now consider the energy balance of the same athlete after energy intake has been restricted to $35 \, \text{kcal} \cdot \text{kg FFM}^{-1} \cdot \text{day}^{-1}$ for a month:

$$EB = EI - (RMR + TEF + NEAT) - EEE$$

$$= 35 - (24 + 3.5 + 9) - 15 \, \text{kcal} \cdot \text{kg FFM}^{-1} \cdot \text{day}^{-1}$$

$$= -16.5 \, \text{kcal} \cdot \text{kg FFM}^{-1} \cdot \text{day}^{-1}$$

Note that the thermic effect of food is still 10% of energy intake and that resting metabolic rate has declined by 20% because reproductive function, bone turnover, and other physiological processes have been suppressed.

By comparison, the athlete's energy availability is:

$$EA = EI - EEE$$

$$= 35 - 15 \, \text{kcal} \cdot \text{kg FFM}^{-1} \cdot \text{day}^{-1}$$

$$= 20 \, \text{kcal} \cdot \text{kg FFM}^{-1} \cdot \text{day}^{-1}$$

By calculating differences in energy balance, the athlete's energy deficiency appears to be:

$$EB_{\text{final}} - EB_{\text{initial}} = -16.5 - 0 \, \text{kcal} \cdot \text{kg FFM}^{-1} \cdot \text{day}^{-1}$$

$$= -16.5 \, \text{kcal} \cdot \text{kg FFM}^{-1} \cdot \text{day}^{-1}$$

but this does not account for the suppression of physiological systems. By calculating differences in energy availability, the athlete's actual energy deficiency is found to be:

$$\text{EA}_{\text{final}} - \text{EA}_{\text{initial}} = 20 - 45 \, \text{kcal} \cdot \text{kg FFM}^{-1} \cdot \text{day}^{-1}$$

$$= -25 \, \text{kcal} \cdot \text{kg FFM}^{-1} \cdot \text{day}^{-1}$$

In this example, energy balance underestimates the athlete's energy deficiency by $100*(25 - 16.5)/25 = 34\%$.

Now, suppose the chronically undernourished athlete consults a nutritionist to correct his or her energy deficiency. If the nutritionist's approach is to measure the athlete's resting metabolic rate and then to multiply that by a factor (F) related to the athlete's level of physical activity, the nutritionist will assess the athlete's physical activity and pick the corresponding activity factor (F) from a standard table, *which was developed from data on adequately nourished individuals*. Therefore, if the nutritionist correctly assesses the athlete's level of physical activity, the nutritionist will pick:

$$F = \text{EI}/\text{RMR}$$

$$= 60 \, \text{kcal} \cdot \text{kg FFM}^{-1} \cdot \text{day}^{-1}/$$

$$\times \, 30 \, \text{kcal} \cdot \text{kg FFM}^{-1} \cdot \text{day}^{-1} = 2.0$$

The nutritionist will then multiply the undernourished athlete's measured resting metabolic rate by this value to arrive at a recommended energy intake of:

$$\text{EI} = F*\text{RMR} = 2.0*24 \, \text{kcal} \cdot \text{kg FFM}^{-1} \cdot \text{day}^{-1}$$

$$= 48 \, \text{kcal} \cdot \text{kg FFM}^{-1} \cdot \text{day}^{-1}$$

which perpetuates the athlete's undernutrition by $100*(60 - 48)/60 = 20\%$.

Sports nutrition by reference to energy availability

The energy availability approach to sports nutrition assumes that energy intake must exceed exercise energy expenditure by $45 \, \text{kcal} \cdot \text{kg FFM}^{-1} \cdot \text{day}^{-1}$ for all physiological systems to function normally, because $45 \, \text{kcal} \cdot \text{kg FFM}^{-1} \cdot \text{day}^{-1}$ is the average energy intake of healthy, young sedentary adults in energy balance.

By this approach, the nutritionist in the above example would measure the undernourished athlete's exercise energy expenditure as $15 \, \text{kcal} \cdot \text{kg FFM}^{-1} \cdot \text{day}^{-1}$ and recommend:

$$\text{EI} = \text{EA} + \text{EEE} = 45 + 15 \, \text{kcal} \cdot \text{kg FFM}^{-1} \cdot \text{day}^{-1}$$

$$= 60 \, \text{kcal} \cdot \text{kg FFM}^{-1} \cdot \text{day}^{-1}$$

which is the amount required to provide sufficient metabolic fuels for all physiological processes.

Data consistent with this example are reported in Myerson *et al.* (1991).

3 Nutrition on match day

CLYDE WILLIAMS AND LUIS SERRATOSA

What players should eat on match day is a frequently asked question in sports nutrition. The recommendation from the available evidence is that players should eat a high-carbohydrate meal about 3 h before the match. This may be breakfast when the matches are played around midday, lunch for late afternoon matches, and an early dinner when matches are played late in the evening. The combination of a high-carbohydrate pre-match meal and a sports drink, ingested during the match, results in a greater exercise capacity than a high-carbohydrate meal alone. There is evidence to suggest that there are benefits to a pre-match meal that is composed of low-glycaemic index (GI) carbohydrate foods rather than high-GI foods. A low-GI pre-match meal results in feelings of satiety for longer and produces a more stable blood glucose concentration than after a high-GI meal. There are also some reports of improved endurance capacity after low-GI carbohydrate pre-exercise meals. The physical demands of soccer training and match-play draw heavily on players' carbohydrate stores and so the benefits of good nutritional practices for performance and health should be an essential part of the education of players, coaches, and in particular the parents of young players.

Keywords: Soccer, football, carbohydrates, glycaemic index, fatigue, exercise capacity

Introduction

"Breakfast is the most important meal of the day" is such a well held belief that it has become a mantra repeated as much to our athletes as to our children. In general, the recommendation not to miss breakfast is sound because it helps replenish the carbohydrate stores that are lost from the liver during the overnight fast as well as replenishing other nutrients and fluid that are necessary for health (Casey et al., 2000; Nilsson, Furst, & Hultman, 1973; Nilsson & Hultman, 1973). In addition, a high-carbohydrate breakfast also helps "top up" muscle glycogen stores within 3–4 h after the meal (Chryssanthopoulos, Williams, Nowitz, & Bogdanis, 2004; Wee, Williams, Tsintzas, & Boobis, 2005). When matches are played between late morning and early afternoon, breakfast may well be the pre-match meal for those players who are not early risers. Most matches are played in the afternoons on a Saturday or Sunday. However, there has been an increase in the number of matches played in the evenings, especially on weekdays (e.g. Champion's League games).

Planning a nutritional strategy for match day begins by first knowing the time and location of the match. Thereafter, the team nutritionist can work out how much time is available for meals and then recommend their composition bearing in mind the culinary likes and dislikes of the players. For example, when the match begins in the afternoon, players may have a light breakfast followed by a main meal around midday. When a match is played in the evening, players may have a late breakfast followed by a light lunch and their pre-match meal during the late afternoon, say about 15.00–16.00 h. To develop a successful nutritional strategy for players on match day, it is important to recognize that in many football clubs the pre-match meal is largely dictated by tradition and routine. For many players, a departure from their favourite pre-match meal is regarded as much a disadvantage as beginning a match with a physical injury. Therefore, any nutritional strategy must be developed in the context of what is custom and practice within a football club and supported by sound evidence.

The standard recommendation is that players should eat an easy-to-digest high-carbohydrate meal no later than about 3 h before a match. This recommendation has not changed since the publication of the last Consensus Statement on Nutrition and Soccer a decade ago (Ekblom & Williams, 1994). Since then there has been further progress in understanding the links between food intake and exercise performance but there have been few studies on football. Nevertheless, laboratory studies that have investigated the links between food intake and exercise performance have helped establish the principles, leaving team nutritionists to translate these principles into practice.

Our aim here is to provide an overview of those studies that have examined the influence of food intake on subsequent exercise performance in order to establish the bases for our recommendations for nutritional strategies on match day.

Pre-exercise meals

Most studies on exercise performance fall into two broad categories: whether the mode of exercise is cycling or running. Exercise tests that require participants to complete a fixed amount of work as quickly as possible or do as much work as possible in a set time, usually when cycling, may be regarded as assessing "exercise performance". Exercise tests that require participants to exercise as long as possible at a fixed power output (cycling) or at a set pace (running) may be regarded as assessing "endurance capacity".

In one of the early endurance performance studies, participants ate a breakfast consisting of bread, cereal, milk, and fruit juice (200 g carbohydrate) 4 h before cycling to exhaustion (Neufer *et al.*, 1987). This meal increased pre-exercise muscle glycogen concentration by about 15% (though this was not statistically significant). The performance test required the participants to cycle for 45 min at 77% of maximal oxygen uptake ($\dot{V}O_{2max}$) and then to cycle as fast as possible for 15 min. The total work accomplished during the last 15 min of the test was greater (22%) after the pre-exercise meal than it was following the no-meal trial. However, not all performance studies have found such marked improvements in performance following the ingestion of a high-carbohydrate pre-exercise meal. In one cycling study, Whitley et al. (1998) found no difference in time-trial performance when participants were provided with a meal containing 215 g of carbohydrate, or no meal, 4 h before a 10 km time-trial. Their cyclists completed 90 min at 70% $\dot{V}O_{2max}$ and then the 10 km as fast as possible, but the 10 km times for the fed (878 s) and the fasted (874 s) trials were almost identical.

These two examples of exercise performance studies are typical of those reported in the early literature and, in general, the benefits of eating a high-carbohydrate meal before an exercise performance test are not as clear as before an exercise endurance capacity test.

In one endurance capacity study, Schabort, Bosch, Weltan and Noakes (1999) provided their participants with a commercially available breakfast cereal (100 g carbohydrate) and milk 3 h before they cycled to exhaustion at 70% $\dot{V}O_{2max}$. They also obtained muscle biopsy samples from the participants before each trial and then again at the end of exercise to assess the use of muscle glycogen. Endurance capacity was significantly greater after the carbo-hydrate breakfast than when the participants exercised to exhaustion after an overnight fast (136 vs. 109 min). There were no differences in the muscle glyco-gen concentrations at the end of exercise in the two trials, but a direct com-parison of the respective rates of glycogenolysis cannot be undertaken because the final biopsy samples were obtained at different times.

The amount of carbohydrate ingested in a pre-exercise meal is also an impor-tant consideration. For example, Sherman et al. (1989) showed that although small amounts of carbohydrate (46 and 156 g) consumed 4 h before intermittent cycling improved endurance capacity, a greater amount (312 g) was even more effective. After this larger amount of carbohydrate, the exercise capacity was 15% greater (56 min) than after the water placebo (48 min) trial.

Footballers' breakfasts usually contain about 100–150 g of carbohydrate (C. Williams, unpublished observations) and so increasing this amount in one meal may lead to abdominal discomfort. Nevertheless, a compromise must be reached between eating sufficient carbohydrate to benefit performance without eating so much that it causes gastrointestinal disturbances during subsequent exercise. Sherman et al. (1989) avoided these potential gastrointestinal problems by liquidizing the pre-exercise meals given to their participants.

If eating a carbohydrate meal 3–4 h before exercise causes gastrointestinal discomfort, one alternative is to drink a carbohydrate solution before exercise. This nutritional strategy even allows athletes to take in carbohydrate to good effect as late as 1 h before exercise. Sherman, Peden and Wright (1991) showed that performance was improved during submaximal cycling lasting more than 90 min, when a solution containing the equivalent of 1.1–2.2 g · kg body mass^{-1} (BM) of carbohydrate was consumed 1 h before exercise. Wright, Sherman and Dernbach (1991) built on these observations by comparing the cycling time to exhaustion while their participants ingested carbohydrate before exercise, during exercise, undertook a combination of both, or exercised without carbohydrate. Endurance capacity increased to a greater extent when the cyclists drank a carbohydrate solution before and during exercise than when they exercised without carbohydrate (18% and 32% more, respectively). However, the greatest increase in endurance capacity (44%) was achieved when the cyclists ingested carbohydrate solutions both before and during exercise.

A similar result was reported when running rather than cycling was used to assess the influence of pre-exercise meals on endurance capacity (Chryssanthopoulos, Williams, Novitz, Kotsipoulou, & Vleck, 2002). When runners ate a high-carbohydrate breakfast (2.5 g carbohydrate $\cdot$ kg BM^{-1}) 3 h before exercise and drank a carbohydrate-electrolyte solution during a subsequent run to exhaustion, their endurance capacity was greater than when they ran after a high-carbohydrate breakfast alone. The pre-exercise carbohydrate meal and the carbohydrate-electrolyte solution increased running time by 9% (125 min) more than when only the meal was consumed (115 min) but 21% more (103 min) than when the runners completed the test without breakfast and had fasted overnight.

One obvious question is whether or not drinking a carbohydrate-electrolyte solution during prolonged running improves endurance capacity more than the combination of a high-carbohydrate pre-exercise meal and a carbohydrate-electrolyte solution during exercise. Chryssanthopoulos and Williams (1997) attempted to answer this question by comparing the endurance running capacity of ten runners who completed three trials. In one trial the participants ate a high-carbohydrate meal (2.5 g $\cdot$ kg BM^{-1}) 3 h before a treadmill run to exhaustion at 70% $\dot{V}O_{2max}$, and in another they consumed a placebo solution as the pre-exercise meal and drank a 6.9% carbohydrate-electrolyte solution throughout the run to exhaustion. In a third trial, they consumed a placebo solution as the pre-exercise meal and drank a placebo solution during the run to exhaustion. Again the most successful combination was the high-carbohydrate pre-exercise meal with a carbohydrate-electrolyte solution during the run. This combination of carbohydrates resulted in a run time to exhaustion of 147 min, whereas when the runners drank the carbohydrate-electrolyte solution during exercise they ran for 125 min. However, in both carbohydrate trials the run times were significantly longer than when the runners had a liquid placebo pre-exercise meal and drank a placebo solution during the run (115 min).

This same high-carbohydrate pre-exercise meal (2.5 g $\cdot$ kg BM^{-1}) was subsequently shown to increase glycogen concentration in the vastus lateralis of runners by 11% just 3 h later (Chryssanthopoulos *et al.*, 2004). However, this increase in muscle glycogen storage could not account for all the carbohydrate consumed. Therefore, it is reasonable to assume that at the end of the 3 h post-prandial period, some of the carbohydrate was still undergoing digestion and absorption and some would have been deposited in the liver as glycogen.

In contrast to the clear benefits of pre-exercise meals plus the ingestion of a carbohydrate-electrolyte solution during constant-paced running to exhaustion (i.e. endurance capacity), compared with ingesting only a carbohydrate-electrolyte solution during exercise, there may not be such clear differences between the nutritional interventions when endurance performance is the criterion of success.

Williams and Chryssanthopoulos (1996) compared the influences of a pre-exercise meal with no-meal on endurance running performance during a 30 km treadmill time-trial. The pre-exercise meal provided the runners with the equivalent of 2 g carbohydrate · kg BM^{-1} in the form of white bread, cereal, sugar, jam, and orange juice. During the time-trial, 4 h later, the runners ingested only water. In the no-meal trial the runners ingested 10 ml · kg BM^{-1} of a liquid placebo instead of breakfast, and immediately before the 30 km time-trial they drank 8 ml · kg BM^{-1} of a commercially available carbohydrate-electrolyte solution. They also drank 2 ml · kg BM^{-1} of this same solution every 5 km during the simulated race. In the fasting trial during which the runners drank the carbohydrate-electrolyte solution, they completed the 30 km in 121.7 min and in the fed trial their run time was an almost identical 121.8 min. Again this is an example of the point made earlier, that the choice of the exercise test has a profound influence on the outcome of studies on carbohydrate feedings and exercise performance.

Nevertheless, the weight of available evidence supports the recommendation that a high-carbohydrate meal before exercise is of greater benefit to performance than undertaking exercise in the fasting state. Thus in trying to optimize muscle and liver glycogen stores in preparation for the game, nutritional interventions should always try to match the individual needs of players by taking into account a player's position, physical characteristics, recent demands of training and competition, as well individual food preferences. The growing evidence in support of the beneficial role of high-carbohydrate diets for prolonged heavy exercise should be communicated to all players and coaches at all levels of the game through appropriate nutritional educational programmes. Education of young players and their parents, and older players as well as coaches, will help establish good nutritional practices that will not only help players realize their physical potential, as a result of a greater capacity to train hard, but also benefit their long-term health.

One of issues that a nutrition education programme should address is the demand of many coaches that their players become as lean as possible. Low-energy and low-carbohydrate diets are often recommended for players who are attempting to lose body fat. However, recommending that players train and compete in negative energy balance ignores the negative consequences for performance and health. A diet low in carbohydrate will fail to resynthesize muscle glycogen stores after training and matches (Bangsbo, Mohr, & Krustrup, 2006). Furthermore, low-carbohydrate diets that do not allow players to cover their daily energy expenditures appear to suppress the immune system and so make them more susceptible to viral infections (Nieman & Bishop, 2006). In summary, the more that players and coaches know about all the physical demands on players during the preparation for, and the participation in, football, the better able they will be to appreciate the needs for well-balanced diets that are high in carbohydrates and contain sufficient energy to cover daily energy expenditures.

Composition of pre-competition meals

Accepting that a high-carbohydrate pre-exercise meal is of benefit to performance, the next question to ask is whether there is an advantage in selecting one type of carbohydrate over another. The ingestion of different types of carbohydrates will produce markedly different changes in plasma glucose and insulin concentrations. These glycaemic and insulinaemic responses following the ingestion of different carbohydrates are the bases of a classification of carbohydrates that is more informative than describing them as simple or complex.

The changes in plasma glucose concentration following the ingestion of 50 g of available carbohydrate when compared with the glycaemic response following the ingestion of 50 g of glucose is used to describe the glycaemic index (GI) of that carbohydrate (Jenkins *et al.*, 1981). For example, white bread has a high value whereas lentils have a low value, reflecting the differences in the size of the glycaemic responses following the ingestion of these two carbohydrates (Foster-Powell & Brand Miller, 1995; Wolever, Jenkins, Jenkins, & Josse, 1991). Although the concept was developed to help prescribe diets for diabetics, it is now being used in studies of the influence of carbohydrate pre-exercise meals on performance (Burke, Collier, & Hargreaves, 1999). One of the potential attractions of consuming low- rather than high-GI carbohydrate foods before exercise is that the normal suppression of fatty acid mobilization is less and so there is a greater contribution of fat to energy metabolism (Wu, Nicholas, Williams, Took, & Hardy, 2003).

In one of the first studies on the influence of high- and low-GI carbohydrate foods on exercise capacity, the low-GI food appeared to improve endurance capacity to a greater extent than the high-GI food. In this study, Thomas, Brotherhood and Brand (1991) used lentils as the low-GI food and potatoes as the high-GI food, and compared the responses to those obtained after drinking a glucose solution or water. The meals and solutions were ingested 1 h before cycling to exhaustion at an exercise intensity of between 65 and 70% $\dot{V}O_{2max}$. The carbohydrate content of the meals and glucose solution was equivalent to $1 \text{ g} \cdot \text{kg BM}^{-1}$ and the volume was adjusted to 400 ml. The exercise times for the lentils, the potato, the glucose, and the water trials were 117, 97, 108, and 99 min, respectively. There was a clear difference in exercise time for the lentils trial, but there were no differences in performance times between the potato, the glucose, or the water trials. Thomas *et al.* (1991) did not address the different rates of digestion and absorption of the three carbohydrates within the hour before the start of exercise, or the fact that they had matched only the amount of carbohydrate ingested in these trials and did not account for the other nutrients in the lentils and potatoes, including protein.

A more recent study addressed the question of whether there are performance benefits to eating low-GI carbohydrate meals before exercise – that is, whether the amount of work done in a fixed time is increased. Febbraio and Stewart (1996) fed their participants instant mashed potatoes (made up in water) as the high-GI carbohydrate and lentils as the low-GI carbohydrate ($1\,g\cdot kg$ BM^{-1}), and they used a low-energy jelly as the control meal. The three conditions were assigned in random order and the "meals" were consumed 45 min before exercise. The exercise test required the six participants to cycle at 70% $\dot{V}O_{2peak}$ for 2 h before they cycled to complete as much work as possible in 15 min. There was no difference in the muscle glycogen concentrations at the start or at the end of exercise on the three test occasions The total amount of work accomplished during the last 15 min period was not different between the three conditions. Although these results do not confirm the benefits of a low-GI carbohydrate diet as reported by Thomas *et al.* (1991), a direct comparison cannot be made because different performance criteria were used in the two studies. Thomas *et al.* (1991) assessed endurance capacity, whereas Febbraio and Stewart (1996) assessed total work done in a fixed time (endurance performance).

Most of the subsequent studies on high- and low-GI carbohydrate pre-exercise foods have used similar cycling performance trials (DeMarco, Sucher, Cisar, & Butterfield, 1999; Febbraio, Keegan, Angus, Campbell, & Garnham, 2000; Goodpaster *et al.*, 1996; Paul, Rokusek, Dykstra, Boileau, & Layman, 1996; Sparks, Selig, & Febbraio, 1998; Stannard, Constantini, & Miller, 2000). In only one of these later studies was there a significant difference in performance times following the ingestion of a low-GI pre-exercise meal. DeMarco *et al.* (1999) reported an improvement in exercise time after their participants had eaten a low-GI meal 30 min before exercise that required them to cycle for 2 h at 70% $\dot{V}O_{2max}$ and then at 100% $\dot{V}O_{2max}$ to exhaustion. The times to exhaustion were 206, 130, and 120 s for the low-GI, high-GI, and water trials, respectively.

The most positive results have been reported when exercise capacity tests have been employed in cycling (Kirwan, O'Gorman, & Evans, 1998) and some (Stevenson, Williams, McComb, & Oram, 2005a; Wu & Williams, 2006) but not all (Wee, Williams, Gray, & Horabin, 1999) running studies.

In most of the studies on high- and low-GI carbohydrate pre-exercise meals, the foods were consumed within 2 h of the start of exercise. Therefore, it is likely that much of the food was in the gastrointestinal tract during exercise and glucose was released into the systemic circulation throughout exercise. In one of the first running studies on this topic, the pre-exercise meals were consumed 3 h before the participants completed a treadmill run to exhaustion at speeds equivalent to 69% $\dot{V}O_{2max}$ (Wee *et al.*, 1999). There were no differences in run times between the high-GI (113 min) and the low-GI (111min) trials, but the rate of fat oxidation was significantly greater in the low trial, both during the 3 h postprandial period and during the run to exhaustion.

In a more recent study, Wu *et al.* (2003) repeated the running study of Wee *et al.* (1999) but used foods that are more commonly eaten at breakfast. In the earlier study (Wee *et al.*, 1999), the low-GI pre-exercise meal consisted entirely of lentils and this was matched for energy and carbohydrate by a selection of high-GI foods. In the more recent study (Wu & Williams, 2006), the pre-exercise meals were matched for energy, carbohydrate, and macronutrient composition (Table 1). The run time to exhaustion at 70% $\dot{V}O_{2max}$ was significantly longer in the low-GI trial (109 min) than in the high-GI trial (101 min). Furthermore, the rate of fat oxidation during the run to exhaustion was greater, and plasma glucose concentrations were more stable, during the low-GI trial (Wu & Williams, 2006). A low-GI diet during recovery from prolonged running has also been shown to result in a greater endurance capacity during a subsequent run to exhaustion than a high-GI recovery diet (Stevenson *et al.*, 2005a).

The metabolic common denominator in those studies that have shown a clear improvement in endurance capacity following the ingestion of a low-GI carbohydrate pre-exercise meal appears to be a combination of a greater rate of fat oxidation and more stable plasma glucose concentrations during exercise than after a high-GI carbohydrate meal. An increased fat oxidation is accompanied by a reduction in the rate of carbohydrate degradation. This might suggest a sparing of the limited glycogen store in skeletal muscles. Some support for this suggestion is provided in a recent study that examined the influences of high- and low-GI carbohydrate pre-exercise meals on glycogen storage and utilization. In this study (Wee *et al.*, 2005), muscle biopsy samples were obtained from seven male runners after an overnight fast, 3 h after high- and low-GI carbohydrate (2 g·kg BM^{-1}) meals, and again after a 30 min treadmill run at 70% $\dot{V}O_{2max}$. Muscle glycogen increased by 15% 3 h after the high-GI meal, but

Table 1. Characteristics of the High and Low GI meals (for a 70 kg subject)

Meal	Description	Macronutrient content
High-GI breakfast	72 g Corn Flakes®, 300 ml skimmed milk, 93 g white bread, 12 g Flora spread, 23 g jam, 181 ml Lucozade Original®	852 kcal 162 g carbohydrate 12 g fat 23 g protein **GI = 78**[*]
Low-GI breakfast	100 g muesli (without raisins), 300 ml skimmed milk, 78 g apple, 120 g tinned peaches, 149 g yoghurt, 300 ml apple juice	855 kcal 162 g carbohydrate 11 g fat 27 g protein **GI = 44**[*]

[*] Calculated by the method of Wolever (1986). Glycaemic index values from Foster-Powell *et al.* (2002).

Registered trade marks: Corn Flakes® (Kellogg's Ltd, Manchester, UK); Lucozade Original® (GlaxoSmithKline, Brentford, UK).

there was no increase after the low-GI meal. During the 30 min treadmill run, the amount of muscle glycogen used was significantly greater after the high- than after the low-GI meal. Again the rate of fat oxidation was greater in the low-GI trial and plasma glucose was more stable during exercise than was the case in the high-GI trial. An explanation for the greater endurance capacity following low- rather than high-GI pre-exercise meals based on glycogen sparing alone would be too simplistic without considering the overall contribution of carbohydrate to energy balance. Although some studies have provided clear evidence of improved exercise capacity coinciding with glycogen sparing (Tsintzas & Williams, 1998), there are older (Coyle, Coggan, Hemmert, & Ivy, 1986) and more recent studies (Claassen *et al.*, 2005) that have reported improvements in endurance capacity that cannot be explained by differences in muscle glycogen at the point of fatigue. The additional exercise time may well be linked to the continued optimum rate of hepatic glucose output late in exercise, and so simply focusing only on differences in muscle glycogen may provide a limited understanding of the mechanisms underpinning these improvements in exercise duration.

Multiple-sprint studies

In most studies of pre-exercise feeding, the exercise used has been cycling or treadmill running, but these types of exercise are not directly applicable to foot- ball. In an attempt to fill this gap in exercise protocols, Nicholas, Nuttall and Williams (2000) designed a shuttle running test that includes activity patterns similar to those that routinely occur in football. The Loughborough Intermit- tent Shuttle Test (LIST) requires the participants to repeatedly run, walk, jog, and sprint between two lines 20 m apart for 15 min, and this is continued, with 3 min rest between blocks, for 90 min (i.e. six blocks; see Figure 1). During the 90 min test, participants perform 66 maximum sprints. The total distance covered while walking, jogging, running, and sprinting is approxi- mately 12 km and participants expend about 1330 kcal, which is similar to the estimated distances (about 11–12 km) and energy expenditures (1360 kcal) in football matches (Nicholas *et al.*, 2000) (Table 2). These performances are similar to those of midfield players who demonstrate high work rates during matches (Bangsbo *et al.*, 2006). Furthermore, this protocol involves turning, acceleration, and deceleration at speed and it is so demanding that all partici- pants report some delayed-onset muscle soreness (Thompson, Nicholas, & Williams, 1999) with clear evidence of muscle damage and decreased function (Thompson *et al.*, 2004).

   This protocol and slightly modified versions of it have been used to assess the efficacy of various nutritional interventions on exercise capacity (Davis, Jackson, Broadwell, Queary, & Lambert, 1997; Davis, Welsh, De Volve, & Alderson, 1999; McGregor, Nicholas, Lakomy, & Williams, 1999; Nicholas, Green, Hawkins, & Williams, 1997; Nicholas, Williams, Boobis, & Little, 1999; Nicholas, Williams, Lakomy, Phillips, & Nowitz, 1995; Welsh, Davis, Burke,

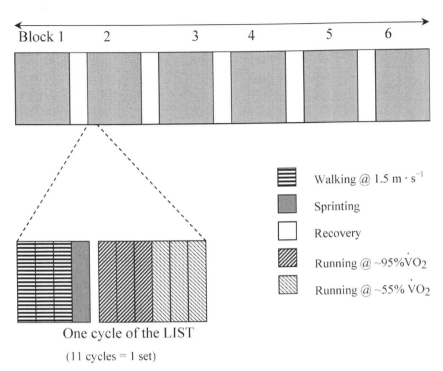

Figure 1. The Loughborough Intermittent Shuttle Test (LIST) is designed to reflect the activity pattern commonly associated with multiple-sprint sports such as soccer. The structure of the protocol is depicted. The LIST is performed in a sports hall on a marked 20 m track. The total exercise time of the LIST is 90 min, with a total rest time of 15 min. The varying running and walking speeds are dictated by an audio signal using a computer program developed at Loughborough University. Sprint times are recorded by a data logger using information from infrared photo-electric cells separated by 15 m. Over the course of the LIST, individuals cover a total distance of 12 km, sprinting approximately 1 km, and changing direction 624 times, with an estimated total energy expenditure of approximately 1330 kcal.

& Williams, 2002). In one study, Nicholas *et al.* (1997) reported that successful recovery of performance from this intermittent high-intensity running protocol was achieved when their participants increased their carbohydrate intake from about 4 to $9 \, g \cdot kg \, BM^{-1}$ during the 24 h between exercise tests. When the participants ate their normal amount of carbohydrate during the recovery period, even though it matched the higher carbohydrate diet for energy, they were unable to repeat their performance of the previous day.

When this study was repeated using iso-energetic meals of either high- or low-GI carbohydrate foods as the 24 h recovery diet, there were no differences in endurance running capacity between trials when the LIST was performed again on the second day (S. Erith *et al.*, unpublished study).

Table 2. Activity pattern and typical physiological responses to the Loughborough Intermittent Shuttle Test

Activity	Percent of time
Walking	49%
Jogging (55% $\dot{V}O_{2max}$)	24%
Running (95% $\dot{V}O_{2max}$)	19%
Sprinting	3%
Recovery	5%
Physiological characteristics	*Response*
Heart rate	165–170 beats $\cdot$ min^{-1}
% $\dot{V}O_{2max}$	$\sim$ 70%
Energy expenditure	$\sim$ 1300 kcal
Rectal temperature	$\sim$ 38.7C
Blood lactate concentration	$\sim$ 5–7 mmol $\cdot$ l^{-1}
Distance covered	$\sim$ 10–12 km
Sprinting	$\sim$ 8% distance
Deceleration after sprints	$\sim$ 4%

The benefits of high- or low-GI carbohydrate pre-exercise meals on performance of a modified version of the LIST have also been explored in male games players (rugby and soccer) (J. Davis & M. Dombo, unpublished study) and elite female football players (S. Chamberlain *et al.*, unpublished study). In these two studies, the high- and low-GI meals contained the same amount of carbohydrate ($2\,g \cdot kg\,BM^{-1}$) and consisted of the same quantities of macronutrients (Table 1). Three hours after the high- or low-GI meal, the participants completed five blocks of the LIST (i.e. 75 min and then ran to fatigue alternating between sprinting and jogging between the 20 m lines that defined the test area. The time to exhaustion was not different between the high-GI (10.3 min) and the low-GI (12.0 min) trials for the elite female football players. Although there were no differences in the overall sprint times between the two dietary trials during the 75 min before the intermittent sprints to exhaustion, the mean sprint times in the first 15 min were faster after the low- than after the high-GI meal.

When the men consumed the high- and the low-GI carbohydrate pre-exercise meals, the mean sprint times for the five blocks of the LIST were faster after the low-GI (2.61 s) than after the high-GI meal (2.66 s). However, there was no difference between the run times to fatigue for the high-GI (11.2 min) and the low-GI trials (10.0 min). It is difficult to offer an explanation for these differences in the responses to the high- and low-GI meals during this prolonged intermittent high-intensity shuttle running test. One consistent and common observation by all the participants in these pre-exercise feeding studies is that they never felt hungry after the low-GI pre-exercise meal during the 3 h postprandial period or during the 90 min of exercise. In contrast, most participants in the studies mentioned above reported that they felt hungry towards the end of the 3 h postprandial period and during prolonged exercise after the high-GI meal.

Therefore, when preparing for a match, ingesting enough carbohydrate in the pre-match meals is probably the most important strategy, because with the present rules the opportunities to consume carbohydrate during the game are limited to the half-time break. The stress of the game and other circumstances during the 10–15 min break may limit the amount of carbohydrate that can be consumed by players. It therefore becomes even more important that the pre-match meal should contain low-GI carbohydrate foods because they result in long-term stable blood glucose concentrations and general feelings of satiety (Stevenson *et al.*, 2005b). Furthermore, stable blood glucose concentrations may delay the onset of fatigue not only by providing substrate for muscle metabolism, but also as a result of positive influences on the central nervous system in general and the brain in particular (Meeussen, Watson, & Dvorak, 2006).

Carbohydrate intake within the hour before exercise

Earlier studies on the influence of ingesting carbohydrate within the hour before exercise suggested that this practice would have a detrimental influence on performance (Costill *et al.*, 1977; Foster, Costill, & Fink, 1979). These studies showed that there was a greater rate of glycogen degradation during exercise after ingesting a concentrated carbohydrate solution (25% w/v) (Costill *et al.*, 1977), and that fatigue occurred sooner (19%) during cycling to exhaustion at 80% $\dot{V}O_{2max}$ (Foster *et al.*, 1979). However, this highly publicised recommendation has not been supported by subsequent studies (Burke, Claassen, Hawley, & Noakes, 1998; Chryssanthopoulos, Hennessy, & Williams, 1994).

These early studies also showed a sharp peak in blood glucose concentrations following the ingestion of the concentrated glucose solution and then a rapid fall at the onset of exercise. For most people, the transient fall in blood glucose concentrations during the first few minutes of exercise appears to go unnoticed and has little influence on subsequent exercise capacity (Chryssanthopoulos *et al.*, 1994). During a match, the half-time interval is an opportunity to replenish some of the fluid lost and also an ideal opportunity to consume some carbohydrate. Therefore, it is unsurprising that well-formulated sports drinks are recommended because they are an effective and convenient way of providing fluid, carbohydrate, and electrolytes during the limited time available.

Carbohydrate intake during exercise

The influence of drinking carbohydrate solutions during exercise on subsequent performance has been extensively studied (for reviews, see Coyle, 2004; Maughan & Murray, 2000). There have also been some field studies on football players during match-play (Kirkendall, 1993). For example, when players were given glucose polymer solutions to ingest before and during matches, they had higher work rates than players who consumed placebo solutions (Kirkendall,

Foster, Dean, Grogan, & Thompson, 1988). Furthermore, there was also evidence that those players who were given the glucose polymer solution used less muscle glycogen during match-play (Leatt & Jacobs, 1989).

The LIST protocol has been used in several recent studies of the effects of drinking carbohydrate-electrolyte solutions on performance during prolonged intermittent high-intensity exercise under controlled conditions (Davis *et al.*, 1997, 1999; Davis, Welsh, & Alderson, 2000; McGregor *et al.*, 1999; Nicholas *et al.*, 1995; Welsh *et al.*, 2002). In the study of Nicholas *et al.* (1995), a group of recreational football players completed five blocks of the LIST and then they began sprinting and jogging back and forth over the 20 m course to the point of fatigue. They found that the distance covered was 33% greater when the football players drank a carbohydrate-electrolyte solution (6.5%) than when they drank a flavoured placebo solution. In a subsequent study, Nicholas *et al.* (1999) examined the amount of glycogen used during the completion of six blocks of the LIST (90 min) and reported that less glycogen was used when their participants consumed the carbohydrate-electrolyte solution than when they consumed flavoured water placebo. Welsh *et al.* (2002) used a similar protocol but gave their participants higher amounts of carbohydrate and found even greater improvements in endurance capacity (50%) than when the participants drank a placebo solution during the test.

It is clear from studies that simulate the demands of match-play that those players who do not eat before a match or eat very little will benefit from drinking a carbohydrate-electrolyte solution during the match (Nicholas *et al.*, 1995; Welsh *et al.*, 2002). For example, players who completed the LIST after an overnight fast but drank a carbohydrate-electrolyte solution during exercise tended to maintain their sprinting ability for longer than if they had ingested water alone (A. Ali *et al.*, unpublished study).

Drinking a carbohydrate-electrolyte solution also appears to improve endurance capacity during intermittent exercise even when players have high pre-exercise muscle glycogen stores. Foskett, Williams, Boobis and Tsintzas (2002) studied the influence of drinking a carbohydrate-electrolyte solution on endurance capacity during intermittent shuttle running after participants had increased their pre-exercise muscle glycogen concentrations by carbohydrate loading in the previous 48 h. Six male recreational footballers were required to continue running repeated 15 min blocks of the LIST to the point of fatigue On one occasion they drank a flavoured placebo and on another they drank a 6.4% carbohydrate-electrolyte solution throughout the exercise test. Muscle biopsy samples were obtained from the participants after an overnight fast (i.e. before exercise), after 90 min of the LIST, and again at the point of fatigue. All six participants ran for longer when they drank the carbohydrate-electrolyte solution (158 min) than when they drank the flavoured placebo solution (131 min). However, there were no differences in the muscle glycogen concentrations after 90 min of running during the two trials, endorsing the important role of blood glucose during the later stages of prolonged exercise (Claassen *et al.*, 2005; Coggan & Coyle, 1989; Coyle *et al.*, 1983, 1986). Of note is that these run times were much longer than when similar participants completed the same exercise protocol in the fasting state but without the prior carbohydrate loading (approximately 105 min, i.e. 90 min of the LIST plus one 15 min block: A. Foskett, unpublished observations). Therefore, it would appear that carbohydrate loading before a match plus drinking a carbohydrate-electrolyte solution during the match may be a worthwhile strategy, especially in the event of the game going into extra time. This strategy might also include a low-GI pre-exercise meal because the sensations of satiety are maintained for longer than after a high-GI meal. However, there is some evidence to suggest that the greater fat metabolism during exercise after a low-GI than after a high-GI meal is abolished when a carbohydrate solution is ingested during subsequent exercise (Burke *et al.*, 1998). Nevertheless, not feeling hungry during a match may have a beneficial influence on a player's performance even though the metabolic differences between low- and high-GI meals are minimized as a consequence of ingesting carbohydrate solutions at suitable breaks during a match.

Carbohydrate intake and skill performance

Unfortunately, too few studies have been conducted on the effects of ingesting carbohydrate on the ability to sustain soccer-specific skills during match-play. Some studies examining soccer-specific skills during match-play have found no differences following the ingestion of a carbohydrate-electrolyte solution (Zeederberg *et al.*, 1996), an improvement (Ostojic & Mazic, 2002), or at least maintenance of skill (Northcott, Kenward, Purnell, & McMorris, 1999). However, in attempting to make the soccer skill tests as real as possible, these studies had to compromise their control of confounding variables. Therefore, it is difficult to obtain a clear consensus on the influence of carbohydrate ingestion on soccer-specific skills from these studies.

In a series of studies on soccer-specific skills, fatigue, and the influence of carbohydrate nutrition, Ali *et al.* (2002) tested the skills of soccer players before, during, and after they had performed the 90 min LIST. The LIST was used to simulate the activity patterns common to soccer in a controlled environment and so focus on the performance of the skills, which is not possible in soccer matches *per se*. They found that the performances of a soccer passing test and a goal shooting test were significantly poorer after the 90 min LIST. However, the decrease in these skills was less when the players ingested a carbohydrate-electrolyte solution immediately before and at 15 min intervals throughout the test than when they ingested a placebo solution. Furthermore, not only were the two soccer-specific skills better maintained during the carbohydrate-electrolyte trial, the accumulated sprint times of the players were also faster than in the placebo trial (Ali *et al.*, 2002). Clearly, more research is required on the effects of carbohydrates (or lack of them) on cognitive performance in general and sports skills in particular before we can formulate more precise nutritional strategies for players.

In summary, the evidence to support the recommendation that players should eat a high-carbohydrate pre-exercise meal has increased since the 1994 Consensus Conference on Nutrition and Soccer. This evidence comes from studies on pre-exercise meals containing high- and low-GI carbohydrate foods that are provided as palatable meals. It would appears that low-GI carbohydrate meals may be of some benefit as pre-match meals if only because they may make players feel "better", which in itself is often the basis of better performance. Therefore, while progress has been made in studying the influences of real foods on performance, there is still a need for more ecologically valid exercise tests that are well controlled and use footballers as their participants.

References

Ali, A., Nicholas, C., Brooks, J., Davison, S., Foskett, A., & Williams, C. (2002). The influence of carbohydrate-electrolyte ingestion on soccer skill performance. *Medicine and Science in Sports and Exercise, 34*, 5.

Bangsbo, J., Mohr, M., & Krustrup, P. (2006). Physical and metabolic demands of training and match-play in the elite player. *Journal of Sports Sciences, 24*, 665–674.

Burke, L., Claassen, A., Hawley, J., & Noakes, T. (1998). Carbohydrate intake during prolonged cycling minimises effect of glycemic index of a preexercise meal. *Journal of Applied Physiology, 85*, 2220–2226.

Burke, L., Collier, G., & Hargreaves, M. (1999). Glycemic index – a new tool in sports nutrition. *International Journal of Sport Nutrition, 8*, 401–415.

Casey, A., Mann, R., Banister, K., Fox, J., Morris, P. G., Macdonald, I. et al. (2000). Effect of carbohydrate ingestion on glycogen resynthesis in human liver and skeletal muscle, measured by ^{13}C MRS. *American Journal of Physiology: Endocrinology and Metabolism, 278*, E65–E75.

Chryssanthopoulos, C., Hennessy, L., & Williams, C. (1994). The influence of pre-exercise glucose ingestion on endurance running capacity. *British Journal of Sports Medicine, 28*, 105–109.

Chryssanthopoulos, C., & Williams, C. (1997). Pre-exercise carbohydrate meal and endurance running capacity when carbohydrates are ingested during exercise. *International Journal of Sports Medicine, 18*, 543–548.

Chryssanthopoulos, C., Williams, C., Nowitz, A., & Bogdanis, G. (2004). Skeletal muscle glycogen concentration and metabolic responses following a high glycacmic carbohydrate breakfast. *Journal of Sports Sciences, 22*, 1065–1071.

Chryssanthopoulos, C., Williams, C., Novitz, C., Kotsipoulou, C., & Vleck, V. (2002). The effect of a high carbohydrate meal on endurance running capacity. *International Journal of Sport Nutrition and Exercise Metabolism, 12*, 157–171.

Claassen, A., Lambert, E., Bosch, A., Rodger, I., Gibson, A., & Noakes, T. (2005). Variability in exercise capacity and metabolic response during endurance exercise after a low carbohydrate diet. *International Journal of Sport Nutrition and Exercise Metabolism, 15*, 97–116.

Coggan, A., & Coyle, E. (1989). Metabolism and performance following carbohydrate ingestion late in exercise. *Medicine and Science in Sports and Exercise, 21*, 59–65.

Costill, D., Coyle, E., Dalsky, G., Evans, W., Fink, W., & Hoopes, D. (1977). Effects of elevated plasma FFA and insulin on muscle glycogen usage during exercise. *Journal of Applied Physiology, 43,* 695–699.

Coyle, E. (2004). Fluid and fuel intake during exercise. *Journal of Sports Sciences, 22,* 39–59.

Coyle, E., Hagberg, J., Hurley, B., Martin, W., Ehsani, A., & Holloszy, J. (1983). Carbohydrate feeding during prolonged strenuous exercise can delay fatigue. *Journal of Applied Physiology, 55,* 230–235.

Coyle, E. F., Coggan, A. R., Hemmert, M. K., & Ivy, J. L. (1986). Muscle glycogen utilization during prolonged strenuous exercise when fed carbohydrate. *Journal of Applied Physiology, 61,* 165–172.

Davis, J., Welsh, R., & Alderson, N. (2000). Effects of carbohydrate and chromium ingestion during intermittent high-intensity exercise to fatigue. *International Journal of Sport Nutrition and Exercise Metabolism, 10,* 476–485.

Davis, M., Jackson, D., Broadwell, M., Queary, J., & Lambert, C. (1997). Carbohydrate drinks delay fatigue during intermittent, high intensity cycling in active men and women. *International Journal of Sport Nutrition, 7,* 261–273.

Davis, M., Welsh, R., De Volve, K., & Alderson, N. (1999). Effects of branched chained amino acids and carbohydrate on fatigue during intermittent, high-intensity running. *International Journal of Sports Medicine, 20,* 309–314.

DeMarco, H., Sucher, K., Cisar, C., & Butterfield, G. (1999). Pre-exercise carbohydrate meals: Application of glycemic index. *Medicine and Science in Sports and Exercise, 31,* 164–170.

Ekblom, B., & Williams, C. (1994). Foods, nutrition and soccer performance: Final consensus statement. *Journal of Sports Sciences, 12,* S3.

Febbraio, M., Keegan, M., Angus, J., Campbell, S., & Garnham, A. (2000). Preexercise carbohydrate ingestion, glucose kinetics, and muscle glycogen use: Effect of the glycemic index. *Journal of Applied Physiology, 89,* 1845–1851.

Febbraio, M., & Stewart, K. (1996). CHO feeding before prolonged exercise: Effect of glycemic index on muscle glycogenolysis and exercise performance. *Journal of Applied Physiology, 82,* 1115–1120.

Foskett, A., Williams, C., Boobis, L., & Tsintzas, K. (2004). Effect of carbohydrate ingestion on muscle glycogen utilisation during exhaustive high-intensity intermittent running after consumption of a high carbohydrate diet. *Journal of Physiology, 555P,* C63.

Foster, C., Costill, D., & Fink, W. (1979). Effects of pre-exercise feedings on endurance performance. *Medicine and Science in Sports and Exercise, 11,* 1–5.

Foster-Powell, K., & Brand Miller, J. (1995). International tables of glycemic index. *American Journal of Clinical Nutrition, 62,* 871S–893S.

Goodpaster, B., Costill, D., Fink, W., Trappe, T., Jozsi, A., Starling, R. *et al.* (1996). The effects of pre-exercise starch ingestion on endurance performance. *International Journal of Sports Medicine, 17,* 366–372.

Jenkins, D. J. A., Thomas, D. M., Wolever, M. S., Taylor, R. H., Barker, H., Fielden, H. *et al.* (1981). Glycemic index of foods: A physiological basis for carbohydrate exchange. *American Journal of Clinical Nutrition, 34,* 362–366.

Kirkendall, D. (1993). Effects of nutrition on performance in soccer. *Medicine and Science in Sports and Exercise, 25,* 1370–1374.

Kirkendall, D., Foster, C., Dean, J., Grogan, J., & Thompson, N. (1988). Effect of glucose polymer supplementation on performance of soccer players. In T. Reilly,

A. Lees, K. Davids, & W. Murphy (Eds.), *Science and football* (pp. 33–41). London: E & FN Spon.

Kirwan, J., O' Gorman, D., & Evans, W. (1998). A moderate glycemic meal before endurance exercise can enhance performance. *Journal of Applied Physiology, 84,* 53–59.

Leatt, P. B., & Jacobs, I. (1989). Effect of glucose polymer ingestion on glycogen depletion during a soccer match. *Canadian Journal of Sports Science, 14,* 112–116.

Maughan, R., & Murray, R. (2000). *Sports drinks: Basic science and practical aspects.* London: CRC Press.

McGregor, S., Nicholas, C., Lakomy, H., & Williams, C. (1999). The influence of intermittent high intensity shuttle running and fluid ingestion on the performance of a soccer skill. *Journal of Sports Sciences, 17,* 895–903.

Meeussen, R., Watson, P., & Dvorak, J. (2006). The brain and fatigue: new opportunities for nutritional interventions. *Journal of Sports Sciences, 24,* 773–782.

Neufer, P. D., Costill, D. L., Flynn, M. G., Kirwan, J., Mitchell, J., & Houmard, J. (1987). Improvements in exercise performance: Effects of carbohydrate feedings and diet. *Journal of Applied Physiology, 62,* 983–988.

Nicholas, C., Green, P., Hawkins, R., & Williams, C. (1997). Carbohydrate intake and recovery of intermittent running capacity. *International Journal of Sport Nutrition, 7,* 251–260.

Nicholas, C., Nuttall, F., & Williams, C. (2000). The Loughborough Intermittent Shuttle Test: A field test that simulates the activity pattern of soccer. *Journal of Sports Sciences, 18,* 97–104.

Nicholas, C., Williams, C., Boobis, L., & Little, N. (1999). Effect of ingesting a carbohydrate-electrolyte beverage on muscle glycogen utilisation during high intensity, intermittent shuttle running. *Medicine and Science in Sports and Exercise, 31,* 1280–1286.

Nicholas, C., Williams, C., Lakomy, H., Phillips, G., & Nowitz, A. (1995). Influence of ingesting a carbohydrate-electrolyte solution on endurance capacity during intermittent, high-intensity shuttle running. *Journal of Sports Sciences, 13,* 283–290.

Nieman, D. C., & Bishop, N. C. (2006). Nutritional strategies to counter stress to the immune system in athletes, with special reference to soccer. *Journal of Sports Sciences, 24,* 763–772.

Nilsson, L. H. S., Furst, P., & Hultman, E. (1973). Carbohydrate metabolism of the liver in normal man under varying dietary conditions. *Scandinavian Journal of Clinical and Laboratory Investigations, 32,* 331–337.

Nilsson, L. H. S., & Hultman, E. (1973). Liver glycogen in man – the effect of total starvation or a carbohydrate-poor diet followed by carbohydrate refeeding. *Scandinavian Journal of Clinical and Laboratory Investigations, 32,* 325–330.

Northcott, S., Kenward, M., Purnell, K., & Mcmorris, T. (1999). Effect of a carbohydrate solution on motor skill proficiency during simulated soccer performance. *Applied Research in Coaching and Athletics Annual, 14,* 105–118.

Ostojic, S., & Mazic, S. (2002). Effects of a carbohydrate-electrolyte drink on specific soccer tests and performance. *Journal of Sports Science and Medicine, 2,* 47–53.

Paul, G., Rokusek, J., Dykstra, G., Boileau, R., & Layman, D. (1996). Oats, wheat or corn cereal ingestion before exercise alters metabolism in humans. *Journal of Nutrition, 126,* 1372–1382.

Schabort, E., Bosch, A., Weltan, S., & Noakes, T. (1999). The effect of a preexercise meal on time to fatigue during prolonged cycling exercise. *Medicine and Science in Sports and Exercise, 31,* 464–471.

Sherman, W., Brodowicz, G., Wright, D., Allen, Wk, A., Simonsen, J., & Dernbach, A. (1989). Effects of 4h preexercise carbohydrate feedings on cycling performance. *Medicine and Science in Sports and Exercise, 21,* 598–604.

Sherman, W., Peden, M., & Wright, D. (1991). Carbohydrate feedings 1 h before exercise improves cycling performance. *American Journal of Clinical Nutrition, 54,* 866–870.

Sparks, M., Selig, S., & Febbraio, M. (1998). Pre-exercise carbohydrate ingestion: Effect of the glycemic index on endurance exercise performance. *Medicine and Science in Sports and Exercise, 30,* 844–849.

Stannard, S., Constantini, N., & Miller, J. (2000). The effect of glycemic index on plasma glucose and lactate levels during incremental exercise. *International Journal of Sport Nutrition and Exercise Metabolism, 10,* 51–61.

Stevenson, E., Williams, C., McComb, G., & Oram, C. (2005a). Improved recovery from prolonged exercise following the consumption of low glycemic index carbohydrate meals. *International Journal of Sport Nutrition and Exercise Metabolism, 15,* 333–349.

Stevenson, E., Williams, C., & Nute, M. (2005b). The influence of glycaemic index of breakfast and lunch on substrate utilisation during postprandial periods and subsequent exercise. *British Journal of Nutrition, 93,* 885–893.

Thomas, D., Brotherhood, J., & Brand, J. (1991). Carbohydrate feeding before exercise: Effect of glycemic index. *International Journal of Sports Medicine, 12,* 180–186.

Thompson, D., Bailey, D., Hill, J., Hurst, T., Powell, J., & Williams, C. (2004). Prolonged vitamin C supplementation and recovery from eccentric exercise. *European Journal of Applied Physiology, 92,* 133–138.

Thompson, D., Nicholas, C., & Williams, C. (1999). Muscle soreness following prolonged intermittent high intensity shuttle running. *Journal of Sports Sciences, 17,* 387–395.

Tsintzas, K., & Williams, C. (1998). Human muscle glycogen metabolism during exercise: Effect of carbohydrate supplementation. *Sports Medicine, 25,* 7–23.

Wee, S.-L., Williams, C., Gray, S., & Horabin, J. (1999). Influence of high and low glycemic index meals on endurance running capacity. *Medicine and Science in Sports and Exercise, 31,* 393–399.

Wee, S., Williams, C., Tsintzas, K., & Boobis, L. (2005). Ingestion of a high-glycemic index meal increases muscle glycogen storage at rest but augments its utilization during subsequent exercise. *Journal of Applied Physiology, 99,* 707–714.

Welsh, R., Davis, M., Burke, J., & Williams, H. (2002). Carbohydrates and physical/mental performance during intermittent exercise to fatigue. *Medicine and Science in Sports and Exercise, 34,* 723–731.

Whitley, H., Humphries, S., Campbell, I., Keegan, M., Jayanetti, T., Sperry, D. et al. (1998). Metabolic and performance relationship during endurance exercise after high fat and high carbohydrate meals. *Journal of Applied Physiology, 85,* 418–424.

Williams, C., & Chryssanthopoulos, C. (1996). Pre-exercise food intake and performance. In A. Simopoulos & K. Pavlou (Eds.), *Nutrition and fitness: Metabolic and behavioural aspects in health and disease* (pp. 33–45). New York: Karger.

Wolever, T., & Jenkins, D. (1986). The use of glycemic index in predicting the blood glucose response to mixed meals. *American Journal of Clinical Nutrition, 43,* 167–172.

Wolever, T., Jenkins, D., Jenkins, A., & Josse, R. (1991). The glycemic index: Methodology and clinical implications. *American Journal of Clinical Nutrition, 54,* 846–854.

Wright, D., Sherman, W., & Dernbach, A. (1991). Carbohydrate feedings before, during, or in combination improve cycling endurance performance. *Journal of Applied Physiology, 71,* 1082–1088.

Wu, C.-L., & Williams, C. (2006). A low glycemic index meal before exercise improves running capacity in man. In *Journal of Sport Nutrition and Exercise Metabolism, 16,* 510–527.

Wu, C.-L., Nicholas, C., Williams, C., Took, A., & Hardy, L. (2003). The influence of high-carbohydrate meals with different glycaemic indices on substrate utilisation during subsequent exercise. *British Journal of Nutrition, 90,* 1049–1056.

Zeederberg, C., Lloyd, L., Lambert, E., Noakes, T., Dennis, S., & Hawley, J. (1996). The effect of carbohydrate ingestion on the motor skill proficiency. *International Journal of Sport Nutrition, 6,* 348–355.

4 Water and electrolyte needs for football training and match-play

SUSAN M. SHIRREFFS, MICHAEL N. SAWKA
AND MICHAEL STONE

The high metabolic rates sustained by soccer players during training and match-play cause sweat to be produced in both warm and temperate environments. There is limited published information available on the effects of this sweat loss on performance in soccer. However, this limited information, together with knowledge of the effects of sweat loss in other sports with skill components as well as endurance and sprint components, suggests that the effects of sweating will be similar to the effects in these other activities. Therefore, the generalization that a body mass reduction equivalent to 2% should be the acceptable limit of sweat losses seems reasonable. This amount, or more, of sweat loss reflected in body mass loss is a common experience for some players. Sodium is the main electrolyte lost in sweat and the available data indicate considerable variability in sodium losses between players due to differences in sweating rate and sweat electrolyte concentration. Additionally, the extent of sodium loss is such that its replacement will be warranted for some of these players during training sessions and matches. Although soccer is a team sport, the great individual variability in sweat and electrolyte losses of players in the same training session or match dictates that individual monitoring to determine individual water and electrolyte requirements should be an essential part of a player's nutritional strategy.

Keywords: Water balance, electrolyte balance, sweating, hydration, sodium

Introduction

In the 1994 Consensus Conference held in Zurich, Maughan and Leiper (1994) reviewed "Fluid loss in soccer", providing information available from soccer players during both training and match-play. They then discussed issues relating to "Fluid and carbohydrate replacement". This discussion was largely from a non-soccer-specific point of view but did cover issues relating to "Fluid replacement for competition", "Fluid replacement in recovery from training and competition", and "Fluid loss and intake in training". The final focus of the review was to consider issues related to "Training and competition in the heat" and to provide "Practical recommendations".

In the 2005 Consensus Conference, the more extensive programme, with twelve rather than eight papers, means that this current update focuses only on the water and electrolyte needs for training and match-play. Data were collected for soccer players during training, match-play or during simulated soccer activity, and when possible only publications from 1994 onwards were used. Readers should consult Maughan and Leiper's (1994) review to gain relevant background information and should consider the paper of Armstrong (1996) on "Nutritional strategies for soccer" in this volume to be of particular relevance.

An in-depth discussion of the rationale and requirements for water and electrolyte intake before, during, and after exercise took place at the June 2003 International Olympic Committee Consensus Conference. The outcomes of the conference were published in the January 2004 edition of the *Journal of Sports Sciences*, with the papers by Coyle (2004) and Shirreffs *et al.* (2004) being especially relevant. Therefore, these topics will not be covered again here as there is no good evidence to suggest that the physiological or nutritional requirements of soccer players, with regard to their water and electrolyte requirements, differ significantly from those of other athletes.

This review focuses on the water and electrolyte needs of soccer players during training and match-play. Data for adult and adolescent male and female players are reviewed and recommendations are proposed. The recommendations can be used by players themselves, coaches, and clubs, or indeed by governing organizations when considering the rules and regulations of the game.

Water and electrolyte losses in soccer

Methods of assessing water loss

It is common practice to use changes in body mass as an index of body water content changes and thus of hydration status. Many publications providing advice to athletes from all types of sports contain statements along the lines that exercise performance is impaired when dehydration exceeds about 2% of the pre-exercise body mass, especially in warm environments. These statements are based on the assumption that 1 kg of mass loss is equal to 1 litre of sweat loss. Clearly, any fluid intake and urine or faecal loss needs to be accounted for and appropriate corrections made. The initial pre-exercise body mass should be obtained from early morning measurements established for several days before any glycogen loading procedures (if used for competition). Glycogen loading can cause water bonding and therefore modest hyperhydration. The dehydration level should be calculated as the reduction below the baseline body weight. The sweating rate should be calculated as the change in body weight (with appropriate corrections) during the training session, regardless if baseline or not.

Potential sources of error in using change in body mass to quantify sweat loss include loss of water and therefore mass from the respiratory tract and mass loss due to substrate oxidation. Although individually these losses may be small, their overall effects are of significance in many exercise contexts. The decision of whether to correct for substrate oxidation and respiratory water loss is usually based on the relative magnitude of the different avenues of mass loss, the precision required in the expression of the data, and the purpose for which it is being determined. Indeed, respiratory water loss and metabolic water produced are generally of similar magnitude and more or less cancel each other, minimizing the need for correction.

Methods of assessing electrolyte loss

The main routes of electrolyte loss from the human body are the urine, faeces, and sweat, although vomiting also results in significant losses. Large amounts of electrolytes are also temporarily secreted from the body into the gastrointestinal tract, but these are largely reabsorbed later in the system. It is sweat electrolyte losses that have the potential to set exercisers apart from non-exercisers and will therefore be the focus for consideration here.

A wide range of values for all of the major sweat electrolytes has been reported in the literature, reflecting variations between individuals, differences due to the experimental conditions, and differences due to the collection methods. The latter may be due to errors caused by contamination or to incomplete collection of the sample, or it may reflect a real difference induced by the collection site (e.g. arm vs. chest). The composition of sweat has been examined using a variety of sampling methods. The crudest method is simply to collect sweat as it drips from the skin surface, meaning there will have been a variable amount of evaporation from the skin surface, leading to an unknown degree of concentration of the sample and the possibility of contamination with skin cells. The two main methods that have been used in attempts to overcome these difficulties involve collection of sweat from a specific body region using some form of enclosing bag, capsule or absorptive patch, or a variation on the whole body-washdown technique. The enclosing bag approach can eliminate the problem of evaporation of water from the skin surface, but the method itself may lower the local sweat rate and thus alter electrolyte composition.

Sweat glands will reabsorb electrolytes (e.g. sodium) as the precursor fluid moves down the duct. The amount of electrolytes reabsorbed is dependent on sweat rate, such that at low sweat rates more sodium is reabsorbed so the secreted sweat sodium concentration is lowered. There also appear to be regional variations in sweat composition, as evidenced by the different values obtained when the composition of sweat obtained from different parts of the body is compared (Costa, Calloway, & Margen, 1969). In addition, regional sweat collection procedures provide higher sweat electrolyte concentrations than from the whole body-washdown technique (Lemon, Yarasheski, & Dolny, 1986; Patterson, Galloway, & Nimmo, 2000; Shirreffs & Maughan, 1997; Van Heyningen & Weiner, 1952). The higher electrolyte concentrations with local sweat collection procedures than whole-body washdown are probably due to an alteration in composition caused by the restriction of sweat evaporation. The difficulties caused by the restriction of evaporation can be overcome by using a ventilated capsule or chamber: the water in the effluent air is trapped in a cold trap, and the electrolytes are recovered at the end of the study period by washing out the enclosing apparatus. This does not, however, help to overcome the difficulties caused by regional differences in the composition of sweat.

A number of variations on the whole-body sweat collection method have been developed. In most of these, total sweat loss is calculated from the change in body mass. In early studies when participants exercised in a desert environment, it was assumed that there was no electrolyte loss from the skin surface due to sweat dripping, so the participants were washed before exercise, the body and the clothes worn were washed after exercise with distilled water, and the electrolyte content of that water was measured. Alternatively, thorough washing and drying of the individual, who then wears an absorbent suit to absorb sweat secreted onto the skin, has been reported. Forced convection has also been used to maximize sweat evaporation, or participants have worn minimal clothing and then been dried at regular intervals with towels that were then added to the washdown water. Enclosing participants within a close-fitting plastic bag and exposing them to a hot humid environment to stimulate sweating is a method that has been used in non-exercise settings. Finally, having participants exercise within a large plastic bag that forms a "small room" around them has been used successfully in laboratory studies (Shirreffs & Maughan, 1997).

Most published data for soccer players have been obtained using absorbent patches to collect sweat. While this is not a particularly difficult technique, clubs and players wanting to determine their sweat electrolyte losses are likely to need specialized help to do so (Burke, 2005). Besides providing approximate sweat electrolyte losses, this approach, at a minimum, identifies those athletes with electrolyte-rich ("salty") sweat and who need to pay particular attention to electrolyte replacement. When it is not possible to determine electrolyte losses in this way, it may be possible to identify subjectively players with very high salt losses. That is, they may complain of the very salty taste of sweat in their mouth, that they experience irritation when salt gets in their eyes, or salt stains may be visible on clothing worn during training or matches.

New data and developments in soccer research since 1994: Adult male players

In recent years, several papers have reported the results of "in-the-field" hydration monitoring, sweat collection, and subsequent estimation of sweat electrolyte losses in adult male professional soccer players (Maughan, Merson, Broad, & Shirreffs, 2004; Maughan, Shirreffs, Merson, & Horswill, 2005; Shirreffs *et al.*, 2005). In this section, the findings from players training with three European professional soccer clubs, all of which were competing in the highest league in their country, are summarized. This represents data from 67 players. Except where otherwise stated, the following methodology has been used to establish fluid and electrolyte losses and guidelines for the replacement. For a more detailed description of the methodologies used, the original papers should be consulted (Maughan *et al.*, 2004, 2005; Shirreffs *et al.*, 2005).

Data were collected during training sessions of approximately 90 min duration. With the exception of goalkeepers, all the players tested within each club completed very similar training sessions. Players were weighed nude or wearing only underpants before and after each training session. Between these two weighing periods, all urine excreted was collected and weighed and all drink consumed was accounted for by weighing drinks bottles. In the few instances when solid food was consumed, the appropriate correction was applied to the player's body mass. Sweat losses were estimated by correcting the change in body mass for drinks consumed and urine passed. After appropriate cleaning of the skin, four absorbent patches were applied to the right side of the player's body on the forearm, thigh, upper back, and chest ($n = 48$). These were removed during or at the end of the training session for subsequent analysis. Researchers attempted to make as few changes as possible to the normal training ground procedures at each club. This ensured that the data collected represented the player's normal behaviour as closely as possible. The environmental conditions in which the training sessions took place are shown in Table 1.

Table 1. Temperature and relativity humidity at each of the three clubs during 90 min training sessions (mean ± *s*)

	Temperature (°C)	Relative humidity (%)
Club 1	5 ± 1	81 ± 6
Club 2	27 ± 2	55 ± 6
Club 3	32 ± 3	20 ± 5

Water balance

The average calculated sweat losses, fluid intake, and percent change in body mass for the players (Table 2) are in agreement with those previously reported in the literature for adult males (Burke, 1997; Burke & Hawley, 1997; Maughan & Leiper, 1994). This translates into mean (± *s*) sweat losses and drinking rates of 1.3 ± 0.3 and $0.6 \pm 0.3 \, l \cdot h^{-1}$ respectively, with a significant relationship between the two ($r^2 = 0.13$, $P = 0.003$; Figure 1). However, these mean values detract from the considerable variation in both sweating response and drinking behaviour within the clubs As shown in Table 3, there is a substantial variation in responses and behaviour between players. This variation was not due to the difference in body size between players as illustrated in Figure 2, where there is no relationship between body mass and either sweat loss ($P = 0.160$) or volume of liquid consumed ($P = 0.770$). Therefore, factors such as activity rate (metabolic rate), heat acclimatization status, and genetic differences probably contribute to this large variability.

Table 2. Sweat loss, fluid intake, and percent change in body mass of players at each of the three soccer clubs during 90 min training sessions (mean ± s)

	Sweat loss (litres)	Fluid intake (ml)	% Decrease in body mass
Club 1 (n = 17)	1.7 ± 0.4	420 ± 220	1.6 ± 0.6
Club 2 (n = 24)	2.0 ± 0.4	970 ± 300	1.4 ± 0.5
Club 3 (n = 26)	2.2 ± 0.4	970 ± 340	1.6 ± 0.6
Overall (n = 67)	2.0 ± 0.4	830 ± 80	1.5 ± 0.5

Table 3. Minimum and maximum sweat loss, fluid intake, and percent change in body mass of players at each of the three soccer clubs during 90 min training sessions

	Sweat loss (litres)		Fluid intake (ml)		% Decrease in body mass	
	min.	max.	min.	max.	min.	max.
Club 1 (n = 17)	1.1	2.6	40	950	0.9	2.8
Club 2 (n = 24)	1.3	2.8	270	1660	0.5	2.6
Club 3 (n = 26)	1.7	3.1	240	1720	0.7	3.2
Overall (n = 67)	1.1	3.1	40	1720	0.5	3.2

The percentage change in body mass was, on average, the same ($P = 0.426$) in the players training in the cool conditions (Club 1) and the temperate (Club 2) and warm (Club 3) conditions. In the cool environment, players sweated only slightly less than those in the temperate and warm environment (1.7 ± 0.4 vs. 2.1 ± 0.4 litres; $P = 0.002$), most likely because of the additional clothing they wore. However, they drank only about half the volume that was consumed by the players in the temperate and warm environments (420 ± 220 vs. 970 ± 320 ml; $P = 0.000$).

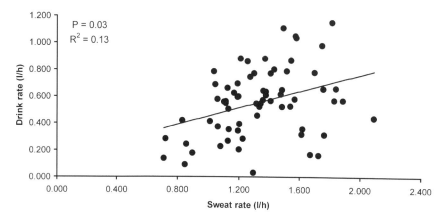

Figure 1. The significant relationship between sweat rate and drinking rate.

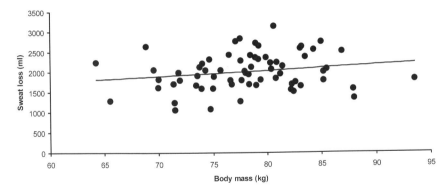

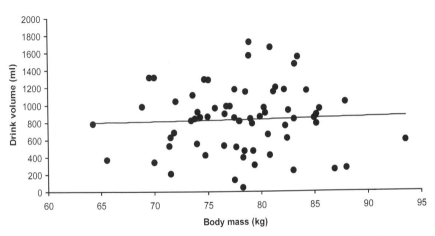

Figure 2. There is no relationship between body mass and either sweat loss (upper panel) or volume of liquid consumed (lower panel).

For 38 of the players, an estimate of pre-training hydration status was obtained by collecting a urine sample and determining its osmolality (Shirreffs & Maughan, 1998). Most of the players appeared to start training in a euhydrated state, with a urine osmolality less than 900 mOsmol·kg^{-1} (Figure 3). However, urine osmolality had no influence on the sweat losses that subsequently occurred during training, although in the players training in a cool environment, high urine osmolality tended to be associated with a greater volume of liquid consumed during training ($r^2 = 0.21$, $P = 0.062$).

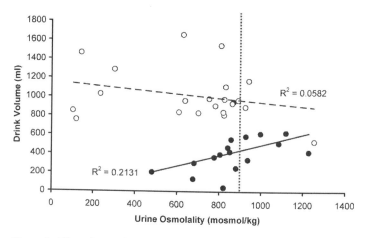

Figure 3. The relationship between pre-training osmolality and volume of liquid consumed during training. The vertical dotted line indicates an osmolality of 900 mOsmol · kg^{-1}; values above this line may indicate pre-training hypohydration (Shirreffs & Maughan, 1998). ●, data for players at Club 1; ○, data for players training in a warm environment.

Electrolyte balance

The main electrolyte lost in sweat is sodium, with chloride being present in slightly smaller amounts. The other electrolytes present (e.g. potassium, calcium, magnesium) are at vastly lower concentrations (Lentner, 1981; Shirreffs & Maughan, 1997). For the purpose of this review, only sodium is considered in detail.

The average sweat sodium concentration measured in players at each of the clubs is shown in Table 4 and did not differ from the normal range reported in the literature. The mean values are similar to those expected for a heat-

Table 4. Sweat sodium concentration and calculated sodium and "salt" (sodium chloride)* losses at each of the three soccer clubs during 90 min training sessions (mean ± s)

	Sweat sodium concentration (mmol · l^{-1})	*Sweat sodium loss (mmol)*	*"Salt" loss (g)*
Club 1 (n = 17)	43 ± 13	73 ± 31	4.3 ± 1.8
Club 2 (n = 24)	49 ± 12	99 ± 24	5.8 ± 1.4
Club 3 (n = 7)	30 ± 19	67 ± 37	3.9 ± 2.2
Overall (n = 48)	44 ± 15	85 ± 32	5.0 ± 1.8

* "Salt" loss is estimated sodium chloride loss based on the assumption that all sodium is lost as sodium chloride.

Table 5. Minimum and maximum sweat sodium concentration and calculated sodium and salt losses at each of the three soccer clubs during 90 min training sessions

	Sweat sodium concentration $(mmol \cdot l^{-1})$		Sweat sodium loss $(mmol)$		"Salt" loss (g)	
	min.	max.	min.	max.	min.	max.
Club 1 ($n = 17$)	16	66	29	121	1.7	7.0
Club 2 ($n = 24$)	26	67	53	133	3.1	7.8
Club 3 ($n = 7$)	16	66	26	129	1.5	7.6
Overall ($n = 48$)	16	67	26	133	1.5	7.8

acclimatized athlete. However, the mean values detract from the considerable variation in sweat sodium concentration and sodium losses between players. As shown in Table 5, some players lose about five times as much sodium as others.

It is important to remember that these data have been determined from localized collection of sweat from four sites on the body. From the limited evidence available, this procedure may lead to an overestimation of whole-body sweat sodium losses by approximately 30–40% (Patterson *et al.*, 2000; Shirreffs & Maughan, 1997). If this is the case, the actual sweat sodium concentrations and losses and estimated salt losses would be more closely represented by the data shown in Table 6, which employs a 35% reduction of local values as a correction to represent whole-body losses.

New data and developments in soccer research since 1994: Adolescent players

There are limited published data on water and electrolyte losses in adolescent players. Broad, Burke, Cox, Heeley and Riley (1996) examined the sweat

Table 6. Minimum and maximum sweat sodium concentration and calculated sodium and salt losses, corrected for the possible 35% overestimation of losses due to the method used at each of the three soccer clubs during 90 min training sessions

	Sweat sodium concentration $(mmol \cdot l^{-1})$		Sweat sodium loss $(mmol)$		"Salt" loss (g)	
	min.	max.	min.	max.	min.	max.
Club 1 ($n = 17$)	10	43	19	79	1.1	4.5
Club 2 ($n = 24$)	17	44	34	86	2.1	5.1
Club 3 ($n = 7$)	10	43	17	84	1.0	4.9
Overall ($n = 48$)	10	44	17	86	1.0	5.1

volume losses and drinking practices of thirty-two 16- to 18-year-old male players. However, this study did allow comparisons to be made between training and competitive games, or between cool winter (9–10°C) and warmer summer (25°C) conditions. The mean sweat rates (winter: $0.7 \pm 0.3 \, l \cdot h^{-1}$ in training, $1.0 \pm 0.3 \, l \cdot h^{-1}$ in a match; summer: $1.0 \pm 0.3 \, l \cdot h^{-1}$ in training, $1.2 \pm 0.3 \, l \cdot h^{-1}$ in a match) and drinking rates (winter: $0.3 \pm 0.3 \, l \cdot h^{-1}$ in training, $0.4 \pm 0.2 \, l \cdot h^{-1}$ in a match; summer: $0.4 \pm 0.3 \, l \cdot h^{-1}$ in training, $0.5 \pm 0.3 \, l \cdot h^{-1}$ in a match) of the players were, on average, slightly lower than those of the adult male players described above.

Mao, Chen and Ko (2001) were concerned with a possible relationship between profuse sweating, sweat iodine losses, and iodine deficiency. They studied thirteen 16- to 18-year-old male players to determine their sweat volume losses during training sessions by monitoring changes in body mass, and also collected sweat samples from the players' chest and back. They reported mean sweat sodium concentrations of $55 \pm 27 \, \text{mmol} \cdot l^{-1}$, with sweat volume losses averaging 1.54 ± 0.57 litres over a one-hour training match. The authors noted that one player lost an estimated $5.9 \, \text{g}$ of salt during this period.

Based on the results of these two studies, it would appear that 16- to 18-year-old male soccer players do not differ significantly from adult male players in terms of their sweat volume and sodium losses during training sessions.

New data and developments in soccer research since 1994: Female players

Broad *et al.* (1996) examined the sweat losses and drinking practices of female soccer players using similar methods to those used for the adolescent male players described above. Although the environmental conditions were slightly warmer (25–30°C), the sweat rates ($0.8 \pm 0.2 \, l \cdot h^{-1}$ in training, $0.8 \pm 0.2 \, l \cdot h^{-1}$ in a match) and drinking rates ($0.4 \pm 0.2 \, l \cdot h^{-1}$ in training, $0.4 \pm 0.2 \, l \cdot h^{-1}$ in a match) tended to be lower. These rates are in general agreement with comparisons showing lower sweat rates in women than men across most activities for which data are available (Burke & Hawley, 1997).

To our knowledge, there are no published data on the electrolyte losses of female players during either training or matches. However, unpublished observations of both under-21 England women players ($n = 14$) during training and senior England women internationals ($n = 25$) during a friendly match concur with Broad *et al.* (1996) that sweat rates and therefore volume losses tend to be lower than for their male counterparts. Additionally, the sweat sodium losses of these players were less than those of their male counterparts, but were due solely to smaller volume losses: the sodium concentrations were similar ($44 \pm 18 \, \text{mmol} \cdot l^{-1}$; mean $\pm s$).

Current practice and practical recommendations

From observations of training sessions and matches at different soccer clubs and discussion with staff and players with different clubs, the impression obtained is that the water and electrolyte requirements of players receive minimal attention. Many clubs have sponsorship agreements with drinks manufacturers, which may limit the range of drinks (sports drinks, soft drinks, and even water) that are available to players either at training or in matches. Furthermore, many players will find different drinks being available to them when they are playing for their club and when they are playing for their country. These different drinks are sometimes not to the liking of players.

Water requirements

There are limited data on the effects of a body water deficit on performance in soccer (McGregor, Nicholas, Lakomy, & Williams, 1999), and there is no information on elite players. From the limited information available, it would appear that there is little likelihood that any negative effects of dehydration on soccer performance would be different from those in other intermittent-activity sports or endurance sports, and indeed there is no reason why this should be so. That is, it is unlikely that any negative effects would be seen until hypohydration reaches a level equivalent to a 2% loss of body mass (Cheuvront, Carter, & Sawka, 2003), and perhaps even greater losses could be tolerated in cool environments (Cheuvront, Carter, Castellani, & Sawka, 2005).

From estimated sweat volume losses, it is apparent that although many players (39 of the 48 adult male players described above) match their drinking sufficiently closely to their sweat losses to restrict their body mass losses to less than 2% of their pre-exercise mass, individual monitoring of players – even in the same training session – is necessary if these guidelines are to be followed correctly. However, the type of intermittent activity during soccer games and training has been shown to slow the rate of gastric emptying of carbohydrate-electrolyte sports drinks (Leiper, Prentice, Wrightson, & Maughan, 2001), raising the possibility that feelings of stomach fullness may limit the volumes players can comfortably consume. Some further practical recommendations are provided in Table 7. It should be noted that no data have been collected in hot weather (>35°C) when sweat losses are likely to be highest. Athletes participating in hot weather competition should not only pay additional attention to drinking, but should undertake a formal heat acclimatization programme (Montain, Maughan, & Sawka, 1996). Heat acclimatization will improve fluid consumption to help match fluid loss requirements.

Electrolyte requirements

Available evidence indicates substantial variation in sweat sodium losses during soccer training. Most players (43 of the 48 adult players, 12 of the 13 male

Table 7. Some practical recommendations to establish water and electrolyte needs in soccer, and some practical recommendations regarding water and electrolyte consumption

Monitoring fluid/electrolyte status in players

- Treat each player is as an individual.
- Measure body mass changes during training and matches as a player-education tool.
- Educate players on their likely individual sweat losses during training and matches.
- Identify salty sweaters (taste, eye irritation, salt stains on clothing) to identify possible problem players.
- If feasible, monitor each player individually (in varying environmental conditions) in training and in match-play to assess water and electrolyte losses.

Water and electrolyte intake

- To ensure adequate hydration during training or matches, drink approximately 500 ml or the equivalent of 6–8 ml per kilogram of body mass (e.g. water, sports drink, or other soft drink) 2 h before the start. Water required by the body will be retained and the excess will be excreted as urine over the 2 h period.
- Consume plain water at this time only if some solid food is consumed with it; this will provide electrolytes and in particular sodium to retain the consumed water.
- When appropriate, ensure each player has suitable drinks available during training and matches.
- During training and matches, limit body mass loss (due to sweat loss) to about 2% of body mass.
- When drinking is deemed necessary, choose a drink with a composition that has a minimal slowing effect on gastric emptying rate.
- During training and matches, consume a drink containing some sodium if significant amounts (3–4 g) are likely to be lost.
- When the environmental conditions are such that large sweat losses are likely in some or most players, consider specific drink break opportunities for all players during each half of the match.
- Between periods provide small salted snacks (e.g. pretzels, crackers) with beverages.

adolescent players, and 36 of the 39 female players described above) had sodium losses of less than 3–4 g during a training session or match, so replacement would not be essential during the training session (Coyle, 2004). For the remaining few players, some consideration must be given to consuming drinks containing sodium during training sessions and matches. Consumption of sports drinks will help to maintain serum sodium concentrations during periods of high sweat losses (Montain, Cheuvront, & Sawka, 2006).

It is clear that high salt losses are a factor in the aetiology of muscle cramps and heat illness in industrial settings and that these can be alleviated by the ingestion of salt-containing drinks (Brockbank, 1929; Oswald, 1925), but it is less clear whether this applies to the generally smaller losses that occur in the sporting environment. There is some limited evidence that American Football players who have high sweat sodium concentrations may be especially susceptible to muscle cramps (Stofan et al., 2003). Bergeron (1996, 2003) has also published reports and case studies suggesting that failure to replace sweat salt losses predisposes to muscle cramps in tennis and that these can be prevented by ensuring an adequate salt intake. Symptomatic hyponatraemia (low serum sodium) has not been reported in soccer players.

Conclusions

Based on knowledge of the effects of water and electrolyte losses on athletes undertaking other forms of activity and sport, it is prudent to recommend that soccer players consider the benefits of limiting their body mass reduction due to water loss during both training sessions and matches to less than about 2%. Body water deficits equivalent to less than 2% of body mass have been clearly associated with reduced aerobic exercise performance. However, the activity pattern in soccer may make this recommendation difficult for players in some circumstances, in which case careful consideration must be given to providing drinks that are palatable and to encouraging drinking.

During matches and training sessions, some players will lose considerable quantities of electrolytes – particularly sodium – and may need to replace these during the match or training session. If sodium-containing beverages do not suffice, athletes may want to consume small amounts of salted snacks between periods to replace salt losses and stimulate drinking.

Finally, the inter-individual variation between players in the same team taking part in the same training session or match is so great that players must be treated as individuals with regard to their water and electrolyte needs.

Disclaimer

The views, opinions, and findings contained in this report are those of the authors and should not be construed as an official Department of the Army position, or decision, unless so designated by other official documentation. Approved for public release; distribution unlimited.

References

Bergeron, M. F. (1996). Heat cramps during tennis: A case report. *International Journal of Sport Nutrition*, 6, 62–68.

Bergeron, M. F. (2003). Heat cramps: Fluid and electrolyte challenges during tennis in the heat. *Journal of Science and Medicine in Sport*, 6, 19–27.

Broad, E. M., Burke, L. M., Cox, G. R., Heeley, P., & Riley, M. (1996). Body weight changes and voluntary fluid intakes during training and competition sessions in team sports. *International Journal of Sports Nutrition*, 6, 307–320.

Brockbank, E. M. (1929). Miner's cramp. *British Medical Journal*, I, 65–66.

Burke, L. M. (1997). Fluid balance during team sports. *Journal of Sports Sciences*, 15, 287–295.

Burke, L. M. (2005). Fluid balance testing for elite team athletes: An interview with Dr. Susan Shirreffs. *International Journal of Sports Nutrition and Exercise Metabolism, 15,* 323–327.

Burke, L. M., & Hawley, J. A. (1997). Fluid balance in team sports: Guidelines for optimal practices. *Sports Medicine, 24,* 38–54.

Cheuvront, S. N., Carter, R., III, & Sawka, N. (2003). Fluid balance and endurance performance. *Current Sports Medicine Reports, 2,* 202–208.

Cheuvront, S. N., Carter, R., III, Castellani, J. W., & Sawka, M. N. (2005). Hypohydration impairs endurance exercise performance in temperate but not cold air. *Journal of Applied Physiology, 99,* 1972–1976.

Costa, F., Calloway, D. H., & Margen, S. (1969). Regional and total body sweat composition of men fed controlled diets. *American Journal of Clinical Nutrition, 22,* 52–58.

Coyle, E. F. (2004). Fluid and fuel intake during exercise. *Journal of Sports Sciences, 22,* 39–55.

Leiper, J. B., Prentice, A. S., Wrightson, C., & Maughan, R. J. (2001). Gastric emptying of a carbohydrate-electrolyte drink during a soccer match. *Medicine and Science in Sports and Exercise, 33,* 1932–1938.

Lemon, P. W. R., Yarasheski, K. E., & Dolny, D. G. (1986). Validity/reliability of sweat analysis by whole-body washdown vs. regional collections. *Journal of Applied Physiology, 61,* 1967–1971.

Lentner, C. (Ed.) (1981). *Geigy scientific tables. Vol. 1. Units of measurement, body fluids, composition of the body, nutrition* (8th edn., pp. 108–112). Basle: Ciba-Geigy.

Mao, I. F., Chen, M. L., & Ko, Y. C. (2001). Electrolyte loss in sweat and iodine deficiency in a hot environment. *Archives of Environmental Health, 56,* 271–277.

Maughan, R. J., & Leiper, J. B. (1994). Fluid replacement requirements in soccer. *Journal of Sports Sciences, 12,* S29–S34.

Maughan, R. J., Merson, S. J., Broad, N. P., & Shirreffs, S. M. (2004). Fluid and electrolyte intake and loss in elite soccer players during training. *International Journal of Sports Nutrition and Exercise Metabolism, 14,* 333–346.

Maughan, R. J., Shirreffs, S. M., Merson, S. J., & Horswill, C. A. (2005). Fluid and electrolyte balance in elite male football (soccer) players training in a cool environment. *Journal of Sports Sciences, 23,* 63–79.

McGregor, S. J., Nicholas, C. W., Lakomy, H. K., & Williams, C. (1999). The influence of intermittent high-intensity shuttle running and fluid ingestion on the performance of a soccer skill. *Journal of Sports Sciences, 17,* 895–903.

Montain, S. J., Cheuvront S. N. and Sawka, M. N. (2006). Exercise-associated hyponatremia: Quantitative analyses for understanding etiology and prevention. *British Journal of Sports Medicine, 40,* 98–106.

Montain, S. J., Maughan R. J., & Sawka, M. N. (1996). Fluid replacement strategies for exercise in hot weather. *Athletic Therapy Today, 1,* 34–37.

Oswald, R. J. W. (1925). Saline drink in industrial fatigue. *Lancet, 1,* 1369.

Patterson, M. J., Galloway, S. D. R., & Nimmo, M. A. (2000). Variations in regional sweat composition in normal human males. *Experimental Physiology, 85,* 869–875.

Shirreffs, S. M., Aragon-Vargas, L. F., Chamorro, M., Maughan, R. J., Serratosa, L., & Zachwieja, J. J. (2005). The sweating response of elite professional soccer players to training in the heat. *International Journal of Sports Medicine, 26,* 90–95.

Shirreffs, S. M., Armstrong, L. E., & Cheuvront, S. N. (2004). Fluid and electrolyte needs for preparation and recovery from training and competition. *Journal of Sports Sciences, 22*, 57–63.

Shirreffs, S. M., & Maughan, R. J. (1997). Whole body sweat collection in man: An improved method with preliminary data on electrolyte content. *Journal of Applied Physiology, 82*, 336–341.

Shirreffs, S. M., & Maughan, R. J. (1998). Urine osmolality and conductivity as indices of hydration status in athletes living and training in the heat. *Medicine and Science in Sports and Exercise, 30*, 1598–1602.

Stofan, J. R., Zachwieja, J. J., Horswill, C. A., Lacambra, M., Murray, R., & Eichner, E. R. (2003). Sweat and sodium losses in NCAA Division 1 football players with a history of whole-body muscle cramping. *Medicine and Science in Sports and Exercise, 35*, S48.

Van Heyningen, R., & Weiner, J. S. (1952). A comparison of arm-bag sweat and body sweat. *Journal of Physiology, 116*, 395–403.

5 Promoting training adaptations through nutritional interventions

JOHN A. HAWLEY, KEVIN D. TIPTON AND MINDY L. MILLARD-STAFFORD

Training and nutrition are highly interrelated in that optimal adaptation to the demands of repeated training sessions typically requires a diet that can sustain muscle energy reserves. As nutrient stores (i.e. muscle and liver glycogen) play a predominant role in the performance of prolonged, intense, intermittent exercise typical of the patterns of soccer match-play, and in the replenishment of energy reserves for subsequent training sessions, the extent to which acutely altering substrate availability might modify the training impulse has been a key research area among exercise physiologists and sport nutritionists for several decades. Although the major perturbations to cellular homeostasis and muscle substrate stores occur during exercise, the activation of several major signalling pathways important for chronic training adaptations take place during the first few hours of recovery, returning to baseline values within 24 h after exercise. This has led to the paradigm that many chronic training adaptations are generated by the cumulative effects of the transient events that occur during recovery from each (acute) exercise bout. Evidence is accumulating that nutrient supplementation can serve as a potent modulator of many of the acute responses to both endurance and resistance training. In this article, we review the molecular and cellular events that occur in skeletal muscle during exercise and subsequent recovery, and the potential for nutrient supplementation (e.g. carbohydrate, fat, protein) to affect many of the adaptive responses to training.

Keywords: AMPK, carbohydrate, glycogen, genes, fat, MAPK, mTOR, protein

Introduction

The capacity of human skeletal muscle to adapt to repeated bouts of physical activity over time so that subsequent exercise capacity is improved is termed "physical training" (Booth & Thomason, 1991). The goal of such training for the soccer player is to induce multiple physiological and metabolic adaptations that enable the working muscles to increase the rate of adenosine triphosphate (ATP) production from both aerobic and oxygen-independent pathways, maintain tighter metabolic control (i.e. match ATP production with ATP hydrolysis), minimize cellular disturbances, and improve fatigue resistance during exercise (for a review, see Hawley 2002a). Although the major perturbations to cellular homeostasis and muscle substrate stores occur during exercise, the activation of several major signalling pathways important for chronic training adaptations take place during the first few hours of recovery, returning to base-line values within 24 h after exercise (Hildebrandt, Pilegaard, & Neufer, 2003; Pilegaard, Ordway, Saltin, & Neufer, 2000). This has led to the paradigm that many chronic training adaptations are generated by the cumulative effects of the transient events that occur during recovery from each (acute) exercise bout (Pilegaard *et al.*, 2000; Widegren, Ryder, & Zierath, 2001; Williams & Neufer, 1996).

Training and nutrition are highly interrelated in that optimal adaptation to the demands of repeated training sessions typically requires a diet that can sustain muscle energy reserves (Coyle, 2000). As nutrient stores (i.e. muscle and liver glycogen) play a predominant role in the performance of prolonged, intense, intermittent exercise (McInerney *et al.*, 2005; Nicholas, Tsintzas, Boobis, & Williams, 1999) typical of the patterns of soccer match-play (Hargreaves, 1994), and in the replenishment of energy reserves for subsequent training sessions (Burke, Kiens, & Ivy, 2004; Jentjens and Jeukendrup, 2003), the extent to which acutely altering substrate availability might modify the training impulse has been a key research area among exercise physiologists and sport nutritionists for several decades. Here we review several nutritional interventions that modify the acute responses to exercise and thus have the potential to influence subsequent training adaptations. Specifically, we discuss the molecular and cellular events that occur in skeletal muscle during exercise and subsequent recovery and show that diet is a potent modulator of many of the adaptive responses to training. The cardiovascular and other adaptations that take place outside the skeletal muscles are not discussed here.

The training stimulus, response, and adaptation

The acute metabolic responses associated with a single bout of exercise and subsequent training-induced adaptations are highly specific to the mode, intensity, and duration of the stimulus (Hildebrandt *et al.*, 2003; Nader & Esser, 2001) and the corresponding pattern of muscle fibre recruitment (Gollnick *et al.*, 1973). Although long-term muscle adaptations are likely to be the result of the cumulative effect of repeated bouts of exercise, the initial responses that lead to these chronic changes occur during and after each training session (Pilegaard *et al.*, 2000; Widegren *et al.*, 2001; Williams & Neufer, 1996). Consideration of the molecular and cellular events that occur in skeletal muscle in response to a single bout of exercise is essential to understand how nutritional interventions might modulate these responses and promote (or inhibit) subsequent training adaptations. When such a view on training is taken, it becomes clear that any chronic training-induced adaptation is merely the consequence of increases in exercise-induced proteins (Hansen *et al.*, 2005). The coordinated series of events that allows for these changes in protein levels is pivotal to any training adaptation.

Figure 1 illustrates the events that take place during and after a single bout of exercise and with repeated exposure to that stimulus. Contractile activity pro-

Acute exercise ➡️ Metabolic adaptation ➡️ Altered phenotype

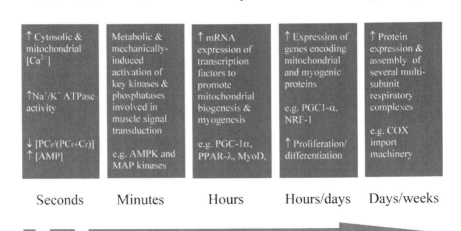

↑ Cytosolic & mitochondrial [Ca²⁺] ↑Na⁺/K⁺ ATPase activity ↓ [PCr/(PCr+Cr)] ↑ [AMP]	Metabolic & mechanically-induced activation of key kinases & phosphatases involved in muscle signal transduction e.g. AMPK and MAP kinases	↑ mRNA expression of transcription factors to promote mitochondrial biogenesis & myogenesis e.g. PGC-1α, PPAR-λ, MyoD,	↑ Expression of genes encoding mitochondrial and myogenic proteins e.g. PGC1-α, NRF-1 ↑ Proliferation/ differentiation	↑ Protein expression & assembly of several multi-subunit respiratory complexes e.g. COX import machinery
Seconds	Minutes	Hours	Hours/days	Days/weeks

Figure 1. Schematic representation of the time-course of selected contraction-induced physiological, biochemical, and molecular responses in skeletal muscle that lead to the training adaptation. Adapted and redrawn from Hood (2001).

duces a multitude of time-dependent physiological, biochemical, and molecular changes within the muscle cells. With sufficient time, and in accordance with the dominant stimulus, this sequence of events produces mitochondrial biogenesis (Hood, 2001), muscle hypertrophy (Glass, 2003), and concomitant alterations in muscle phenotype that serve to improve cellular function and thereby enhance exercise capacity.

At the onset of exercise there are rapid (within milliseconds) increases in cytosolic and mitochondrial [Ca²⁺] and Na⁺/K⁺ ATPase activity and, depending on the relative intensity, changes in metabolite concentrations (i.e. increases in [ADP] and [AMP]). There may also be increases in muscle [lactate], accompanied by decreased muscle (and blood) pH, and impaired oxygen flux. With an increase in exercise duration, endogenous muscle substrates (principally glycogen) become depleted. These contraction-induced metabolic disturbances in muscle, together with the accompanying mechanical stress (particularly muscle damage caused by physical contact and/or eccentric work), activate several key kinases and phosphatases involved in signal transduction. Chief among these are the 5′-adenosine monophosphate-activated protein kinases (AMPK), several of the mitogen-activated protein kinases (MAPK), and the mammalian target of rapamycin (mTOR).

AMPK is a critical signalling protein involved in the regulation of multiple metabolic and growth responses in skeletal muscle in response to exercise. This "fuel-sensing" enzyme is involved in acute exercise-induced events and also plays an obligatory role in adapting skeletal muscles to repeated bouts of exercise during training programmes (for reviews, see Ashenbach, Sakamoto,

& Goodyear, 2004; Winder, 2001). The AMPK cascade is turned on by cellular stresses that deplete ATP (and consequently elevate AMP) either by accelerating ATP consumption (e.g. muscle contraction) or by inhibiting ATP production (e.g. hypoxia, ischaemia). Once activated, the AMPK cascade switches on catabolic processes both acutely (by phosphorylation of downstream metabolic enzymes such as acetyl coenzyme A carboxylase) and chronically (by effects on gene expression), while concomitantly switching off ATP-consuming processes (Hardie & Hawley, 2001). Activation of AMPK is rapid (< 30 s) and occurs in an intensity-dependent and isoform-specific fashion (Chen *et al.*, 2003; Fujii *et al.*, 2000; Wojtaszewski, Nielsen, Hansen, Richter, & Kiens, 2000). Pharmacological activation of AMPK (an "exercise-like" effect) enhances the protein expression of GLUT4, hexokinase, and several oxidative enzymes, as well as increasing mitochondrial density and muscle glycogen content (Aschenbach *et al.*, 2004). Accordingly, many of the chronic training-induced adaptations in skeletal muscle have been proposed to involve AMPK. In this regard, cross-sectional studies have revealed that muscle from endurance-trained athletes shows increased AMPK protein levels (Nielsen *et al.*, 2003), while AMPK activation during exercise is blunted in highly trained individuals compared with untrained individuals when exercising at the same relative intensity (Frosig *et al.*, 2004; Nielsen *et al.*, 2003; Yu *et al.*, 2003), an observation consistent with the maintenance of a better phosphorylation potential of the muscle (as reflected by the difference in [PCr]/[PCr + Cr] ratios) in trained muscle. Muscle glycogen content also modulates the AMPK response to exercise. Low muscle glycogen stores elevate resting AMPK activity compared with normal glycogen stores (Wojtaszewski *et al.*, 2003). AMPK is also likely to mediate the contraction-induced increase in glucose uptake (Hayashi, Hirshman, Kurth, Winder, & Goodyear, 1998) and thus may play a role in promoting post-exercise glycogen accumulation in skeletal muscle (Barnes *et al.*, 2005; Carling & Hardie, 1989; Sakoda *et al.*, 2005).

The MAPK signal transduction cascade has been identified as a candidate system that converts contraction-induced biochemical perturbations into appropriate intracellular responses (for reviews, see Hawley & Zierath, 2004; Widegren *et al.*, 2001). Exercise is a powerful and rapid activator of several MAP kinases and numerous downstream enzymes (Widegren *et al.*, 1998; Wretman *et al.*, 2001). Both local and systemic factors mediate phosphorylation of the MAPK signalling cascades (Aronson *et al.*, 1997; Widegren *et al.*, 1998), which have been implicated in transcriptional regulation of important genes in skeletal muscle in response to exercise (Widegren *et al.*, 2001). In this regard, exercise-induced activation of the MAPK pathway has recently been demonstrated to play a role in aerobic muscle adaptation by promoting specific co-activators involved in mitochondrial biogenesis and slow-twitch muscle fibre formation (Akimoto *et al.*, 2005). Crucially, MAPK activation can result not only in the production of transcription factors mediating gene expression, but can also stimulate the activity of the translational stage of protein synthesis. Muscle hypertrophy through increased protein synthesis may also require activation of the MAPK signalling cascades (Williamson, Gallagher, Harber, Hollon, & Trappe, 2003).

The specific cascades linking growth stimuli to the activation of protein synthesis in skeletal muscle are not fully resolved. However, they involve phosphorylation of mTOR and sequential activation of S6 protein kinase (p70^{S6k}) (Glass, 2003; Proud, 2002). Both insulin and amino acids are potent activators of mTOR. While the mechanisms of action of insulin on mTOR are well documented (for a review, see Bolster, Jefferson, & Kimball, 2004), the precise pathways by which amino acids act are presently unclear. In rodents, exercise-induced p70^{S6k} activation correlates with increased skeletal muscle mass after 6 weeks of resistance training (Baar & Esser, 1999). Thus, changes in p70^{S6k} phosphorylation in skeletal muscle after exercise may partially account for increases in protein synthesis during the early recovery phase. Exercise and amino acid supplementation recruit different signalling pathways upstream of mTOR: exercise seems to activate partially the same pathways as insulin, whereas amino acids may act directly on the mTOR complex itself (for reviews, see Deldicque, Theisen, & Francaux, 2005; Kimball, Farrell, & Jefferson, 2002). Activation of AMPK inhibits mTOR, either directly or indirectly (Bolster, Crozier, Kimball, & Jefferson, 2002; Cheng, Fryer, Carling, & Shepherd, 2004), making mTOR less active in promoting protein synthesis. The practical implication of this observation is obvious when planning the order of training sessions that include both endurance and strength/resistance components. There is some evidence to suggest that simultaneous endurance and strength training inhibits the normal adaptation to either training regimen when performed alone (Nelson, Arnall, Loy, Silverster, & Conlee, 1990).

With regard to the effects of contraction on gene expression, many studies have reported that mRNA abundance for several metabolic and stress-related genes is acutely and transiently elevated in muscle after a single bout of exercise (Cluberton, McGee, Murphy, & Hargreaves, 2005; Kraniou, Cameron-Smith, Misso, Collier, & Hargreaves, 2000; Neufer & Dohm, 1993; Pilegaard et al., 2000). Indeed, it appears that for many exercise-related genes, the time-course of transcriptional activation occurs during the first few hours of recovery (Pilegaard et al., 2000), and may be linked by common signalling and/or regulatory mechanisms to the restoration of muscle energy stores, predominantly glycogen (Richter, Derave, & Wojtaszewski, 2001). As gene expression and its associated phenotypic/functional manifestations do not occur until there is an increase in the concentration of the protein encoded by the gene, the extent to which a protein will increase in response to an adaptive stimulus cannot be predicted from the increase in mRNA. This makes the measurement of protein concentrations critical when studying the adaptive responses to exercise training or other stimuli (Baar et al., 2002). Physical preparation for soccer requires several divergent yet interdependent types of training incorporating sprint, endurance, and resistance training (Bangsbo, 1994). Under conditions in which the training inputs (intensity, duration, and frequency) are held constant, any training programme must be of sufficient length for the cellular proteins to reach their new "steady-state" concentration and the biochemical/metabolic adaptations to develop fully (Hildebrandt *et al.*, 2003; Terjung & Hood, 1986).

Modification of the training response/adaptation via dietary interventions

Changes in dietary intake that alter the concentration of blood-borne nutrients and hormones can regulate the short-term macronutrient oxidative and storage profile of skeletal muscle. Perturbations in muscle and blood substrates (especially carbohydrate and fat) alter the uptake and flux of these fuel-specific intermediates within related metabolic pathways (i.e. skeletal muscle). This response serves to redirect enzymatic processes involved in substrate metabolism and the subsequent concentration of particular proteins critical for metabolic pathway function. Altering substrate availability affects not only resting energy metabolism and subsequent fuel utilization during exercise, but also regulatory processes underlying gene expression (Arkinstall, Tunstall, Cameron-Smith, & Hawley, 2004; Hargreaves & Cameron-Smith, 2002; Tunstall & Cameron-Smith, 2005). To bring about such modifications, a number of highly coordinated processes occur, including gene transcription, RNA transport from the nucleus, protein synthesis, and, in some cases, post-translational modification of the protein (Figure 2). However, the initiation of gene transcription is strongly related to both acute and chronic changes in dietary intake and composition (Jump & Clarke, 1999) and thus has the potential to modulate many of the adaptive responses to training.

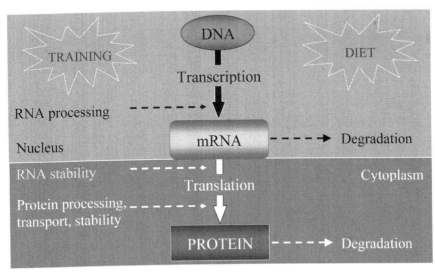

Figure 2. Steps at which gene expression can be controlled/regulated. The effect of diet/training interactions on these processes is largely unknown. Adapted and redrawn from Williams and Neufer (1996).

Dietary interventions that modify the training adaptation

Carbohydrate availability

It has long been recognized that there is a close association between dietary carbohydrate intake, muscle glycogen concentration, and endurance capacity (Bergstrom, Hermansen, Hultman, & Saltin, 1967). For this reason, it is recommended that individuals training for sports in which carbohydrate is the most heavily metabolized fuel (including football) should consume a diet rich in carbohydrate (Balsom, Wood, Olsson, & Ekblom, 1999; Clark,1994; Hargreaves, 1994; Hawley, Dennis, & Noakes, 1994; Kirkendall 1993; Rico-Sanz et al., 1998; Rico-Sanz, Zehnder, Buchli, Dambach, & Boutellier, 1999). However, it should be noted that only a few researchers have chronically manipulated dietary carbohydrate intake in well-trained individuals and examined the effect on subsequent training responses/adaptations and performance (for a review, see Hawley, Dennis, Lindsay, & Noakes, 1995).

Sherman, Doyle, Lamb and Strauss (1993) compared the effects of 7 days of two diets (5 or 10 g carbohydrate per kilogram of body mass [BM] per day) on training capacity and performance in trained endurance athletes. Training incorporated both sprint and endurance workouts typical of those that might be encountered during soccer training. Athletes on the high-carbohydrate diet maintained basal muscle glycogen concentrations over the training period, but those on the moderate-carbohydrate regimen had a 33% reduction by day 5. Despite this decline in glycogen stores, all athletes were able to successfully complete the prescribed training sessions and had a similar (endurance) exercise performance on day 7. Lamb, Rinehardt, Bartels, Sherman and Snook (1990) determined the effects of a "moderate" ($6.5 \, \text{g} \cdot \text{kg BM}^{-1} \cdot \text{day}^{-1}$) or high ($12 \, \text{g} \cdot \text{kg BM}^{-1} \cdot \text{day}^{-1}$) carbohydrate diet during 9 days of intense interval training. Although muscle glycogen was not measured in that study, the high-carbohydrate diet did not permit the athletes to maintain a higher intensity of training compared with the "moderate"-carbohydrate diet. These workers concluded that "there may be an upper limit of carbohydrate intake (perhaps $500–600 \, \text{g} \cdot \text{day}^{-1}$) beyond which additional carbohydrate does not contribute significantly to muscle glycogen storage and athletic performance" (Lamb et al., 1990), a hypothesis originally proposed by Costill and co-workers (1981).

In contrast, the results of other studies demonstrate improved performance following increased dietary carbohydrate during training. Achten and colleagues (2004) reported that consumption of a high- ($8.5 \, \text{g} \cdot \text{kg BM}^{-1} \cdot \text{day}^{-1}$) versus a moderate-carbohydrate($5.4 \, \text{g} \cdot \text{kg BM}^{-1} \cdot \text{day}^{-1}$) diet sustained higher rates of carbohydrate oxidation during exercise and that this was associated with a better maintenance of physical performance and mood state during 11 days of intensified training in competitive athletes. Increasing the ad libitum daily intake of carbohydrate from 6.5 to $9 \, \text{g} \cdot \text{kg BM}^{-1} \cdot \text{day}^{-1}$ during a week of training improved run time to exhaustion at 90% maximal oxygen uptake ($\dot{V}O_{2max}$) following a 90 min pre-load in trained athletes (Millard-Stafford, Cureton, & Ray, 1988). Balsom et al. (1999) observed that soccer players performed more high-intensity movement during a simulated 90 min four-a-side game when fed a high versus a low (65% or 30% of energy intake) carbohydrate diet, presumably because the high-carbohydrate intake resulted in higher pre-game muscle glycogen content. Of note was that other technical measures of the game were not impacted by the dietary regimen.

To date, the longest study to examine the interaction of daily diet and training in athletes was undertaken by Simonsen *et al.* (1991). In contrast to the results of Sherman *et al.* (1993), consuming a moderate ($5 \, g \cdot kg \, BM^{-1} \cdot day^{-1}$) carbohydrate diet maintained muscle glycogen concentrations ($\sim 120 \, mmol \cdot kg$ wet weight^{-1}) over 4 weeks of twice-daily workouts in rowers. However, athletes consuming the high-carbohydrate diet ($10 \, g \cdot kg \, BM^{-1} \cdot day^{-1}$) had a progressive (65%) increase in glycogen stores by the end of the fourth week (to $\sim 155 \, mmol \cdot kg$ wet weight^{-1}). While all participants were able to successfully complete the prescribed training sessions, athletes consuming the high-carbohydrate diet showed greater improvements (11%) in power output in time-trials performed three times weekly than those consuming the moderate-carbohydrate diet (2%). This study provides evidence that while a moderate-carbohydrate diet may not reduce the ability of trained athletes to complete rigorous training sessions for up to a month, consumption of a high-carbohydrate diet optimizes improvements in performance of these individuals. Taken collectively, the results of these studies (Achten *et al.*, 2004; Balsom *et al.*, 1999, Lamb *et al.*, 1990; Millard-Stafford *et al.*, 1988; Sherman *et al.*, 1993; Simonsen *et al.*, 1991) demonstrate that trained athletes benefit from a high carbohydrate intake during periods of intensified training, probably due to the maintenance (or an increase) in muscle glycogen stores and an ability to sustain higher rates of carbohydrate oxidation sustained during exercise. Certainly, there are no reports in the literature of impairments in training capacity and performance when athletes ingest a high-carbohydrate diet. Soccer players engaged in strenuous training and competition should be encouraged to consume a diet that provides a minimum of $7 \, g \cdot kg \, BM^{-1} \cdot day^{-1}$.

While the available evidence suggests that a high-carbohydrate intake during training allows athletes to train faster/harder and for longer to achieve a superior training response, it has recently been proposed that a "cycling" of muscle glycogen stores may be desirable to further promote the training response/adaptation (Chakravarthy & Booth, 2004). Indeed, Hansen *et al.* (2005) recently reported that *untrained* participants who completed 10 weeks of training with low muscle glycogen levels had a more pronounced increase in resting glycogen content and citrate synthase activity compared to when the same volume of training was undertaken with normal glycogen concentrations. Remarkably, this "train-low, compete-high" approach also resulted in a two-fold increase in exercise time to fatigue compared with when participants commenced training sessions with normal glycogen levels. These results suggest that under certain conditions, a lack of substrate (i.e. carbohydrate) might trigger selected training adaptations that would be viewed as beneficial for performance. Certainly, there is accumulating evidence to demonstrate that commencing endurance exercise with low muscle glycogen content enhances the transcription rate of several genes involved in the training adaptation (Febbraio et al., 2003; Keller et al., 2001; Pilegaard et al., 2002). This is probably because several transcription factors include glycogen-binding domains, and when muscle glycogen is low, these factors are released and become free to associate with different targeting proteins (Printen, Brady, & Saltiel, 1997). Coaches and athletes should be careful not to draw practical consequences of these studies with regard to training regimens. In the real world, training with a high muscle glycogen content may allow the athlete to train for longer periods and thereby obtain better results.

With regard to intracellular signalling, muscle glycogen content is a potent modulator of both resting and contraction-induced AMPK and MAPK responses (Chan, McGee, Watt, Hargreaves, & Febbraio, 2004; Wojtaszewski et al., 2003). Well-trained individuals have been studied under conditions of low- and high-glycogen content (160 vs. 900 mmol·kg dry weight^{-1}), at rest, and subsequently during 1 h of endurance exercise (Wojtaszewski et al., 2003). At rest, AMPK activity was approximately 2.5-fold higher in the low- versus the high-glycogen states. Low pre-exercise glycogen content also increased AMPKα-2 activity during subsequent submaximal exercise. Altering dietary carbohydrate intake to reduce muscle glycogen content also leads to an increased MAPK signalling response (Chan et al., 2004). In contrast to the up-regulation of signalling cascades when endurance exercise is commenced with low muscle glycogen stores, resistance exercise undertaken in a glycogen-depleted state may disrupt mechanisms involved in protein translation and blunt the normal adaptive response. Creer et al. (2005) recently reported that when endurance-trained individuals performed a bout of moderate-intensity resistance exercise (similar to that likely to be undertaken by soccer players) with low (~175 mmol·kg dry weight^{-1}) muscle glycogen content, phosphorylation of Akt, a critical signalling mediator of cell growth and metabolism (Glass 2003), was diminished compared with when they undertook the same workout with normal (~600 mmol·kg dry weight^{-1}) glycogen stores.

Glucose availability has been shown to modulate metabolic regulation within skeletal muscle (Arkinstall, Bruce, Nikolopoulos, Garnham, & Hawley, 2001; Coyle, Coggan, Hemmert, & Ivy, 1986) and to exert effects on gene expression (Cheng et al., 2005; Civitarese, Hesselink, Russell, Ravussin, & Schrauwen, 2005; Cluberton et al., 2005; Febbraio et al., 2003). In this regard, it has been proposed that carbohydrate ingestion during and after exercise could inhibit long-term adaptation to training (Åkerstrom, Wojtaszewski, Plomgaard, & Pedersen, 2005; Febbraio et al., 2003). To test this hypothesis, Åkerstrom et al. (2005) determined the effects of chronic oral glucose supplementation (or placebo) in untrained individuals on substrate metabolism, training responses, and performance during 10 weeks of endurance-training (2 h per day, 5 days per week). Training induced large improvements in performance for both experimental conditions. However, glucose ingestion during training did not alter patterns of substrate metabolism or alter a variety of muscle markers of training adaptation (i.e. metabolic enzymes, glycogen content, and GLUT4 protein). Accordingly, it would appear prudent to recommend that athletes maximize carbohydrate availability during and after training sessions, in line with current sports nutrition guidelines (Burke, 2003). Clearly, the role of carbohydrate availability in modifying the activation of transcription factors and signalling responses to contraction requires further research. Whether chronic perturbations in glycogen and/or glucose availability can translate into improved training adaptations in *well-trained individuals* is currently not known.

Fat availability

Another nutritional strategy that might enhance the training adaptation, presumably by allowing athletes to train for longer, would be to utilize an alternative fuel source to carbohydrate and/or to slow its normal rate of utilization during exercise. Such a fuel is fat, and there has been recent interest in the effects of both acute and chronic fat supplementation on metabolism and exercise performance (for reviews, see Burke & Hawley, 2002; Hawley, 2002b). Of interest here is whether such dietary modification can enhance the adaptive response to training. Certainly, when well-trained individuals consume a high-fat/low-carbohydrate diet for 5–7 days, there is a rapid and marked capacity for these changes in macronutrient availability to modulate the expression of mRNA-encoding proteins that are necessary for fatty acid transport and oxidative metabolism (Cameron-Smith *et al.*, 2003). Accompanying these changes are large shifts in substrate metabolism in favour of fat, and a sparing of muscle glycogen (Burke *et al.*, 2000). Even when carbohydrate availability is increased following "fat adaptation", by the restoration of muscle glycogen stores and provision of exogenous carbohydrate during exercise, the enhanced capacity for muscle fat oxidation persists (Burke *et al.*, 2002).

In terms of the effect of such metabolic perturbations on the training response, Stepto *et al.* (2002) reported that competitive endurance athletes are able to perform intense (40 min at 86% $\dot{V}O_{2max}$) interval training during short-term (<5 days) exposure to a high-fat diet. Such training was associated with rates of fat oxidation that are among the highest reported in the literature (i.e. $>60\,\mu\text{mol}\cdot\text{kg}^{-1}\cdot\text{min}^{-1}$). However, compared with a high-carbohydrate diet, training sessions were associated with increased ratings of perceived exertion. Recently, Stellingwerff *et al.* (2006) examined the effects of 5 days of a high-fat diet while training, followed by 1 day of carbohydrate restoration (and rest), on the regulation of key regulatory enzymes in the pathways of skeletal muscle fat and carbohydrate metabolism during sprint exercise. Resting pyruvate dehydrogenase (PDH) activity was lower at rest and estimated rates of glycogenolysis were reduced upon the completion of a standardized 1 min sprint after fat-adaptation compared with control (high carbohydrate). These results suggest that the muscle glycogen "sparing" observed in previous studies of fat-adaptation may actually be an impairment of glycogenolysis (due to a down-regulation of PDH). Such an adaptation would not be favourable to athletes in a sport such as soccer that requires repeated bouts of maximal sprint activity.

Protein availability

Although insulin, amino acids, and exercise individually activate multiple signal transduction pathways in skeletal muscle, one pathway, the phosphatidy-linositol 3-kinase- (PI3K-) mTOR signalling pathway, is a common target of all three. Activation of the PI3K-mTOR signal pathways results in both acute (i.e. minutes to hours) and long-term (i.e. hours to days) up-regulation of protein synthesis through modulation of multiple steps involved in mediating the initiation of mRNA translation and ribosome biogenesis respectively. In addition, changes in gene expression through altered patterns of mRNA translation promote cell growth, which in turn promotes muscle hypertrophy.

Protein availability is critical for optimizing many of the adaptations that take place in muscle in response to both endurance and resistance training. The main determinants of an athlete's protein needs are their training regimen and habitual nutrient intake (Tipton & Wolfe, 2004). However, the optimal amount of protein required by athletes to enhance the training adaptation is unclear. While some researchers suggest that during periods of intense training, protein requirements should be increased to $\sim 2.0 \, g \cdot kg \, BM^{-1} \cdot day^{-1}$ (Lemon, 2000), others maintain that athletes should consume the same amount recommended for the general population (i.e. $\sim 1.0 \, g \cdot kg \, BM^{-1} \cdot day^{-1}$) (Rennie & Tipton, 2000; Tipton & Wolfe, 2004). The discrepancy is probably due to the difficulty in determining true protein requirements for athletes, and the disparate methods used for such determination. Of note is that the scientific evidence is probably immaterial for the vast majority of athletes, because most individuals, including soccer players (Rico Sanz *et al.*, 1998), consume sufficient protein to accommodate even the highest estimates of protein needs.

Increased muscle protein results from a positive net muscle protein balance (i.e. when protein synthesis is greater than protein breakdown). At rest and in the fasted state, net protein balance is negative because protein breakdown exceeds the rate of synthesis. Following exercise in the fasted state, the rates of both protein synthesis and breakdown are increased but, compared with resting conditions, the net (negative) balance is attenuated because the increase in protein synthesis is greater than the increase in protein breakdown (Biolo, Maggi, Williams, Tipton, & Wolfe, 1995; Phillips, Tipton, Aarsland, Wolf, & Wolfe, 1997). Ingesting a mixture of carbohydrate and amino acids before or immediately after completion of a training session (Tipton *et al.*, 2001) counteracts this catabolic state by increasing amino acid availability and transport into muscle (Biolo, Tipton, Klein, & Wolfe, 1997). In this situation, protein synthesis is increased (Biolo *et al.*, 1997; Borsheim, Tipton, Wolf, & Wolfe, 2002), while the increase in protein breakdown is attenuated (Biolo *et al.*, 1997) resulting in a net positive protein balance.

Acute protein ingestion near the time of exercise appears to have the greatest potential impact on training adaptation. Recently, Karlsson *et al.* (2004) examined the effect of resistance exercise alone or in combination with oral intake of branch-chain amino acids (BCAA) on the signalling pathways responsible for translational control of protein synthesis. In that study, a single bout of resistance training led to a robust and persistent (2–3 h) increase in $p70^{S6k}$ phosphorylation that was further enhanced by BCAA ingestion. These workers speculated that BCAA supplementation enhances protein synthesis during recovery from resistance training through a $p70^{S6k}$-dependent signalling cascade (Karlsson *et al.*, 2004). It is noteworthy that the effect of post-exercise amino acid supplementation on protein balance is enhanced by co-ingestion of carbohydrate (Miller, Tipton, Chinkes, Wolf, & Wolfe, 2003), possibly via the elevated insulin concentrations. After resistance exercise, a mixture of whey protein, amino acids, and carbohydrate stimulated muscle protein synthesis to a greater extent and for a longer duration than isoenergetic carbohydrate alone (Borsheim, Aarsland, & Wolfe, 2004). This has been demonstrated for both casein and whey protein added to carbohydrate (Tipton *et al.*, 2004). The amount of protein necessary for ingestion immediately after exercise to elicit this effect appears to be quite modest (~6 g) (Tipton, Ferrando, Phillips, Doyle, & Wolfe, 1999; Tipton *et al.*, 2001). Furthermore, net muscle protein synthesis may be greater when a carbohydrate–amino acid solution is consumed immediately before resistance exercise than when the same solution is consumed after exercise, primarily because of an increase in muscle protein synthesis as a result of increased delivery of amino acids to the leg (Tipton *et al.*, 2001).

While the impact of protein ingestion (alone or co-ingested with carbohydrate) before or after resistance training appears to enhance net muscle protein balance, the effects on endurance exercise responses are not as clear. When consumed immediately after prolonged, glycogen-depleting exercise, protein co-ingested with carbohydrate may improve net protein balance in the early post-exercise period (Koopman *et al.*, 2004) and possibly enhance glycogen re-synthesis (Ivy *et al.*, 2002, Williams, Raven, Fogt, & Ivy, 2003; Zawadzki, Yaspelkis, & Ivy, 1992). Marked improvements (>40%) in exercise capacity during a subsequent bout of exercise have been demonstrated when protein was added to carbohydrate (Saunders, Kane, & Todd, 2004; Williams *et al.*, 2003), but neither of these studies used an isoenergetic carbohydrate comparison treatment. When an isocaloric carbohydrate recovery drink is compared with carbohydrate + protein, subsequent running performance is not improved (Millard-Stafford *et al.*, 2005) and rates of muscle glycogen synthesis are similar (Carrithers *et al.*, 2000; Jentjens, 2001; Van Hall, Shirreffs, & Calbet, 2000; Van Loon, Saris, Kruijshoop, & Wagenmakers, 2000). Therefore, improved performance and/or muscle glycogen observed after the co-ingestion of protein and carbohydrate may be attributed to the greater energy intake *per se* rather than any proven physiological effect. It has also been reported that the co-ingestion of protein with carbohydrate immediately after endurance exercise attenuates muscle soreness (Saunders *et al.*, 2004) and plasma creatine kinase responses to high-intensity exercise (Millard-Stafford *et al.*, 2005; Saunders *et al.*, 2004).

Two recent reports offer evidence that habitual daily protein intake may influence muscle protein metabolism and thus the adaptations to training. Harber, Schenk, Barkham and Horowitz (2005) reported that muscle protein synthesis in the basal state (i.e. resting, post-absorptive) was increased following 7 days of high (35% of total energy intake) protein intake. Presumably, such increased protein synthesis would lead to gains in muscle protein. However, no measurements of muscle protein turnover were made by Harber *et al.* (2005). Since increased muscle protein breakdown is usually associated with increased synthesis (Tipton & Wolfe, 1998), the actual accretion of muscle protein is unlikely to be as high as the increased rate of synthesis would suggest (Harber *et al.*, 2005). Presumably, the increased protein synthesis was mediated by increased signalling of the translation initiation pathways. However, increased muscle protein synthesis occurred without increased phosphorylation of two proteins downstream of mTOR (ribosomal protein S6 and eIF4G). This finding suggests that muscle protein synthesis is enhanced by high protein intake, but may not be associated with a chronic alteration in components of the mTOR signalling pathway. Accordingly, any acute up-regulation of selected signalling pathways after protein feeding may simply be a transient change in phosphorylation state and would not necessarily be evident at a time when increased muscle protein synthesis takes place.

Following exercise, the response of muscle protein synthesis to high protein intake seems to be different than at rest (Bolster *et al.*, 2005). After treadmill running, rates of muscle protein synthesis were higher in athletes who consumed 0.8 and 1.8 g protein $\cdot$ kg BM$^{-1}\cdot$ day^{-1} for 2 weeks (Bolster *et al.*, 2005) than in athletes who consumed ~3.6 g protein $\cdot$ kg BM$^{-1}\cdot$ day^{-1}. In fact, rates of muscle protein synthesis following exercise in athletes who consumed the chronic high-protein diet were similar to those generally measured in resting (untrained) participants (Volpi, Sheffield-Moore, Rasmussen, & Wolfe, 2001). These data suggest that a high-protein diet may actually inhibit the response of muscle protein synthesis to exercise. Accordingly, such high levels of protein intake would not be recommended for individuals during training. There is preliminary evidence to suggest that the decreased level of protein synthesis after high protein intake is accompanied by decreased muscle protein breakdown, thus further reducing the effect on net muscle protein balance (Bolster *et al.*, 2005). Taken collectively, there does not seem to be any reason to suggest that soccer players need to consume greater daily protein than currently recommended for most athletes. While the signalling cascades that stimulate muscle protein synthesis are undoubtedly complex, an understanding of how these pathways respond to exercise and specific nutritional interventions could provide sports scientists and coaches with information that may lead to modification of training/recovery processes and maximize training adaptations.

Summary and directions for future research

It is clear from the preceding discussion that nutrient supplementation can serve as a potent modulator of many of the acute responses to both endurance and resistance training. In this regard, recent scientific enquiry has focused on the role of specific nutrition strategies in promoting optimal biological adaptations to training. Research has focused on the role of carbohydrate availability before, during, and after exercise to amplify the training response, while there has been an emerging interest in the role of protein intake to enhance muscle hypertrophy after resistance exercise and possibly facilitate recovery from endurance exercise when co-ingested with carbohydrate. With advances in molecular biology, several techniques are now available that allow for the investigation of the interactive effects of exercise and diet on skeletal muscle gene expression and the early signalling responses to these different interventions. The greatest challenge for the exercise physiologist and sport nutritionist in the forthcoming years will be to link early gene and signalling responses in skeletal muscle that occur after exercise to chronic training-induced adaptations in already highly trained athletes. This task is complicated because many of these pathways are not linear, but rather constitute a complex network, with a high degree of cross-talk, feedback regulation, and transient activation (Hawley & Zierath, 2004). Nevertheless, several lines of inquiry may yield useful practical information concerning the interaction between nutrient intake and training adaptation. It is currently unclear whether periods of endurance training in the face of low glycogen stores can further drive the training adaptation in already well-trained athletes (the so-called "train-low/compete-high" approach). However, the muscle glycogen "sparing" observed in early studies of fat-adaptation may actually be an impairment of glycogenolysis, and such a nutritional strategy is not recommended for athletes involved in high-intensity activities such as soccer. While protein synthesis in strength-trained athletes may be increased by protein ingestion before or after training, it is not presently known if carbohydrate supplementation *alone* during recovery from resistance or endurance exercise can enhance gene, protein, and signalling responses to a greater/lesser degree than protein, or a combination of the two macronutrients. Furthermore, the efficacy of protein and/or protein plus carbohydrate ingestion following intense, intermittent exercise in promoting recovery (e.g. increasing muscle protein synthesis and muscle glycogen storage) and attenuating muscle damage and soreness during days of multiple training sessions and/or tournament play requires additional investigation. At present, the following recommendations are made:

- daily CHO intake during intense training should approach $7\,g \cdot kg\, BM^{-1} \cdot day^{-1}$;
- nutrient timing before, during, and after training can affect many of the adaptive responses to training;

- the provision of calories (in the form of carbohydrate and/or protein) before and within the hour after training are recommended.

Acknowledgements

The work undertaken in the principal author's laboratory on the interaction of exercise and diet is funded by GlaxoSmithKline, Consumer Healthcare (UK), and the Australian Institute of Sport.

References

Achten, J., Halson, S. L., Moseley, L., Rayson, M. P., Casey, A., & Jeukendrup, A. E. (2004). Higher dietary carbohydrate content during intensified running training results in better maintenance of performance and mood state. *Journal of Applied Physiology*, 96, 1331–1340.

Åkerstrom, T. C. A., Wojtaszewski, J. F. P., Plomgaard, P., & Pedersen, B. K. (2005). Effect of oral glucose ingestion on endurance training adaptation in human skeletal muscle. *Proceedings of the European College of Sport Sciences*, OS12-2, 76.

Akimoto, T., Pohnert, S. C., Li, P., Zhang, M., Gumbs, C., Rosenberg, P. B. et al. (2005). Exercise stimulates PGC-1α transcription in skeletal muscle through activation of the p38 MAPK pathway. *Journal of Biological Chemistry*, 280, 19587–19593.

Arkinstall, M. J., Bruce, C. R., Nikolopoulos, V., Garnham, A. P., & Hawley, J. A. (2001). Effect of carbohydrate ingestion on metabolism during running and cycling. *Journal of Applied Physiology*, 91, 2125–2134.

Arkinstall, M. J., Tunstall, R. J., Cameron-Smith, D., & Hawley, J. A. (2004). Regulation of metabolic genes in human skeletal muscle by short-term exercise and diet manipulation. *American Journal of Physiology: Endocrinology and Metabolism*, 287, E25–E31.

Aronson, D, Violan, M. A., Dufresne, S. D., Zangen, D., Fielding, R. A., & Goodyear, L. J. (1997). Exercise stimulates the mitogen-activated protein kinase pathway in human skeletal muscle. *Journal of Clinical Investigation*, 99, 1251–1257.

Aschenbach, W. G., Sakamoto, K., & Goodyear, L. J. (2004). 5′ adenosine monophosphate-activated protein kinase, metabolism and exercise. *Sports Medicine*, 34, 91–103.

Balsom, P. D., Wood, K., Olsson, P., & Ekblom, B. (1999). Carbohydrate intake and multiple sprint sports: With special reference to football (soccer). *International Journal of Sports Medicine*, 20, 48–52.

Baar, K., & Esser, K. (1999). Phosphorylation of p70(S6k) correlates with increased skeletal muscle mass following resistance exercise. *American Journal of Physiology*, 276, C120–C127.

Baar, K., Wende, A. R., Jones, T. E., Marison, M., Nolte, L. A., Chen, M. et al. (2002). Adaptations of skeletal muscle to exercise: Rapid increase in the transcriptional coactivator PGC-1. *FASEB Journal*, 16, 1879–1886.

Bangsbo, J. (1994). The physiology of soccer – with special reference to intense intermittent exercise. *Acta Physiologica Scandinavica*, 619 (suppl.), 1–155.

Barnes, B. R., Glund, S., Long, Y. C., Hjalm, G., Andersson, L., & Zierath, J. R. (2005). 5′-AMP-activated protein kinase regulates skeletal muscle glycogen content and ergogenics. *FASEB Journal*, 19, 773–779.

Bergstrom, J., Hermansen, L., Hultman, E., & Saltin, B. (1967). Diet, muscle glycogen and physical performance. *Acta Physiologica Scandinavica, 71*, 140–150.

Biolo, G., Maggi, S. P., Williams, B. D., Tipton, K. D., & Wolfe, R. R. (1995). Increased rates of muscle protein turnover and amino acid transport after resistance exercise in humans. *American Journal of Physiology: Endocrinology and Metabolism, 268*, E514–E520.

Biolo, G., Tipton, K. D., Klein, S., & Wolfe, R. R. (1997). An abundant supply of amino acids enhances the metabolic effect of exercise on muscle protein. *American Journal of Physiology: Endocrinology and Metabolism, 273*, 122–129.

Bolster, D. R., Crozier, S. J., Kimball, S. R., & Jefferson, L. S. (2002). AMP-activated protein kinase suppresses protein synthesis in rat skeletal muscle through down-regulated mammalian target of rapamycin (mTOR) signalling. *Journal of Biological Chemistry, 277*, 23977–23980.

Bolster, D. R., Jefferson, L. S., & Kimball, S. R. (2004). Regulation of protein synthesis associated with skeletal muscle hypertrophy by insulin-, amino acid- and exercise-induced signalling. *Proceedings of the Nutrition Society, 63*, 351–356.

Bolster, D. R., Pikosky, M. A., Gaine, P. C., Martin, W., Wolfe, R. R., Tipton, K. D. *et al.* (2005). Dietary protein intake impacts human skeletal muscle protein fractional synthetic rates following endurance exercise. *American Journal of Physiology: Endocrinology and Metabolism, 289*, E678–E683.

Booth, F. W., & Thomason, D. B. (1991). Molecular and cellular adaptation of muscle in response to exercise: Perspectives of various models. *Physiological Reviews, 71*, 541–585.

Borsheim, E., Aarsland, A., & Wolfe, R. R. (2004). Effect of an amino acid, protein, and carbohydrate mixture on net muscle protein balance after resistance exercise. *International Journal of Sport Nutrition and Exercise Metabolism, 14*, 255–271.

Borsheim, E., Tipton, K. D., Wolf, S. E., & Wolfe, R. R. (2002). Essential amino acids and muscle protein recovery from resistance exercise. *American Journal of Physiology: Endocrinology and Metabolism, 283*, E648–E657.

Burke, L. M. (2003). The IOC consensus on sports nutrition 2003: New guidelines for nutrition for athletes. *International Journal of Sport Nutrition and Exercise Metabolism, 13*, 549–552.

Burke, L. M., Angus, D. J., Cox, G. R., Cummings, N. K., Febbraio, M. A., Gawthorn, K. *et al.* (2000). Effect of fat adaptation and carbohydrate restoration on metabolism and performance during prolonged cycling. *Journal of Applied Physiology, 89*, 2413–2421.

Burke, L. M., & Hawley, J. A. (2002). Effects of short-term fat adaptation on metabolism and performance of prolonged exercise. *Medicine and Science in Sports and Exercise, 34*, 1492–1498.

Burke, L. M., Hawley, J. A., Angus, D. J., Cox, G. R., Clark, S. A., Cummings, N. K. *et al.* (2002). Adaptations to short-term high-fat diet persist during exercise despite high carbohydrate availability. *Medicine and Science in Sports and Exercise, 34*, 83–91.

Burke, L. M., Kiens, B., & Ivy, J. L. (2004). Carbohydrates and fat for training and recovery. *Journal of Sports Sciences, 22*, 15–30.

Carling, D., & Hardie, D. G. (1989). The substrate and sequence specificity of the AMP-activated protein kinase: Phosphorylation of glycogen synthase and phosphorylase kinase. *Biochimica Biophysica Acta, 1012*, 81–86.

Cameron-Smith, D., Burke, L. M., Angus, D. J., Tunstall, R. J., Cox, G. R., Bonen, A. *et al.* (2003). A short-term, high-fat diet up-regulates lipid metabolism and gene expression in human skeletal muscle. *American Journal of Clinical Nutrition, 77*, 313–318.

Carrithers, J. A., Williamson, D. L., Gallagher, P. M., Godard, M. P., Schulze, K. E., & Trappe, S. W. (2000). Effects of postexercise carbohydrate–protein feedings on muscle glycogen restoration. *Journal of Applied Physiology, 88*, 1976–1982.

Chakravarthy, M. V., & Booth, F. W. (2004). Eating, exercise, and "thrifty" genotypes: Connecting the dots toward an evolutionary understanding of modern chronic diseases. *Journal of Applied Physiology, 96*, 3–10.

Chan, M. H., McGee, S. L., Watt, M. J., Hargreaves, M., & Febbraio, M. A. (2004). Altering dietary nutrient intake that reduces glycogen content leads to phosphorylation of nuclear p38 MAP kinase in human skeletal muscle: Association with IL-6 gene transcription during contraction. *FASEB Journal, 18*, 1785–1787.

Chen, Z. P., Stephens, T. J., Murthy, S., Canny, B. J., Hargreaves, M., Witters, L. A. *et al.* (2003). Effect of exercise intensity on skeletal muscle AMPK signaling in humans. *Diabetes, 52*, 2205–2212.

Cheng, I. S., Lee, N. Y., Liu, K. L., Liao, S. F., Huang, C. H., & Kuo, C. H. (2005). Effect of postexercise carbohydrate supplementation on glucose uptake-associated gene expression in the human skeletal muscle. *Journal of Nutritional Biochemistry, 16*, 267–271.

Cheng, S. W., Fryer, L. G., Carling, D., & Shepherd, P. R. (2004). Thr^{2446} is a novel mammalian target of rapamycin (mTOR) phosphorylation site regulated by nutrient status. *Journal of Biological Chemistry, 279*, 15719–15722.

Civitarese, A. E., Hesselink, M. K., Russell, A. P., Ravussin, E., & Schrauwen, P. (2005). Glucose ingestion during exercise blunts exercise induced gene expression of skeletal muscle fat oxidative genes. *American Journal of Physiology: Endocrinology and Metabolism, 289*, E1023–E1029.

Clark, K. (1994). Nutritional guidance to soccer players for training and competition. *Journal of Sports Sciences, 12*, S43–S50.

Cluberton, L. J., McGee, S. L., Murphy, R. M., & Hargreaves, M. (2005). Effect of carbohydrate ingestion on exercise-induced alterations in metabolic gene expression. *Journal of Applied Physiology, 99*, 1359–1363.

Costill, D. L., Sherman, W. M., Fink, W. J., Maresh, C., Witten, M., & Miller, J. M. (1981). The role of dietary carbohydrates in muscle glycogen resynthesis after strenuous running. *American Journal of Clinical Nutrition, 34*, 1831–1836.

Coyle, E. F. (2000). Physical activity as a metabolic stressor. *American Journal of Clinical Nutrition, 72*, 512S–520S.

Coyle, E. F., Coggan, A. R., Hemmert, M. K., & Ivy, J. L. (1986). Muscle glycogen utilization during prolonged strenuous exercise when fed carbohydrate. *Journal of Applied Physiology, 61*, 165–172.

Creer, A., Gallagher, P., Slivka, D., Jemiolo, B., Fink, W., & Trappe, S. (2005). Influence of muscle glycogen availability on ERK1/2 and Akt signaling following resistance exercise in human skeletal muscle. *Journal of Applied Physiology, 99*, 950–956.

Deldicque, L., Theisen, D., & Francaux, M. (2005). Regulation of mTOR by amino acids and resistance exercise in skeletal muscle. *European Journal of Applied Physiology, 94*, 1–10.

Febbraio, M. A., Steensberg, A., Walsh, R., Koukoulas, I., van Hall, G., & Saltin, B. (2003). Reduced glycogen availability is associated with an elevation in HSP72 in contracting human skeletal muscle. *Journal of Physiology, 538*, 911–917.

Frosig, C., Jorgensen, S. B., Hardie, D. G., Richter, E. A., & Wojtaszewski, J. F. (2004). 5'-AMP-activated protein kinase activity and protein expression are regulated by endurance training in human skeletal muscle. *American Journal of Physiology: Endocrinology and Metabolism, 286*, E411–E417.

Fujii, N., Hayashi, T., Hirshman, M. F., Smith, J. T., Habinowski, S. A., Kaijser, L. *et al.* (2000). Exercise induces isoform-specific increase in 5'-AMP-activated protein kinase activity in human skeletal muscle. *Biochemical and Biophysical Research Communications, 273*, 1150–1155.

Glass, D. J. (2003). Signalling pathways that mediate skeletal muscle hypertrophy and atrophy. *Nature Cell Biology, 5*, 87–90.

Gollnick, P. D., Armstrong, R. B., Saltin, B., Saubert, C. W., Sembrowich, W. L., & Shepherd, R. E. (1973). Effect of training on enzyme activity and fiber composition of human skeletal muscle. *Journal of Applied Physiology, 34*, 107–111.

Hansen, A. K., Fischer, C. P., Plomgaard, P., Andersen, J. L., Saltin, B., & Pedersen, B. K. (2005). Skeletal muscle adaptation: Training twice every second day vs. training once daily. *Journal of Applied Physiology, 98*, 93–99.

Harber, M. P., Schenk, S., Barkham, A. L., & Horowitz, J. F. (2005). Effects of dietary carbohydrate restriction with high protein intake on protein metabolism and the somatotropic axis. *Journal of Clinical Endocrinology and Metabolism, 90*, 5175–5181.

Hardie, D. G., & Hawley, S. A. (2001). AMP-activated protein kinase: The energy charge hypothesis revisited. *Bioessays, 23*, 1112–1119.

Hargreaves, M. (1994). Carbohydrate and lipid requirements of soccer. *Journal of Sports Sciences, 12*, S13–S16.

Hargreaves, M., & Cameron-Smith, D. (2002). Exercise, diet, and skeletal muscle gene expression. *Medicine and Science in Sports and Exercise, 34*, 1505–1508.

Hawley, J. A. (2002a). Adaptations of skeletal muscle to prolonged, intense endurance training. *Clinics in Experimental Pharmacology and Physiology, 29*, 218–222.

Hawley, J. A. (2002b). Effect of increased fat availability on metabolism and exercise capacity. *Medicine and Science in Sports and Exercise, 34*, 1485–1491.

Hawley, J. A., Dennis, S. C., Lindsay, F. H., & Noakes, T. D. (1995). Nutritional practices of athletes: Are they sub-optimal? *Journal of Sports Sciences, 13*, S75–S81.

Hawley, J. A., Dennis, S. C., & Noakes, T. D. (1994). Carbohydrate, fluid, and electrolyte requirements of the soccer player: A review. *International Journal of Sport Nutrition, 4*, 221–236.

Hawley, J. A., & Zierath, J. R. (2004). Integration of metabolic and mitogenic signal transduction in skeletal muscle. *Exercise and Sport Science Reviews, 32*, 4–8.

Hayashi, T., Hirshman, M. F., Kurth, E. J., Winder, W. W., & Goodyear, L. J. (1998). Evidence for 5' AMP-activated protein kinase mediation of the effect of muscle contraction on glucose transport. *Diabetes, 47*, 1369–1373.

Hildebrandt, A. L., Pilegaard, H., & Neufer, P. D. (2003). Differential transcriptional activation of select metabolic genes in response to variations in exercise intensity and duration. *American Journal of Physiology: Endocrinology and Metabolism, 285*, E1021–E1027.

Hood, D. A. (2001). Invited review: Contractile activity-induced mitochondrial biogenesis in skeletal muscle. *Journal of Applied Physiology, 90*, 1137–1157.

Ivy, J. L., Goforth, H. W., Damon, B. M., McCauley, T. R., Parsons, E. C., & Price, T. B. (2002). Early post-exercise muscle glycogen recovery is enhanced with a carbohydrate-protein supplement. *Journal of Applied Physiology, 93*, 1337–1344.

Jentjens, R., & Jeukendrup, A. E. (2003). Determinants of post-exercise glycogen synthesis during short-term recovery. *Sports Medicine, 33,* 117–144.

Jentjens, R. L., van Loon, L. J., Mann, C. H., Wagemakers, A. J., & Jeukendrup, A. E. (2001). Addition of protein and amino acids to carbohydrates does not enhance postexercise muscle glycogen synthesis. *Journal of Applied Physiology, 91,* 832–846.

Jump, D. B., & Clarke, S. D. (1999). Regulation of gene expression by dietary fat. *Annual Reviews of Nutrition, 19,* 63–90.

Karlsson, H. K., Nilsson, P. A., Nilsson, J., Chibalin, A. V., Zierath, J. R., & Blomstrand, E. (2004). Branched-chain amino acids increase p70S6k phosphorylation in human skeletal muscle after resistance exercise. *American Journal of Physiology: Endocrinology and Metabolism, 287,* E1–E7.

Keller, C., Steensberg, A., Pilegaard, H., Osada, T., Saltin, B., Pedersen, B. K. *et al.* (2001). Transcriptional activation of the IL-6 gene in human contracting skeletal muscle: Influence of muscle glycogen content. *FASEB Journal, 15,* 2748–2750.

Kimball, S. R., Farrell, P. A., & Jefferson, L. J. (2002). Invited review: Role of insulin in translational control of protein synthesis in skeletal muscle by amino acids or exercise. *Journal of Applied Physiology, 93,* 1168–1180.

Kirkendall, D. T. (1993). Effects of nutrition on performance in soccer. *Medicine and Science in Sports and Exercise, 25,* 1370–1374.

Koopman, R., Pannemans, D. L. E., Jeukendrup, A. E., Gijsen, A. P., Senden, J. M. G., Halliday, D. *et al.* (2004). Combined ingestion of protein and carbohydrate improves protein balance during ultra-endurance exercise. *American Journal of Physiology, Endocrinology & Metabolism, 287,* E712–E720.

Kraniou, Y., Cameron-Smith, D., Misso, M., Collier, G., & Hargreaves, M. (2000). Effects of exercise on GLUT-4 and glycogenin gene expression in human skeletal muscle. *Journal of Applied Physiology, 88,* 794–796.

Lamb, D. R., Rinehardt, K. F., Bartels, R. L., Sherman, W. M., & Snook, J. T. (1990). Dietary carbohydrate and intensity of interval swim training. *American Journal of Clinical Nutrition, 52,* 1058–1063.

Lemon, P. W. (2000). Beyond the zone: Protein needs of active individuals. *Journal of the American College of Nutrition, 19,* 513S–521S.

McInerney, P., Lessard, S. J., Burke, L. M., Coffey, V. G., Lo Giudice, S. L., Southgate, R. J. *et al.* (2005). Failure to repeatedly supercompensate muscle glycogen stores in highly trained men. *Medicine and Science in Sports and Exercise, 37,* 404–411.

Millard-Stafford, M. L., Cureton, K. J., & Ray, C. A. (1988). Effect of glucose polymer diet supplement on responses to prolonged successive swimming, cycling and running. *European Journal of Applied Physiology, 58,* 327–333.

Millard-Stafford, M. L., Warren, G. L., Thomas, L. M., Doyle, J. A., Snow, T. K., & Hitchcock, K. M. (2005). Recovery from run training: Efficacy of a carbohydrate-protein beverage? *International Journal of Sports Nutrition and Exercise Metabolism, 15,* 610–624.

Miller, S. L., Tipton, K. D., Chinkes, D. L., Wolf, S. E., & Wolfe, R. R. (2003). Independent and combined effects of amino acids and glucose after resistance exercise. *Medicine and Science in Sports and Exercise, 35,* 449–455.

Nader, G. A., & Esser, K. A. (2001). Intracellular signaling specificity in skeletal muscle in response to different modes of exercise. *Journal of Applied Physiology, 90,* 1936–1942.

Nelson, A. G., Arnall, D. A., Loy, S. F., Silvester, L. J., & Conlee, R. K. (1990). Consequences of combining strength and endurance training regimens. *Physical Therapy*, 70, 287–294.

Neufer, P. D., & Dohm, G. L. (1993). Exercise induces a transient increase in transcription of the GLUT-4 gene in skeletal muscle. *American Journal of Physiology*, 265, C1597–C1603.

Nicholas, C. W., Tsintzas, K., Boobis, L., & Williams, C. (1999). Carbohydrate-electrolyte ingestion during intermittent high-intensity running. *Medicine and Science in Sports and Exercise*, 31, 1280–1286.

Nielsen, J. N., Mustard, K. J., Graham, D. A., Yu, H., MacDonald, C. S., Pilegaard, H. et al. (2003). 5′-AMP-activated protein kinase activity and subunit expression in exercise-trained human skeletal muscle. *Journal of Applied Physiology*, 94, 631–641.

Phillips, S. M., Tipton, K. D., Aarsland, A., Wolf, S. E., & Wolfe, R. R. (1997). Mixed muscle protein synthesis and breakdown after resistance exercise in humans. *American Journal of Physiology*, 273, E99–E107.

Pilegaard, H., Keller, C., Steensberg, A., Helge, J. W., Pedersen, B. K., Saltin, B. et al. (2002). Influence of pre-exercise muscle glycogen content on exercise-induced transcriptional regulation of metabolic genes. *Journal of Physiology*, 541, 261–271.

Pilegaard, H., Ordway, G. A., Saltin, B., & Neufer, P. D. (2000). Transcriptional regulation of gene expression in human skeletal muscle during recovery from exercise. *American Journal of Physiology*, 279, E806–E814.

Printen, J. A., Brady, M. J., & Saltiel, A. R. (1997). PTG, a protein phosphatase 1-binding protein with a role in glycogen metabolism. *Science*, 275, 1475–1478.

Proud, C. G. (2002). Regulation of mammalian translation factors by nutrients. *European Journal of Biochemistry*, 269, 5338–5349.

Rennie, M. J., & Tipton, K. D. (2000). Protein and amino acid metabolism during and after exercise and the effects of nutrition. *Annual Reviews of Nutrition*, 20, 457–483.

Richter, E. A., Derave, W., & Wojtaszewski, J. F. (2001). Glucose, exercise and insulin: emerging concepts. *Journal of Physiology*, 535, 313–322.

Rico-Sanz, J., Frontera, W. R., Mole, P. A., Rivera, M. A., Rivera-Brown, A., & Meredith, C. N. (1998). Dietary and performance assessment of elite soccer players during a period of intense training. *International Journal of Sport Nutrition*, 8, 230–240.

Rico-Sanz, J., Zehnder, M., Buchli, R., Dambach, M., & Boutellier, U. (1999). Muscle glycogen degradation during simulation of a fatiguing soccer match in elite soccer players examined noninvasively by ^{13}C-MRS. *Medicine and Science in Sports and Exercise*, 31, 1587–1593.

Sakoda, H., Fujishiro, M., Shojima, N., Ogihara, T., Kushiyama, A., Fukushima, Y. et al. (2005). Glycogen debranching enzyme association with b-subunit regulates AMP-activated protein kinase activity. *American Journal of Physiology*, 289, E474–E481.

Saunders, M. J., Kane, M. D., & Todd, M. K. (2004). Effects of a carbohydrate-protein beverage on cycling endurance and muscle damage. *Medicine and Science in Sports and Exercise*, 36, 1233–1238.

Sherman, W. M., Doyle, J. A., Lamb, D. R., & Strauss, R. H. (1993). Dietary carbohydrate, muscle glycogen, and exercise performance during 7 d of training. *American Journal of Clinical Nutrition*, 57, 27–31.

Simonsen, J. C., Sherman, W. M., Lamb, D. R., Dernbach, A. R., Doyle, J. A., & Strauss, R. (1991). Dietary carbohydrate, muscle glycogen, and power output during rowing training. *Journal of Applied Physiology, 70,* 1500–1505.

Stellingwerff, T., Spriet, L. L., Watt, M. J., Kimber, N. E., Hargreaves, M., Hawley, J.A. *et al.* (2006). Decreased PDH ativation and glycogenolysis during exercise following fat adaptation with carbohydrate restoration. *American Journal of Physiology, Endocrinology & Metabolism, 290,* E380–E388.

Stepto, N. K., Carey, A. L., Staudacher, H. M., Cummings, N. K., Burke, L. M., & Hawley, J. A. (2002). Effect of short-term fat adaptation on high-intensity training. *Medicine and Science in Sports and Exercise, 34,* 449–455.

Terjung, R. L., & Hood, D. A. (1986). Biochemical adaptations in skeletal muscle induced by exercise training. In D. K. Layman (Ed.), *Nutrition and aerobic exercise* (pp. 8–27). Washington, DC: American Chemical Society.

Tipton, K. D., Elliott, T. A., Cree, M. G., Wolf, S. E., Sanford, A. P., & Wolfe, R. R. (2004). Ingestion of casein and whey proteins result in muscle anabolism after resistance exercise. *Medicine and Science in Sports and Exercise, 36,* 2073–2081.

Tipton, K. D., Ferrando, A. A., Phillips, S. M., Doyle, D., & Wolfe, R. R. (1999). Postexercise net protein synthesis in human muscle from orally administered amino acids. *American Journal of Physiology, 276,* E628–E634.

Tipton, K. D., Rasmussen, B. B., Miller, S. L., Wolf, S. E., Owens-Stovall, S. K., Petrini, B. E. *et al.* (2001). Timing of amino acid-carbohydrate ingestion alters anabolic response of muscle to resistance exercise. *American Journal of Physiology, 281,* E197–E206.

Tipton, K. D., & Wolfe, R. R. (1998). Exercise-induced changes in protein metabolism. *Acta Physiologica Scandinavica, 162,* 377–387.

Tipton, K. D., & Wolfe, R. R. (2004). Protein and amino acids for athletes. *Journal of Sports Sciences, 22,* 65–79.

Tunstall, R. J., & Cameron-Smith, D. (2005). Effect of elevated lipid concentrations on human skeletal muscle gene expression. *Metabolism, 54,* 952–959.

Van Hall, G., Shirreffs, S. M., & Calbet, J. A. L. (2000). Muscle glycogen resynthesis during recovery from cycle exercise: No effect of additional protein ingestion. *Journal of Applied Physiology, 88,* 1631–1636.

Van Loon, L. J. C., Saris, W. H. M., Kruijshoop, M., & Wagenmakers, A. J. M. (2000). Maximizing postexercise muscle glycogen synthesis: Carbohydrate supplementation and the application of amino acid or protein hydrolysate mixtures. *American Journal of Clinical Nutrition, 72,* 106–111.

Volpi, E., Sheffield-Moore, M., Rasmussen, B. R., & Wolfe, R. R. (2001). Basal muscle amino acid kinetics and protein synthesis in healthy young and older men. *Journal of the American Medical Association, 286,* 1206–1212.

Widegren, U., Jiang, X. J., Krook, A., Chibalin, A. V., Bjornholm, M., Tally, M. *et al.* (1998). Divergent effects of exercise on metabolic and mitogenic signaling pathways in human skeletal muscle. *FASEB Journal, 12,* 1379–1389.

Widegren, U., Ryder, J. W., & Zierath, J. R. (2001). Mitogen-activated protein kinase signal transduction in skeletal muscle: Effects of exercise and muscle contraction. *Acta Physiologica Scandinavica, 172,* 227–238.

Williams, M. B., Raven, P. B., Fogt, D. L., & Ivy, J. L. (2003). Effects of recovery beverages on glycogen restoration and endurance exercise performance. *Journal of Strength and Conditioning Research, 17,* 12–19.

Williams, R. S., & Neufer, P. D. (1996). Regulation of gene expression in skeletal muscle by contractile activity. In *Handbook of physiology. Exercise: Regulation and integration of multiple systems* (Section 12, pp. 1124–1150). Bethesda, MD: American Physiological Society.

Williamson, D., Gallagher, P., Harber, M., Hollon, C., & Trappe, S. (2003). Mitogen-activated protein kinase (MAPK) pathway activation: Effects of age and acute exercise on human skeletal muscle. *Journal of Physiology*, 547, 977–987.

Winder, W. W. (2001). Energy-sensing and signaling by AMP-activated protein kinase in skeletal muscle. *Journal of Applied Physiology*, 91, 1017–1028.

Wojtaszewski, J. F., MacDonald, C., Nielsen, J. N., Hellsten, Y., Hardie, D. G., Kemp, B. E. *et al.* (2003). Regulation of 5′AMP-activated protein kinase activity and substrate utilization in exercising human skeletal muscle. *American Journal of Physiology*, 284, E813–E822.

Wojtaszewski, J. F., Nielsen, P., Hansen, B. F., Richter, E. A., & Kiens, B. (2000). Isoform-specific and exercise intensity-dependent activation of 5′-AMP-activated protein kinase in human skeletal muscle. *Journal of Physiology*, 528, 221–226.

Wretman, C., Lionikas, A., Widegren, U., Lannergren, J., Westerblad, H., & Henriksson, J. (2001). Effects of concentric and eccentric contractions on phosphorylation of MAPK(ERK1/2) and MAPK(p38) in isolated rat skeletal muscle. *Journal of Physiology*, 535, 155–164.

Yu, M., Stepto, N. K., Chibalin, A. V., Fryer, L. G., Carling, D., Krook, A. *et al.* (2003). Metabolic and mitogenic signal transduction in human skeletal muscle after intense cycling exercise. *Journal of Physiology*, 546, 327–335.

Zawadzki, K. M., Yaspelkis, B. B., & Ivy, J. L. (1992). Carbohydrate-protein supplement increases the rate of muscle glycogen storage post exercise. *Journal of Applied Physiology*, 72, 1854–1859.

6 Nutritional strategies for football: Counteracting heat, cold, high altitude, and jet lag

LAWRENCE E. ARMSTRONG

Environmental factors often influence the physical and mental performance of football players. Heat, cold, high altitude, and travel across time zones (i.e. leading to jet lag) act as stressors that alter normal physiological function, homeostasis, metabolism, and whole-body nutrient balance. Rather than accepting performance decrements as inevitable, well-informed coaches and players should plan strategies for training and competition that offset environmental challenges. Considering the strength of scientific evidence, this paper reviews recommendations regarding nutritional interventions that purportedly counterbalance dehydration, hyperthermia, hypothermia, hypoxia, acute or chronic substrate deficiencies, sleep loss, and desynchronization of internal biological clocks.

Keywords: Metabolism, carbohydrate, glycogen, fat, protein, hydration

Background

The energy requirement for competitive football is large and is influenced by many factors. The mean rate of aerobic energy production for elite players is 70–80% of maximal aerobic power ($\dot{V}O_{2max}$) during the course of a 90 min match. The energy cost of an entire match is 5–6 MJ (1195–1434 kcal), depending on the total distance covered (~10–11 km) and the style of play (Bangsbo, 1994; Ekblom, 1986). These values reflect environmental, physiological, tactical, and technical factors (Kuzon *et al.*, 1990; Mohr, Krustrup, & Bangsbo, 2003; Shephard, 1999).

The metabolic responses and substrate utilization that occur during football are difficult to study because play involves intermittent exercise, varied intensities, and rest periods. In attempts to reproduce match-play, some investigators have designed laboratory simulations, whereas others have conducted controlled studies involving intermittent exercise based on match characteristics (Bangsbo, Norregaard, & Thorsoe, 1991). In general, these research studies indicate that football places great demands on both aerobic and anaerobic energy-producing systems (Balsom, 1995; Shephard, 1999). For example, the liver must mobilize stored glycogen to maintain blood glucose during a match. Also, a pronounced utilization of stored muscle glycogen occurs during a match, indicating that (at a high exercise intensity) substrate availability for anaerobic energy production may be a limiting factor for performance (Balsom, 1995), as evidenced by frequent reports of peak blood lactate concentrations in the range of 4–10 mmol·l^{-1} (Bangsbo, 1994). Regarding lipid metabolism, the concentration of plasma free fatty acids rises (probably due to effects of increased catecholamines and suppressed insulin) during the later stages of a contest, with only a minor increase of plasma glycerol (Shephard, 1999). This suggests a large uptake of glycerol by various tissues, likely as a precursor of gluconeogenesis (Bangsbo, 1994). The roles of intramuscular lipolysis, circulating ketone bodies, and protein as energy sources are not well described (Bangsbo, 1994; Essen, 1978).

Further complicating scientific investigations, football is played in a variety of extreme environments around the world, including heat, cold, and high altitude (Askew, 1995). As athletes move into these environments and travel across time zones, metabolism and substrate utilization change, as does human performance (Armstrong, 2000; Committee on Military Nutrition Research, 1996, 1999a, 1999b; Shephard, 1999; Wilbur, 2004). Today, physiologists and dietitians view nutrition as a key factor to offset the physical and cognitive performance decrements that occur in stressful environments (Askew, 1996). Therefore, the purposes of this review are to: (a) describe the effects of four environmental factors on exercise metabolism, whole-body nutrient balance, and performance; (b) review nutritional interventions that may counteract these effects; (c) evaluate the strength of evidence regarding nutritional interventions; and (d) recommend directions for future research. This review does not consider pharmacological interventions or banned substances (FIFA, 2004).

Environmental influences on metabolism

Previous publications have described the metabolic changes induced by living in stressful environments. For example, two classic studies utilized animals to explore the effects of heat (>35°C), cold (<5°C), and high-altitude (>5500 m, 25°C) stresses on metabolism. After being exposed to each environment for 4 weeks, rats exhibited changes of food and water intake, as well as altered excretion rates for electrolytes and nitrogen (i.e. representing protein and non-protein compounds) (Mefferd, Hale, & Martens, 1958), compared with a control group. The rate of food intake and the rate of waste excretion were considerably greater in the cold-exposed group than the heat-exposed group, reflecting an elevated metabolic rate (i.e. shivering) in the cold. Furthermore, none of the animals had normal weight gains, in comparison to the control group, suggesting that their metabolism did not adapt to these environmental extremes within 4 weeks (Mefferd *et al.*, 1958).

Table 1 presents the four environmental factors that are considered in this review, and the human physiological outcomes that result from each. The primary threats to homeostasis are dehydration, hyperthermia, hypothermia, hypoxia, acute or chronic substrate deficiencies, sleep loss, and desynchronization of internal biological clocks. Table 1 also describes the specific effects

Table 1. Effects of four environmental factors on metabolism and performance

Environmental factors	Physiological outcomes of environmental stress[a]	Effects on human metabolism and performance[b]
Heat	• increased skin and core body temperature • increased cardiovascular strain[c] • increased sweating may lead to fluid-electrolyte deficit (i.e. sodium)	• increased anaerobic metabolism • increased plasma lactate accumulation • increased rate of glycogen depletion • reduced $\dot{V}O_{2max}$ • reduced endurance, strength, and power performance • increased perceived exertion • increased resting metabolic rate[d]
Cold	• decreased skin and core body temperature	• increased heat production (1–4 times resting metabolism) due to shivering • increased metabolism without shivering[e] • increased appetite • decreased utilization of free fatty acids • increased utilization of plasma glucose and muscle glycogen • increased plasma lactate concentration • increased diuresis • reduced maximal aerobic power ($\dot{V}O_{2max}$) • reduced endurance exercise performance • reduced muscular strength and power when muscle temperature decreases[f] • reduced memory and cognitive function
High altitude	• low barometric pressure results in arterial blood hypoxia (reduced partial pressure of oxygen) • increased resting ventilation	• reduced maximal aerobic power ($\dot{V}O_{2max}$) • reduced endurance performance[g] • reduced reaction time and motor coordination

- breathlessness during exercise or activities
- reduced cardiac output (rest and exercise)
- reduced oxygen saturation of haemoglobin and reduced oxygen delivery to tissues
- increased incidence of sleep disturbance and sleep apnoea

- aerobic metabolism is unable to provide adequate energy; this is partially offset by increased anaerobic metabolism
- increased carbohydrate utilization
- increased plasma lactate accumulation
- increased water loss via diuresis and respiratory water loss (acute); decreased muscle and fat mass (chronic)[h]
- impaired mood and appetite
- reduced cognitive performance (i.e. memory, decision making, calculations)
- reduced vigour and increased fatigue
- increased oxidative stress (i.e. free radical formation)[i]

Jet lag
- travel across time zones disrupts the coordination of environmental cues (i.e. light–dark cycle, social activities) with internal biological clocks
- disrupted sleep cycle, sleep loss

- disturbed mood
- increased daytime fatigue
- reduced daytime alertness
- disturbed gastrointestinal function
- altered schedule of eating and drinking

Note: This table was compiled from the following references: Aerospace Medical Association (1996), Ahlers, Thomas, Schrot and Shurtleff (1994), Armstrong (2000), Committee on Military Nutrition Research (1996), Doubt (1991), Ferretti (1992), Fulco and Cymerman (1988), Galloway and Maughan (1997), Normand, Vargas, Bordachar, Benoit and Raynaud (1992), Sawka and Wenger (1988), Stephenson and Kolka (1988), Toner and McArdle (1988), Wenger (1988), Wilbur (2004), Young (1988), Youngstedt and Buxton (2003).

a 8–14 days of acclimatization to heat, cold and altitude alters these effects favourably, in response to specific stresses imposed on the body.
b These effects increase as environmental stress increases.
c Due to simultaneous needs to supply blood flow to exercising muscle to support metabolism, and skin to dissipate internal heat.
d In a hot environment (>35°C), resting energy expenditure increases up to 5%, due to the energetic cost of sweating, hyperventilation, circulatory strain, or the Q_{10} effect (Consolazio & Schnakenberg, 1977).
e Probably because of secretion of hormones (i.e. adrenal catecholamines, thyroxine).
f Muscle temperature may be normal or elevated, even in very cold air, depending on clothing insulation and exercise-induced heat production (Bergh & Ekblom, 1979; Blomstrand, Bergh, Essen-Gustavsson, & Ekblom, 1984).
g The results of studies regarding anaerobic performance are equivocal.
h Chronic body mass loss may be due to a combination of increased resting metabolic rate, increased activity level, decreased appetite and food intake.
i Due to the electron transport chain, hypoxia and ultraviolet radiation.

of heat, cold, high altitude, and transmeridian air travel on metabolism and performance.

Dehydration affects metabolism and performance

The four environmental factors in Table 1 encourage dehydration. Heat exposure is the most obvious, due to sweat losses. Exposure to cold and high-altitude environments stimulates diuresis (i.e. transient increase of urine production), predisposing athletes to dehydration. Also, during lengthy airline flights, dry cabin air and restricted access to food and water result in mild-to-moderate dehydration.

In recent years, numerous studies led to a theory regarding the role that cell shrinkage (i.e. dehydration) plays in cellular metabolism and hormonal responses. This theory states that, when cells shrink, metabolism becomes predominantly catabolic and, when cells swell, metabolism becomes anabolic. Thus, cell shrinkage and swelling lead to opposite effects on protein, carbohydrate, and lipid metabolism. For example, measurements involving humans and animals (Ritz *et al.*, 2003) have shown that cell shrinkage signals the cleavage of glycogen, lysing of proteins, and a temporary halt to the formation of both glycogen and protein. This makes glucose and amino acids available for alternative metabolic pathways. Changes in cell size also theoretically mediate lipolysis, via the hormonal effects of insulin, glucagons, and catecholamines (Keller, Szinnai, Bilz, & Berneis, 2003). If these concepts are supported by future research, the dehydration that often occurs in hot, cold, and high-altitude environments (and the resultant cell shrinkage) may be viewed as an important aspect of metabolic regulation.

Dehydration (i.e. due to heat, cold, or high-altitude exposure) need not be severe to alter mental and physical performance (Maughan, 2003b). Mild dehydration (i.e. equivalent to 1–2% of body mass), for even a brief period, leads to (a) a reduction of the subjective perception of alertness and ability to concentrate, (b) an increase of self-reported tiredness, and (c) an increase of headache pain. Mild dehydration also impairs high-intensity endurance exercise performance (Armstrong, Costill, & Fink, 1985; Maughan, 2003b) and intermittent supramaximal running performance (Maxwell, Gardner, & Nimmo, 1999), although maximal muscle strength and power appear to be relatively unaffected (Maughan, 2003b; Watson *et al.*, 2005).

Nutrition for football in all environments

Three nutritional strategies, to optimize performance and minimize fatigue, are recommended for football players in any environment. First, at least 3 h before a contest and during the half-time of a football match, provide 100–300 g of carbohydrate (Williams & Serrasota, 2006). Ample dietary carbohydrate intake approximately doubles normal muscle glycogen reservoirs (Shephard, 1999) and can result in a 5–6% increase of the ability to perform multiple sprints after

45 min of simulated football (Bangsbo, Norregaard, & Thorsoe, 1992). When left without guidance, most players fail to ingest the necessary quantity and type of carbohydrates during the hours after exercise (Shephard, 1999). As long as a 70 kg person consumes 500–600 g of carbohydrate, glycogen resynthesis is similar whether eaten in two meals or several small meals (Costill *et al.*, 1981); both simple and complex carbohydrates are effective (Coyle, 1995). Even when recovery periods are brief (i.e. 4 h), players can benefit from consuming carbohydrate (Burke, Coyle, & Maughan, 2003; Williams, 1995). Interestingly, one study demonstrated that a carbohydrate-protein solution (7.75% carbohydrate and 1.94% protein) enhanced continuous cycling endurance performance beyond that of a 7.75% carbohydrate solution alone (Ivy, Res, Sprague, & Widzer, 2003). Although the effects of a carbohydrate-protein solution on high-intensity, intermittent exercise are unknown, this project provides a testable hypothesis for future investigations.

Second, because low intramuscular glycogen becomes an important cause of fatigue as a game progresses, players should optimize muscle glycogen resynthesis after exercise (Bangsbo, 1991; Saltin, 1973) by consuming 8–11 g of carbohydrate per kilogram of body mass per day (Sherman, 1992). Third, ensure that total energy, carbohydrate, and protein levels are adequate, as provided by a well-balanced daily diet. After reviewing numerous studies, Shephard (1999) provided the following dietary recommendations for male football players: daily energy intake, 14–15 MJ $\cdot$ day^{-1} (3346–3585 kcal $\cdot$ day^{-1}); carbohydrate, 8 g $\cdot$ kg body mass^{-1} $\cdot$ day^{-1}; protein, 1.5 g $\cdot$ kg body mass^{-1} $\cdot$ day^{-1}. Further information regarding nutritional practices can be found in Williams and Serratosa (2006) and Burke, Loucks and Broad (2006).

Nutritional interventions for specific environments

Physiologists and dietitians have prescribed specific nutritional interventions and supplements that purportedly diminish the effects of environmental stressors (Table 2). Although these recommendations have not been tested for high-intensity, intermittent exercise, they are supported by reports of dietary deficiencies among German and Dutch football teams (Tiedt, Grimm, & Unger, 1991; Van Erp-Baart *et al.*, 1989). The decision to utilize the recommendations in Table 2 may be difficult or even controversial because some health care professionals discourage the use of all ergogenic aids; most professionals suggest that they be used with caution and only after careful examination of safety, efficacy, potency, and legality (ACSM, 2000; FIFA, 2004). Therefore, column 3 of Table 2 provides guidance regarding the strength of scientific evidence for each.

Table 3 considers other nutritional supplements and strategies. Although not specifically recommended for heat, cold, high altitude, and jet lag, these may enhance performance or alter metabolism favourably. The strength of supporting scientific evidence is presented in column 3 of Table 3.

Table 2. Recommended nutritional interventions that counteract environmental stressors, as they appear in publications. Most studies (column 4 did not involve football specifically

Environmental factors	Nutritional interventions and associated effects on performance	Strength of scientific evidence [a]	References
Heat	• Water and carbohydrate-electrolyte replacement fluids counteract the detrimental effects of dehydration	A	Armstrong and Maresh (1996b), Armstrong et al. (1997), Coyle (1991, 1995), Hawley et al. (1994), Shirreffs et al. (1996)
	• Sodium chloride supplementation offsets a whole-body sodium deficiency	D	
	• Post-exercise rehydration fluids should contain sodium; tvolume should equal 150% of the fluid deficit incurred during exercise	A	
Cold	• Tyrosine [b] reduces cognitive deficits, adverse moods, and performance impairments due to cold exposure	B	Ahlers et al. (1994), Baker-Fulco et al. (2001), Bandaret and Lieberman (1989), Berglund and Hemmingsson (1982), Doubt (1991), Fulco et al. (1989), Lieberman (1994), Lieberman and Shukitt-Hale (1996), Reynolds (1996), Schmidt et al. (2002)
	• Caffeine improves endurance performance at low (300 m), moderate (2900 m), and high (4300 m) altitudes	B	
	• Vitamins E, C, β-carotene, pantothenic acid, zinc, selenium, and other antioxidants reduce the oxidative stress of individuals with low initial antioxidant status	D	

Environment	Recommendation		References
High altitude[c]	• Tyrosine[b] reduces cognitive deficits, adverse moods, performance impairments, and the symptoms of altitude illness	B	Baker-Fulco et al. (2001), Bandaret and Lieberman (1989), Committee on Military Nutrition Research (1996), Fulco et al. (2005), Hoyt and Honig (1996), Lieberman (1994), Lieberman and Shukitt-Hale (1996), Simon-Schnass (1996), Wright, Klawitter, Iscru, Merola and Clanton (2005), Zuo and Clanton (2005)
	• Easily consumed liquid or solid carbohydrate foods maintain performance and macronutrient balance[d]	B	
	• Consume ample energy (MJ, kcal) each day to maintain body mass	B	
	• Ensure that iron status is normal and that the recommended daily allowance for iron is consumed	B	
	• Supplement diet with vitamins C, E, and other antioxidants if altitude exposure is prolonged	D	
Jet lag	• Caffeine temporarily reverses sleepiness and cognitive deficits due to sleep deprivation	B	Aerospace Medical Association (1996), Penetar (1994), Reilly, Atkinson and Waterhouse (1997c)
	• Alter, timing, size, and composition of meals to reduce the negative effects of jet lag	C	
All environments	• Consume a high-carbohydrate diet; maximize pre-exercise glycogen levels in muscle and liver[f]; enhances performance[g] during brief high-intensity, repeated-sprint, and endurance exercise[h]	A	Armstrong and Maresh (1996a), Bembden and Lamont (2005), Branch and Williams (2002), Coyle (1991), Fulco et al. (2005), Hawley & Burke (1997), Ivy (1994), Maughan (2002), Shepard (1999), Sherman (1992), Wagenmakers (1999)
	• Consume a fluid-electrolyte replacement beverage during training and competition[g]; provides carbohydrates; sodium supports extracellular (i.e. plasma) volume; flavouring encourages drinking and reduces dehydration	A	

continued on next pages

Table 2. (continued)

Environmental factors	Nutritional interventions and associated effects on performance	Strength of scientific evidence[a]	References
	• Creatine enhances anaerobic performance (maximal force or strength) for events lasting less than 4 min, with no ergogenic effect for endurance exercise	A	

[a] Modification of an evidentiary model (National Heart, Lung, & Blood Institute, 1998) designed to evaluate the strength of scientific evidence. *Level A*: randomized controlled trials (rich body of data) with a substantial number of well-designed studies, substantial number of participants, and consistent pattern of findings. *Level B*: randomized controlled trials (limited body of data) that include post-hoc field studies, subgroups, or meta-analyses; participant populations differ from the target population (i.e. animals vs. humans). *Level C*: evidence arises from uncontrolled/non-randomized trials, clinical observations, or case studies. *Level D*: expert judgement that is based on a synthesis of published evidence, panel consensus, clinical experience, and/or laboratory observations; used when guidance is needed but the published literature is lacking. *Level E*: studies suggest that this intervention may be appropriate for football, but the amount of scientific evidence (i.e. randomized controlled trials) is small.

[b] Increased catecholamine release may counteract various environmental stressors and tyrosine is a catecholamine precursor (i.e. agonist).

[c] Each effect may occur at a different altitude.

[d] Body weight and nitrogen balance are maintained when the energy requirement is met and the diet provides the recommended daily allowance for macronutrients (Butterfield et al., 1992).

[e] Consumed as a fluid (10% carbohydrate solution; 14 g per serving for a male weighing 80 kg; 6–8 servings per trial) (Fulco et al., 2005).

[f] The timing of replacement is important, with optimal muscle glycogen and protein synthesis occurring 1–3 h after exercise (Baker-Fulco et al., 2001; Sherman, 1992).

[g] Endurance performance in a cold environment may not be improved by consumption of a carbohydrate-electrolyte replacement fluid (Galloway & Maughan, 1998; Galloway et al., 2001).

[h] Endurance exercise that is continuous and more than 50–60 min at > 70% $\dot{V}O_{2max}$.

Further complicating our understanding of nutritional interventions, female football players may experience subtle changes of exercise metabolism at different phases of the menstrual cycle, as shown by recent investigations that administered exogenous hormones. These data (D'Eon *et al.*, 2002) suggest that estrogen alone reduced total carbohydrate oxidation during exercise by decreasing the use of both blood glucose and glycogen. Administration of progesterone further reduced blood glucose use but increased glycogen utilization. These findings indicate that substrate utilization across the menstrual cycle is dependent on the relative changes of both estrogen and progesterone. However, their effects on the magnitude and direction of these changes, on mental and physical performance, or their interactions with environmental factors (Table 1), are not known.

Heat exposure

High ambient temperatures (>35°C) increase the strain that an athlete's body experiences. This strain is observed as an increased core body temperature, decreased cardiac stroke volume, increased heart rate, and increased perceived exertion. Dehydration *per se* also increases cardiovascular strain, in an additive manner, and increases muscle glycogen utilization (i.e. versus a euhydrated state) (Shirreffs, 2005). Endurance exercise performance declines when the body water deficit reaches approximately 2–3% of body mass (Armstrong *et al.*, 1985; Cheuvront, Carter, & Sawka, 2003; Shirreffs, 2005). Regarding muscular strength, power, and sprint performance, authorities disagree on the exact level of dehydration that elicits a performance decrement; this threshold apparently occurs at a loss of 5–8% of body mass (Sawka & Pandolf, 1990; Watson *et al.*, 2005). Thus, a body water deficit of 1% or 2% during a football match in the heat is tolerable and ordinarily unavoidable (Maughan, Shirreffs, Merson, & Horswill, 2005).

Field observations of sweat losses and body temperatures during football matches and training sessions provide additional insights. These indicate that the mean sweat losses of elite footballers range from 1.06 to 2.65 litres (mean = 1.69 litres) during a 90 min practice session in cool air (5°C, 81% relative humidity), from 1.67 to 3.14 litres (mean = 2.91 litres) during a 90 min practice session in warm air (33°C, 20% relative humidity), and from 1.48 to 3.93 litres (mean = 2.32 litres) during Olympic qualifying matches (26°C, 78% relative humidity and 33°C, 40% relative humidity) (Maughan *et al.*, 2005; Mustafa & Mahmoud, 1979; Shirreffs *et al.*, 2005). By consuming fluids during exercise and rest periods, these players replaced 25%, 45%, and 9–31% of sweat losses, respectively. This exemplifies voluntary dehydration, a well-known phenomenon that occurs among athletes, labourers, and military personnel. Independent of weather conditions, fluid replacement lags behind fluid lost as sweat by at least 50% (Burke & Hawley, 1997).

Physiological research provides useful fluid consumption guidelines for athletes, to ensure that they begin each morning well hydrated (Shirreffs,

Table 3. Selected nutritional supplements. Although not recommended for football specifically, these may enhance football performance or alter metabolism favourably. The scientific studies in column 4 generally were conducted in non-stressful environments

Nutritional supplement/strategy	General effect on performance or metabolism (all environments)	Strength of scientific evidence[a]	References
Caffeine	Enhances performance during intense aerobic exercise, but not brief power events of less than 90 s. Improves perception of effort, alertness, wakefulness, vigilance, and mood. When consumed in moderation (3–6 mg · kg body mass^{-1}), caffeine does not dehydrate the body	A	Armstrong (2002), Armstrong et al. (2005), Ivy (1994), Magkos and Kavouras (2005), Maughan (2002), Nehlig and Debry (1994), Penetar (1994), Spriet (2002)
Iron	When iron deficiency anaemia[b] exists, iron supplements are necessary to maintain exercise performance and health; the immune system is sensitive to iron deficiency	A	Burke et al. (2003, 2006), Committee on Military Nutrition Research (1999a), Gleeson and Bishop (2000)
Calcium	Important for healthy bones, especially in adolescent and female athletes; not known to affect exercise performance when whole-body balance is normal	A	Armstrong and Maresh (1996a), Burke et al. (2003, 2006)
Carbohydrate and protein-rich diet or solutions[d]	Encourages recovery (i.e. protein synthesis and muscle glycogen resynthesis) after strenuous exercise[c]. Carbohydrates and protein induce different endocrine responses (i.e. plasma insulin, glucagons, growth hormone); when consumed together, they encourage an anabolic state	B	Chandler, Byrne, Patterson and Ivy (1994), Earnest and Rudolph (2001), Ivy (1994), Ivy et al. (2003), Miller et al. (2002)
Choline	Improves endurance performance time in individuals whose plasma choline levels are reduced (i.e. due to prolonged exercise or environmental stress). When choline is available in near-physiologic concentrations, choline supplementation increases acetylcholine release from nerves, enhancing neurotransmission	C	Wurtmen (1994), Zeisel (1994)

Tryptophan	The brain neurotransmitter serotonin, which theoretically is involved in central fatigue, may be modulated by diet or plasma levels of its precursor tryptophan, an amino acid; evidence for this effect is limited	E	Maughan (2002), Newsholme and Castell (2000), Wilson and Maughan (1992)
Vitamin C, vitamin E, selenium, and β-carotene	Although these antioxidants do not enhance performance, they may offer protection (to individuals who exercise strenuously) from intracellular free radical damage, optimize recovery of skeletal muscle, and enhance health in general	D	Committee on Military Nutrition Research (1999a), Gleeson and Bishop (2000), Kalman (2002)
High-fat diet	A few studies have indicated that several weeks of adaptation to a high-fat diet enhances endurance exercise performance, with or without phases of high carbohydrate intake. However, for athletes who participate in high-intensity exercise, there is little support for this approach	E	Coleman and Steen (2002), Coyle (1995), Maughan (2002), Williams (1995)
Glutamine	A glucose precursor that may encourage recovery after intense training, especially in support of the immune system	E	Coleman and Steen (2002), Earnest and Rudolph (2001), Gleeson and Bishop (2000), Wagenmakers (1999)
Sodium bicarbonate	Buffers intramuscular and blood pH, blunting the acidity produced during intense anaerobic exercise lasting 30s to a few minutes. Effects on exercise performance are equivocal	E	Maughan (2002), Webster (2002)
D-Ribose	Observed to preserve body pools of ATP in rats; theoretically, this could maintain maximal functional capacity in humans, but controlled human studies indicate that ribose supplementation has no effect on anaerobic exercise capacity and maximal intermittent exercise performance	E	Brault and Terjung (1999), Coleman and Steen (2002), Kreider et al. (2003), Op't Eijnde et al. (2001), Tullson and Terjung (1991)
Branched-chain amino acids	May limit fatigue at the level of the central nervous system by increasing brain serotonin (i.e. a neurotransmitter that modulates central fatigue). Human performance studies are equivocal	E	Coleman and Steen (2002), Newsholme and Castell (2000), Wagenmakers (1999), Williams (1995)

---

[a] Modified from the evidentiary model described in Table 2 (National Heart, Lung, and Blood Institute, 1998).

[b] Iron deficiency anaemia is defined as a serum ferritin concentration of less than 12 $\mu g \cdot ml^{-1}$ in combination with a haemoglobin concentration of less than 120 $g \cdot l^{-1}$.

[c] Includes amino acid supplements mixed with carbohydrates.

Armstrong, & Cheuvront, 2004). These guidelines arise from rehydration studies that evaluated several combinations of fluid volume and composition (Shirreffs, Taylor, Leiper, & Maughan, 1996). First, players should consume a volume of fluid equal to 150% of the sweat lost during exercise throughout the remainder of the day. Water retention will be greater if the fluid or food contains a moderately high sodium content (i.e. $60 \, \text{mmol} \cdot l^{-1}$). After encountering a 2% body weight loss, these recommendations will result in normal hydration status within 6 h.

Regarding body temperature, Ekblom (1986) reported an average rectal temperature of 39.5°C in players at the end of a Swedish First Division football match. The corresponding average for players of a lower division was 39.1°C, reflecting a slower overall pace of play. Maughan and Lieper (1994) summarized similar data from six other publications, indicating that rectal temperatures reached 39.2–39.6°C at the end of 90 min games contested in environmental conditions ranging from 12 to 38°C.

Because football players may experience large sweat losses, especially when engaged in two training sessions per day, electrolyte losses should also be considered. A whole-body deficit of sodium chloride predisposes players to heat cramps and heat exhaustion (Armstrong, 2003). Two of the previously mentioned studies measured salt losses in the sweat of elite male footballers. The sweat sodium concentration averaged $42 \, \text{mmol} \cdot l^{-1}$ in cool air (5°C) (Maughan *et al.*, 2005) and $30 \, \text{mmol} \cdot l^{-1}$ in warm air (33°C) (Shirreffs *et al.*, 2005). These salt losses totalled 73 and 67 mmol per 90 min, respectively. Given the fact that competitive athletes consume an average of 231 mmol of sodium per day (Kies, 1995), and active college students consume 91–205 mmol of sodium per day (Armstrong *et al.*, 2005; Kies, 1995), it is unlikely that a whole-body sodium deficit will occur in most footballers. Indeed, Maughan, Leiper and Shirreffs (1996) compared post-exercise rehydration via a meal and a commercial fluid-electrolyte replacement beverage. Although the quantity of water was identical for both methods, a single meal provided considerably more electrolytes (63 mmol sodium, 21 mmol potassium) than the sports drink, and approximated the total salt losses calculated above. A similar conclusion can be made for potassium (data not shown).

The few players who have both a high sweat rate and a high sweat sodium concentration (i.e. $>3 \, \text{litres} \cdot h^{-1}$ and $>60 \, \text{mmol Na}^{+}/\text{L}$) should receive individualized nutritional guidance (i.e. sodium, potassium, and fluid intake), and should be monitored regularly by the sports medicine staff (Bergeron, 2003). Some authors recommend salt supplements (i.e. $8–10 \, \text{g} \cdot \text{day}^{-1}$ by adding salt to food) for athletes with a history of heat illness, and for all individuals during the initial days of chronic heat exposure (Wenger, 1988).

Heat acclimatization is important for every athlete who competes in warm or hot ambient temperatures. This process requires 8–14 days of exposure to heat, and results in several physiological adaptations that make exercise in the heat easier to perform (Wenger, 1988). Three interesting acclimatization facts are seldom appreciated. First, dehydration reduces or nullifies the benefits of heat acclimatization, in a progressive manner, as dehydration becomes more severe (Cadarette, Sawka, Toner, & Pandolf, 1984). Second, heat acclimatization affects sweat glands by increasing the amount of sweat that is produced (Wenger, 1988). Although beneficial (i.e. it ensures wet skin and evaporative cooling), this adaptation also increases the water requirement of an athlete exercising in the heat. Both of these facts reinforce the goal of minimizing body water loss (see above). Third, in studies conducted among South African miners, ascorbic acid (vitamin C) supplements of $250-500 \, mg \cdot day^{-1}$ were given during a 10 day ($4 \, h \cdot day^{-1}$) laboratory heat acclimation protocol (Strydom, Kotze, Van der Walt, & Rogers, 1976). As a result, vitamin C reduced rectal temperature and total sweat loss. However, the miners in this study may have been deficient in vitamin C due to their poor dietary habits (Askew, 1995). Although it is unclear whether supplementation benefits individuals who are adequately nourished, this study suggests that adequate dietary vitamin C (and perhaps other antioxidants) is important for normal heat acclimatization to occur.

The foregoing paragraphs point to the primary nutritional needs in hot environments: fluid, carbohydrate, and electrolytes. In hot environments, therefore, footballers should ensure that muscle and liver glycogen are optimal by reducing the volume and intensity of training in the 48–72 h before an important contest and by consuming up to 10 g of carbohydrate per kilogram of body mass per day (Sherman & Wimer, 1991). Before, during, and after a contest, they should consume carbohydrates in a systematic way to maintain exercise metabolism and performance. Specific details are available in the review of this topic by Hawley, Dennis and Noakes (1994). There is no evidence to indicate an increased requirement for protein or fat during exposure to a hot environment (Committee on Military Nutrition Research, 1999b).

Contracting skeletal muscle produces more free radicals when muscle temperature exceeds 42°C, and high free radical production contributes to muscle fatigue (Zuo *et al.*, 2000). Similarly, studies of isolated rat livers, perfused at normal and elevated temperatures (Bowers *et al.*, 1984), demonstrated that leakage of transaminase enzymes did not occur until the perfusion temperature reached 42°C. At this temperature, structural integrity degraded and signs of membrane destabilization occurred; both are consistent with the liver damage that occurs with human and animal heat stroke (Hubbard & Armstrong, 1988). These observations suggest that (a) heat stress stimulates intracellular and extracellular superoxide production, which may contribute to the physiological responses to severe exercise and hyperthermia, and (b) antioxidant intake may some day be shown to protect cells from the stress and damage that hyperthermia induces.

A glycerol-water solution has been shown to be an effective hyperhydrating agent at rest. Although some researchers have demonstrated that ingesting 1.0–1.5 g of glycerol per kg body mass, together with a large volume of water (e.g. $20 \, ml \cdot kg \, body \, mass^{-1}$), significantly increases temporary water retention and cycling time to fatigue, and decreases circulatory and thermal strain

(Anderson, Cotter, Garnham, Casley, & Febbraio, 2001), others have observed no difference in physiological responses or performance (Shirreffs *et al.*, 2004). None of these studies involved high-intensity, intermittent exercise (i.e. similar to a football match), and several reported unwanted side-effects in a small percentage of participants (Latzka & Sawka, 2000). When considered collectively, these studies suggest that the efficacy of pre-exercise hyperhydration with glycerol is uncertain, especially if hydration is maintained during exercise (Latzka & Sawka, 2000; Shirreffs *et al.*, 2004). The present scientific literature does not support a recommendation for the use of glycerol in football.

Cold environments

Although not widely recognized by players and coaches, chronic exposure to very cold air ($<5°C$) can lead to dehydration (i.e. 2–5% of body mass) due to cold-induced diuresis that is accompanied by reduced blood and plasma volumes. Sweating, respiratory water loss, reduced intake of fluids (Committee on Military Nutrition Research, 1996), and diminished thirst (Freund & Sawka, 1996) also contribute to this dehydration Respiratory water loss has been estimated as 0.9 litres $\cdot 24\,h^{-1}$ in 0°C air and 1.0 litres $\cdot 24\,h^{-1}$ in −20°C air. Sweat loss for moderate-to-heavy exercise has been estimated as 0.9–1.9 litres $\cdot 24\,h^{-1}$ in air at 0°C and 0.4–1.9 litres $\cdot 24\,h^{-1}$ in air at −20°C (Freund & Sawka, 1996). This dehydration may contribute to the changes of performance, appetite, and emotions that are observed when humans are exposed to very cold environments (see section headed "Dehydration affects metabolism and performance").

Although the optimal air temperature for endurance exercise is about 11°C (versus 4, 21, and 31°C) (Galloway & Maughan, 1997), it appears that the severity of dehydration and the nature of the exercise performed (i.e. mode, intensity, duration) determine whether physical performance will be affected by cold exposure. For example, a research group led by McConnel (McConnel, Stephens, & Canny, 1999) reported no effect of 1.9% dehydration on cycling exercise (45 min at 80% $\dot{V}O_{2max} + 15$ min sprint) in a 21°C environment, whereas Cheuvront *et al.* (2003) observed a significant decline in performance (30 min at 50% $\dot{V}O_{2peak} + 30$ min sprint) in a 20°C environment subsequent to 3% dehydration. Kenefick, Mahood, Hazzard, Quinn and Castellani (2004) incorporated a 4°C environment, brisk treadmill walking (60 min at 50% $\dot{V}O_{2peak}$), and 4% dehydration but observed no differences in performance, thermoregulatory responses, or cardio vascular strain versus a mild 25°C environment. Regarding muscular power, deep muscle temperature influences performance. When muscle temperature falls, power output declines by virtue of the effects of cold on the rate of adenosine triphosphate (ATP) hydrolysis and/or resynthesis (Ferretti, 1992).

Living outdoors in a very cold environment increases the resting energy requirement by 2–10% above that measured in a mild environment, largely due to muscular shivering. However, the utilization of fats and glucose as fuels differs during shivering and exercise (Tipton, Franks, Meneilly, & Mekjavic, 1997). This suggests that the metabolic substrates utilized by two football players may be quite different during a game in a cold/wet environment, depending on whether they are actively competing or playing a passive part in a game. Furthermore, exercise in cold air requires more energy than exercise performed in a thermoneutral environment. This has been attributed to the increased energy demands of thermoregulation, the preferential use of carbo-hydrate as a substrate (see below), and the restrictive effect of multi-layered clothing (Armstrong, 2000; Committee on Military Nutrition Research, 1996; Gray, Consolazio, & Kark, 1951; Welch, Buskirk, & Iampietro, 1958). It is not known if footballers will expend more energy in cold versus neutral or mild environments, in that they live in climate-controlled buildings and experi-ence one or two daily exposures to cold air (i.e. 1–3 h each).

Chronic exposure to cold air stimulates cold acclimatization. The patterns of response are unique, depending on the duration of exposure, insulation of the clothing, the amount of skin exposed to the air, and extent of core body cooling. Physiological adaptations include altered heat production, skin vasoconstriction (i.e. reduced flow in skin blood vessels), muscle blood flow, and a change of the preferred metabolic substrate. Once cold acclimatization has been established, an athlete uses less of the available muscle glycogen stores in response to a given exercise cold exposure (Shephard, 1993). This change is important because exercise metabolism is fuelled primarily by endogenous carbohydrate (i.e. muscle glycogen) during continuous voluntary exercise in a cold environ-ment (i.e. 84–103 min at 80% $\dot{V}O_{2max}$; 10°C) (Galloway & Maughan, 1998). Exogenous carbohydrate, supplied in fluids, has little or no influence on perfor-mance in the cold (Galloway & Maughan, 1998; Galloway, Wootton, Murphy, & Maughan, 2001). If ample carbohydrate is not consumed during periods of prolonged exercise, glycogen resynthesis during recovery will be reduced. Thus, if footballers consume a diet that is high in dietary fat and low in carbo-hydrate, they may experience decreased mental and physical performance in the cold because their pre-exercise muscle glycogen stores are low (Phinney, Bistrian, Wolfe, & Blackburn, 1983).

The requirement for protein is not increased by chronic exposure to a cold environment *per se* (Committee on Military Nutrition Research, 1999b), and the volitional preference for macronutrients (i.e. carbohydrate versus fat in the diet) does not change when humans freely select foods. For players who consume a well-balanced diet, are healthy, and live in a temperate climate, there is no evidence to suggest that vitamin and mineral supplementation will enhance mental or physical performance (Armstrong & Maresh, 1996b). How-ever, if exposure to cold is prolonged (i.e. one 12 h period or several hours on repeated days) and severe, players may benefit from supplementing their diets with selected antioxidants (Table 2) to counteract oxidative stress (Reynolds, 1996).

High-altitude environments

The 1986 Football World Cup was contested at various sites in Mexico, with elevations to 2607 m (8554 ft) above sea level. During acute exposure to such high altitudes, human appetite decreases and food preferences change (Westerterp-Plantenga et al., 1999; Wilbur, 2004). However, chronic body mass loss can be avoided if adequate energy is consumed (Butterfield, 1996; Butterfield et al., 1992).

Most studies have reported that the absolute and relative dietary carbohydrate intake increases, at the expense of fat and protein, with both acute and chronic altitude exposure (Butterfield, 1996; Gill & Pugh, 1964; Rose et al., 1988). Measurements of arterial-venous substrate differences have also shown that altitude acclimatization decreases free fatty acid consumption in the legs, while glucose uptake increases, during rest and exercise (Roberts et al., 1996). Endurance exercise performance is adversely affected when dietary composition is manipulated to decrease carbohydrate intake at altitude (Butterfield, 1996). Thus, adequate carbohydrate intake is an important nutritional objective for players who train and compete at high altitude.

Interestingly, women may not adjust their substrate oxidation in the same manner as men. Carbohydrate utilization decreases when women are exposed to high altitude acutely and chronically (Beidleman et al., 2002; Braun et al., 2000). Similarly, the blood glucose response to a meal is lower for women than for men at high altitude (Braun et al., 1998). Although the mechanism responsible has yet to be identified, it is possible that women are more sensitive to insulin at high altitude, or that glucose output from the liver is suppressed in women (i.e. suggesting greater reliance on non-glucose fuel sources). Despite these unique responses, the strong influence that exercise intensity exerts on utilization of carbohydrate, as the limiting substrate during football training and competition, suggests that adequate carbohydrate intake is a sound nutritional objective for female players.

Total daily water turnover increases by 1 litre (i.e. from about 2.9 to 3.9 litres $\cdot$ day^{-1}) by moving from a sea-level training site to one at high altitude (Pugh, 1962). Because respiratory water losses average about 600 ml $\cdot$ day^{-1} (Westerterp, Kayser, Brouns, Herry, & Saris, 1992) and increase at very high altitudes (Simon-Schnass, 1996), and because sweat losses range from 1.3 to 2.8 litres per 90 min training session in a 24–29°C environment (Maughan, Merson, Broad, & Shirreffs, 2004), provision of adequate fluids remains a primary nutritional goal in football.

These two objectives agree well with the recommendation for a high-carbohydrate, low-fat, liquid supplement as the preferred ration for individuals who live in high-altitude environments (Cymerman, 1996). Also in concert with these two objectives, Hoyt and Honig (1996) recommended that a specialized diet be consumed during the first 3 days of high-altitude exposure, which is rich in carbohydrates and low in sodium chloride. This diet discourages water and salt retention, which is believed to be a key aetiological factor in acute mountain sickness, high-altitude cerebral oedema, and high-altitude pulmonary oedema (Committee on Military Nutrition Research, 1996). Thus, if ample water, salt-free fluid, tea, and coffee are consumed, physiologic natriuresis will be fostered. Unfortunately, exercise at high altitude favours retention of water and salt (Anand & Chandrashekhar, 1996). This suggests that athletes may be more susceptible to acute mountain sickness if they exercise during the first 3 days of exposure to high altitude; it also suggests that they should limit dietary intake of salt. At low or moderate altitudes, these precautions may not be necessary. For athletes who experience symptoms of acute mountain sickness, a bland, low-fat diet (i.e. crackers, bread, cookie bars, mashed potatoes, rice, cereals, pudding) is generally tolerated well when eaten in small portions every 2 h; dietary fat is not tolerated well (Baker-Fulco, Patton, Montain, & Lieberman, 2001). After the initial days of altitude acclimatization, typical sea-level diet and exercise programmes may be resumed (Hoyt & Honig, 1996).

Although the daily total protein requirement is not increased (Committee on Military Nutrition Research, 1999b) in a high-altitude environment (> 5500 m), limited evidence indicates that adults oxidize leucine and excrete proteins at a slightly greater rate than at sea level (Srivastava & Kumar, 1992). This change of protein metabolism (Cymerman, 1996) suggests that protein and amino acids are utilized as energy sources, although the magnitude of this contribution may be small in comparison to carbohydrates and fats. Furthermore, animal research suggests that free radical production within skeletal muscle is increased in a high-altitude environment, probably because of hypoxia (Zuo & Clanton, 2005). Future research may determine that antioxidant supplements offset the stress of exercise at high altitude.

Two controlled, double-blind studies involving outdoor cross-country skiing trials (at 300 and 2900 m; Berglund & Hemmingsson, 1982) and cycling performance (79–85% of altitude-specific $\dot{V}O_{2max}$) within a high-altitude field laboratory (2 week residence at 4300 m; Fulco et al., 1989) found that submaximal exercise was maintained significantly longer after consuming caffeine (6 mg and 4 mg · kg body mass^{-1}, respectively). The mechanism for this effect is unknown, but theoretically may involve (a) increased lipid mobilization and utilization, (b) stimulation of the central nervous system resulting in altered perception of effort, (c) increased cardiac output, (d) enhanced motor unit recruitment, (e) decreased metabolic products that produce fatigue, (f) altered ion movements (Na^+, K^+, Ca^{2+}) into and within skeletal muscle, (g) an increased sensitivity to the effects of caffeine at altitude, or (h) altered ventilatory characteristics that influence oxygen delivery (Berglund & Hemmingsson, 1982; Spriet, 2002). The measurements recorded during the cycling performance study (Fulco et al., 1989) ruled out mechanisms (a), (b), and (c) above. However, tidal volume (i.e. the volume of air inhaled at each breath during normal breathing), not breathing frequency, increased (versus placebo) during the caffeine experiments at altitude but not at sea level. This paradox was probably due to the small advantage of increased tidal volume at sea level and the large advantage at an elevation of 4300 m (i.e. greater oxygen saturation of haemoglobin and greater oxygen delivery to skeletal muscles). Interestingly, repeated tests indicated that the acute improvement in performance (54% after 1 h exposure; 22.0 to 35.0 min) decreased after chronic exposure (24% after 2 weeks; 30.8 to 38.5 min), in concert with a decrease of the magnitude of the caffeine-stimulated increase in tidal volume (Fulco *et al.*, 1989).

Jet lag: Transmeridian travel

Regular biological rhythms have been observed in animals, plants, and uni-cellular organisms. These rhythms are expressed as oscillations in physiological systems with durations that range from minutes to months. Circadian rhythms last approximately 24 h (derived from the Latin phrase *circa diem*, "about a day") and are synchronized to the Earth's light–dark cycle, social interactions, and various other environmental factors. The following physiological processes exhibit circadian rhythms: breathing, heart rate, body temperature, oxygen consumption, blood plasma volume, plasma protein concentration, sweat rate, flexibility, grip strength, muscular endurance, physical work capacity, neuro-muscular coordination, reaction time, growth hormone, and cortisol (Luce, 1970; Winget, DeRoshia, & Holley, 1985). These and other rhythms are regu-lated by the hypothalamus in coordination with the brain neurotransmitter serotonin and the pineal gland hormone melatonin (Reilly, Atkinson, & Budgett, 1997b).

Of great relevance to football, circadian rhythms exist for all body systems that respond to exercise training, including metabolism, central nervous system arousal, circulation, body temperature, muscular performance, and endocrine function. Systematic studies of these sport-significant rhythms have shown that organ function and performance generally peak at similar times each day (Winget *et al.*, 1985). For example, simple measurements recorded throughout the day indicate that grip strength, flexibility, and exercise tolerance are greatest between 14.00 and 18.00 h. Sport-specific mental factors (i.e. vigour, mood, speed of psychomotor responses) peak between 12.00 and 15.00 h each day.

Because circadian rhythms are intimately linked to the light–dark cycle that results from the Earth's rotation, it may be possible to desynchronize the body's rhythms, reduce organ function, and decrease performance by altering an athlete's normal light–dark cycle and daily schedules. Although other environ-mental stressors may also disrupt the body's normal rhythms, crossing time zones (jet lag) is the most common means by which this occurs. Jet lag reflects a tem-porary desynchronization of the traveller's "biological time" based upon the point of departure and the local time (i.e. light–dark cycle) at the destination. The symptoms of jet lag include periodic tiredness during the day, disturbed concentration, increased irritability, loss of vigour, and irregular sleep at night (Reilly *et al.*, 1997b). The number of time zones crossed, cumulative sleep loss, and the intensity of environmental cues are the most important modulators of the severity of jet-lag symptoms in humans (Aerospace Medical Association, 1996).

Although at least one research team believes that jet lag does not affect athletic performance (Youngstedt & Buxton, 2003), British Olympic squad members exhibited impairments of several performance measures over 5 days, following travel across five time zones from London to Tallahassee, Florida (Reilly *et al.*, 1997a). American football players experienced similar effects due to jet lag when travelling eastward, performance was suppressed more than when travelling westward (Jehue *et al.*, 1993); this directional tendency was not observed in other studies with similar experimental designs (Youngstedt & Buxton, 2003).

Because food components affect the central nervous system in various ways, nutritional interventions have been proposed to counteract the effects of jet lag. Reilly *et al.* (1997b) described several dietary strategies involving meal timing and macronutrient composition. They concluded that the scientific literature does not allow inferences to be formed regarding these practices. The Aerospace Medical Association (1996) advises that small meals before and during flights are better tolerated than large meals, and that caffeine and physical activity may be used strategically at the destination to help control day sleepiness.

Sleep loss

Jet lag often results in sleep loss. Two human studies have reported that sleep loss mildly reduces the body's ability to regulate core temperature (Kolka & Stephenson, 1988; Sawka *et al.*, 1984). Both investigations involved cross-over experimental designs in which participants were tested after periods of normal sleep and sleep loss. The latter experiments demonstrated a loss of thermosensitivity (i.e. effector response per degree rise of oesophageal temperature) of forearm sweating and blood flow, without a change of the hypothalamic threshold for the onset of these thermoregulatory responses. These findings suggest that heat storage may be slightly greater, for a specified amount of exercise, after sleep loss. The effects of jet lag *per se* on thermoregulation have not been studied in footballers.

The amount and type of food may affect the duration of subsequent sleep (Pozos, Roberts, Hackney, & Feith, 1996) by increasing the incidence of indigestion, pattern of food intake, and subjective responses to food (Waterhouse *et al.*, 2005). Also, several animal studies have demonstrated that a high-protein meal triggers the release of somatostatin, which increases rapid eye movement (REM) sleep (i.e. important for a restful night). A meal rich in carbohydrates triggers the release of insulin, which increases the duration of non-REM sleep. Interestingly, these findings contradict a widely publicised strategy that links diet and jet lag; it recommends high-protein meals for breakfast (supposedly to provide substrate for catecholamines) and high-carbohydrate meals for dinner (to furnish substrate for serotonin and hence promote sleep) (Reilly *et al.*,

1997a). Again, the available literature does not allow conclusive statements for or against these strategies.

One non-nutritional strategy to offset the negative effects of jet lag, involving altering the time of football training sessions for a few days before departure to reflect the time of competition in the other time zone, was found to be beneficial (Jehue *et al.*, 1993). Other non-nutritional techniques have been used, with varying success, including mild exercise, bright light therapy, napping, and oral melatonin supplements (Arendt, Aldhous, English, Marks, & Ardent, 1987; Reilly *et al.*, 1997b). Although none of these seems to be effective for all persons in all circumstances, numerous studies support the judicious use of oral melatonin to overcome the negative consequences of jet lag (Cardinali *et al.*, 2002). Reductions in jet-lag symptoms also have been reported when oral melatonin was combined with slow-release caffeine (Pirard *et al.*, 2001) or an altered light–dark schedule (Cardinali *et al.*, 2002). The interactions between jet lag, melatonin, and exercise have not been studied in a sample of athletes.

Counteracting multiple concurrent stressors

Although environmental factors exert unique physiological effects (Table 1), the similarities of cold and high-altitude environments (i.e. low ambient temperatures, initial diuresis, increased energy requirements for work and exercise, carbohydrate is tolerated well) (Askew, 1996) suggest that common elements may exist in the responses of the central nervous system to these stressors. Thus, it may be beneficial to seek a single nutritional strategy that serves as an intervention for the adverse effects of two or more environments.

During stressful situations, highly active neurons may require additional precursor so that neurotransmitter synthesis can keep pace with the increased amount of neurotransmitter being released (Bandaret & Lieberman, 1989). Theoretically, the behavioural deficits caused by acute environmental stress (i.e. influencing alertness, anxiety, motor activity) may be reversed by provision of neurotransmitter precursors. Tyrosine, a large amino acid found in dietary proteins, is a precursor of catecholamines (i.e. noradrenaline, dopamine, and adrenaline). The provision of oral tyrosine in capsule form is known to reverse many adverse effects that are produced by exposure to cold and hypoxia (15°C and 4200–4500 m). The positive effects include improved symptoms (i.e. headache, coldness, distress, fatigue, sleepiness, discomfort), reduced number of adverse emotions (i.e. confusion, unhappiness, hostility, tension), and improved cognitive performance (i.e. pattern recognition, vigilance, choice reaction time) (Bandaret & Lieberman, 1989). Several animal research studies support these findings (Lieberman & Shukitt-Hale, 1996).

Immune function, oxidative stress

Many studies have shown that strenuous exercise suppresses immune function (Pedersen & Bruunsgaard, 1995). Considering Table 1 and the high-intensity intermittent nature of football, immune system function may be compromised when teams play in stressful environments. This concept is supported by observations of Belgian First Division football club players, who exhibited depressed neutrophil function throughout a season (Bury, Marechal, Mahieu, & Pirnay, 1998). Limited evidence from human and animal studies (Committee on Military Nutrition Research, 1999b; Gleeson & Bishop, 2000) suggests that the following nutrients play a role in the optimal function of the immune system during periods of stress: protein; the minerals iron, zinc, copper, and selenium; vitamins A, C, E, B_6, and B_{12}; the amino acids glutamine and arginine; carbohydrates; and the polyunsaturated fatty acids. Even a mild deficiency of a single nutrient or trace element (i.e. iron, selenium, copper) can result in an altered immune response (Chandra, 1997; Gleeson & Bishop, 2000). Furthermore, it is widely accepted that an inadequate intake of protein impairs host immunity with particularly detrimental effects on the T-cell system, resulting in an increased incidence of opportunistic infections (Gleeson & Bishop, 2000). These observations suggest that future research should focus on the relationship between nutrition and immune function.

Provided that energy intake is adequate, there is no evidence that nutritional supplements improve innate antioxidant protection beyond normal/optimal levels (Butterfield, 1999). However, research suggests that a cold, moderate-altitude environment (i.e. 14–24 days of field training; mean low temperature of $-6.9°C$; 2546–3048 m altitude) increases oxidative stress, as indicated by six biochemical markers (Chao, Askew, Roberts, Wood, & Perkins, 1999). Authorities believe that this stress may be ameliorated in individuals with low initial antioxidant status, by an antioxidant mixture (i.e. vitamins C and E, selenium, $β$-carotene) that is consumed as a dietary supplement (Committee on Military Nutrition Research, 1999a; Gleeson & Bishop, 2000; Kalman, 2002; Schmidt et al., 2002). Also, it is reasonable to hypothesize that a deficiency of antioxidants (a) compromises immune function or (b) reduces defences against oxidative stress when intense, intermittent exercise is coupled with environmental stress (Table 1). Utilizing this rationale, authors recommend that antioxidants be provided as dietary supplements prophylactically (Committee on Military Nutrition Research, 1999b; Schmidt et al., 2002; Simon-Schnass, 1992) because there appears to be little harm in doing so. However, it is important to recognize that excessive amounts of specific nutrients (e.g. iron, zinc, polyunsaturated fatty acids) may suppress immune function (Gleeson & Bishop, 2000).

Summary

Football performance depends upon many physiological, psychological, tactical, and technical factors. This review focused on the effects of four environmental factors on metabolism, whole-body nutrient balance, and physiological function. The principle that nutritional interventions offset environmentally induced performance decrements (Table II) serves as the foundation of this paper. Pharmacological interventions and banned substances were not considered. In all stressful environments, football players will find these interventions useful: a high intake of carbohydrates, fluid-electrolyte replacement of sweat losses, and creatine. In hot environments, it is important to replace water and sodium deficits. In cold ambient conditions, caffeine and tyrosine may enhance performance. At high altitudes, evidence supports emphasizing total energy intake, iron and tyrosine consumption. When athletes experience jet lag, caffeine consumption and adjustments of meal size/composition may be helpful. Several other nutritional strategies (Table 3) may offset performance deficits but cannot be recommended presently because of limited scientific evidence. Because relatively few of the aforementioned published investigations involved footballers, future research regarding any of these strategies and supplements is encouraged.

References

Aerospace Medical Association (1996). Medical guidelines for air travel. *Aviation, Space and Environmental Medicine, 67* (suppl.), B1–B16.

Ahlers, S. T., Thomas, J. R., Schrot, J., & Shurtleff, D. (1994). Tyrosine and glucose modulation of cognitive deficits resulting from cold stress. In B. M. Marriott (Ed.), *Food components to enhance performance* (pp. 277–299). Washington, DC: National Academy Press.

American College of Sports Medicine (2000). Nutrition and athletic performance. *Medicine and Science in Sports and Exercise, 32*, 2130–2145.

Anand, I. S., & Chandrashekhar, Y. (1996). Fluid metabolism at high altitudes. In B. M. Marriott & S. J. Carlson (Eds.), *Nutritional needs in cold and in high altitude environments* (pp. 331–356). Washington, DC: National Academy Press.

Anderson, M. J., Cotter, J. D., Garnham, A. P., Casley, D. J., & Febbraio, M. A. (2001). Effect of glycerol-induced hyperhydration on thermoregulation and metabolism during exercise in the heat. *International Journal of Sport Nutrition and Exercise Metabolism, 11*, 315–333.

Arendt, J., Aldhous, M., English, J., Marks, J., & Ardent, J.H. (1987). Some effects of jet lag and their alteration by melatonin. *Ergonomics, 30*, 1379–1394.

Armstrong, L. E. (2000). *Performing in extreme environments.* Champaign, IL: Human Kinetics.

Armstrong L. E. (2002). Caffeine: Body fluid–electrolyte balance and exercise performance. *International Journal of Sport Nutrition and Exercise Metabolism, 12*, 189–206.

Armstrong, L. E. (2003). *Exertional heat illnesses.* Champaign, IL: Human Kinetics.

Armstrong, L. E., Costill, D. L., & Fink, W. J. (1985). Influence of diuretic-induced dehydration on competitive running performance. *Medicine and Science in Sports and Exercise, 17*, 456–461.

Armstrong, L. E., & Maresh, C. M. (1996a). Fluid replacement during exercise and recovery from exercise. In E. R. Buskirk & S. M. Puhl (Eds.), *Body fluid balance in exercise and sport* (pp. 267–289). Boca Raton, FL: CRC Press.

Armstrong, L. E., & Maresh, C. M. (1996b). Vitamin and mineral supplements as aids to performance and health. *Nutrition Reviews, 54*, S149–S158.

Armstrong, L. E., Maresh, C. M., Gabaree, C. V., Hoffman, J. R., Kavouras, S. A., Kenefick, R. W. *et al.* (1997). Thermal and circulatory responses during exercise: Effects of hypohydration, dehydration, and water intake. *Journal of Applied Physiology*, 82, 2028–2035.

Armstrong, L. E., Pumerantz, A. C., Roti, M. W., Judelson, D. A., Watson, G., Dias, J. C. *et al.* (2005). Fluid-electrolyte and renal indices of hydration during eleven days of controlled caffeine consumption. *International Journal of Sport Nutrition and Exercise Metabolism*, 15, 252–265.

Askew, E. W. (1995). Environmental and physical stress and nutrient requirements. *International Journal of Clinical Nutrition*, 61 (suppl. 3), 631S–637S.

Askew, E. W. (1996). Cold-weather and high-altitude nutrition: Overview of the issues. In B. M. Marriott & S. J. Carlson (Eds.), *Nutritional needs in cold and in high altitude environments* (pp. 83–94). Washington, DC: National Academy Press.

Baker-Fulco, C. J., Patton, B. D., Montain, S. J., & Lieberman, H. R. (2001). *Nutrition for health and performance, 2001. Nutritional guidance for military operations in temperate and extreme environments* (pp. 1–4). Natick, MA: US Army Research Institute of Environmental Medicine.

Balsom, P. D. (1995). *High intensity intermittent exercise: Performance and metabolic responses with very high intensity short duration work periods*. Stockholm: Karolinska Institute.

Bandaret, L. E., & Lieberman, H. R. (1989). Treatment with tyrosine, a neurotransmitter precursor, reduces environmental stress in humans. *Brain Research Bulletin*, 22, 759–762.

Bangsbø, J. (1991). Energy demands in competitive football. *Journal of Sports Sciences*, 12, S5–S12.

Bangsbø, J. (1994). The physiology of football – with special reference to intense intermittent exercise. *Acta Physiologica Scandinavica*, 619, 1–155.

Bangsbø, J., Nørregaard, L., & Thorsøe, F. (1991). Activity profile of competition football. *Canadian Journal of Sport Sciences*, 16, 110–116.

Bangsbø, J., Nørregaard, L., & Thorsøe, F. (1992). The effect of carbohydrate diet on intermittent exercise performance. *International Journal of Sports Medicine*, 13, 152–157.

Beidleman, B. A., Rock, P. B., Muza, S. R., Fulco, C. S., Gibson, L. L., Kaminori, G. H. *et al.* (2002). Substrate oxidation is altered in women during exercise upon acute altitude exposure. *Medicine and Science in Sports and Exercise*, 34, 430–437.

Bemben, M. G., & Lamont, H. S. (2005). Creatine supplementation and exercise performance. *Sports Medicine (New Zealand)*, 35, 107–125.

Bergeron, M. (2003). Exertional heat cramps. In L. E. Armstrong (Ed.), *Exertional heat illnesses* (pp. 91–102). Champaign, IL: Human Kinetics.

Bergh, U., & Ekblom, B. (1979). Influence of muscle temperature on maximal muscle strength and power output in human skeletal muscle. *Acta Physiologica Scandinavica*, 107, 33–37.

Berglund, B., & Hemmingsson, P. (1982). Effects of caffeine ingestion on exercise performance at low and high altitudes in cross-country skiers. *International Journal of Sports Nutrition*, 3, 234–236.

Blomstrand, E., Bergh, U., Essen-Gustavsson, B., & Ekblom, B. (1984). Influence of low muscle temperature on muscle metabolism during intense dynamic exercise. *Acta Physiologica Scandinavica*, 120, 229–236.

Bowers, W., Leav, I., Daum, P., Murphy, M., Williams, P., Hubbard, R. W. *et al.* (1984). Insulin and cortisol improve heat tolerance in isolated perfused rat liver. *Laboratory Investigation, 51,* 675–681.

Branch, J. D., & Williams, M. H. (2002). Creatine as an ergogenic supplement. In M. S. Bahrke & C. E. Yesalis (Eds.), *Performance-enhancing substances in sport and exercise* (pp. 175–195). Champaign, IL: Human Kinetics.

Brault, J. J., & Terjung, R. L. (1999). Purine salvage rates differ among skeletal muscle fiber types and are limited by ribose supply. *Medicine and Science in Sports and Exercise, 31* (suppl. 5), S1365 abstracts.

Braun, B., Butterfield, G. A., Dominick, S. B., Zamudio, S., McCullough, R. G., Rock, P. B. *et al.* (1998). Women at altitude: Changes in carbohydrate metabolism at 4,300-m elevation and across the menstrual cycle. *Journal of Applied Physiology, 85,* 1973–1998.

Braun, B., Mawson, J. T., Muza, S. R., Dominick, S. B., Brooks, G. A., Horning, M. A. *et al.* (2000). Women at altitude: Carbohydrate utilization during exercise at 4,300 m. *Journal of Applied Physiology, 88,* 246–256.

Burke, L. M, Coyle, E., & Maughan, R. (2003). *Nutrition for athletes.* Lausanne, Switzerland: International Olympic Committee.

Burke, L. M., & Hawley, J. A. (1997). Fluid balance in team sports. *Sports Medicine (New Zealand), 24,* 38–54.

Burke, L. M, Loucks, A. B., & Broad, N. (2006). Energy and carbohydrate for training and recovery. *Journal of Sport Sciences, 24,* 675–685.

Bury, T., Marechal, R., Mahieu, P., & Pirnay, F. (1998). Immunological status of competitive football players during the training season. *International Journal of Sports Medicine, 19,* 364–368.

Butterfield, G. E. (1996). Maintenance of body weight at altitude: In search of 500 kcal/ day. In B. M. Marriott & S. J. Carlson (Eds.), *Nutritional needs in cold and in high altitude environments* (pp. 357–378). Washington, DC: National Academy Press.

Butterfield, G. E. (1999). Nutritional aspects of exercise: Nutrient requirements at high altitude. *Clinics in Sports Medicine, 18,* 607–621.

Butterfield, G. E., Gates, J., Fleming, S., Brooks, G. A., Sutton, J. R., & Reeves, J. T. (1992). Increased energy intake minimizes weight loss in men at high altitude. *Journal of Applied Physiology, 72,* 1741–1748.

Cadarette, B. S., Sawka, M. N., Toner, M. M., & Pandolf, K. B. (1984). Aerobic fitness and the hypohydration response to exercise-heat stress. *Aviation, Space and Environmental Medicine, 55,* 507–512.

Cardinali, D. P., Bortman, G. P., Liotta, G., Lloret, S. P., Albornoz, L. E., Cutrera, R. A. *et al.* (2002). A multifactorial approach employing melatonin to accelerate resynchronization of sleep–wake cycle after a 12 time-zone westerly transmeridian flight in elite football athletes. *Journal of Pineal Research, 32,* 41–46.

Chandler, R. M., Byrne, H. K., Patterson, J. G., & Ivy, J. L. (1994). Dietary supplements affect the anabolic hormones after weight-training exercise. *Journal of Applied Physiology, 76,* 839–845.

Chandra, R. K. (1997). Nutrition and the immune system: An introduction. *American Journal of Clinical Nutrition, 66,* 460S–463S.

Chao, W. H., Askew, E. W., Roberts, D. E., Wood, S. M., & Perkins, J. B. (1999). Exidative stress in humans during work at moderate altitude. *Journal of Nutrition, 129,* 2009–2012.

Cheuvront, S. N., Carter, R., III, & Sawka, M. N. (2003). Fluid balance and endurance exercise performance. *Current Sports Medicine Reports, 2*, 202–208.

Coleman, E., & Steen, S. N. (2002). Macronutrients and metabolic intermediates. In M. S. Bahrke & C. E. Yesalis (Eds.), *Performance-enhancing substances in sport and exercise* (pp. 157–174). Champaign, IL: Human Kinetics.

Committee on Military Nutrition Research (1996). Review of the physiology and nutrition in cold and in high-altitude environments by the Committee on Millitary Nutrition Research. In B. M. Marriott & S. J. Carlson (Eds.), *Nutritional needs in cold and in high altitude environments* (pp. 3–57). Washington, DC: National Academy Press.

Committee on Military Nutrition Research (1999a). Committee responses to questions. In *Military strategies for sustainment of nutrition and immune function in the field* (pp. 99–124). Washington, DC: National Academy Press.

Committee on Military Nutrition Research (1999b). Committee overview. In *The role of protein and amino acids in sustaining and enhancing performance* (pp. 19–75). Washington, DC: National Academy Press.

Consolazio, C. F., & Schnakenberg, D. D. (1977). Nutrition and the responses to extreme environments. *Federation Proceedings, 36*, 1673–1678.

Costill, D. L., Sherman, W. M., Fink, W. J., Maresh, C., Witten, M., & Miller, J. M. (1981). The role of dietary carbohydrates in muscle glycogen resynthesis after strenuous running. *American Journal of Clinical Nutrition, 34*, 1831–1836.

Coyle, E. (1991). Timing and method of increased carbohydrate intake to cope with heavy training, competition and recovery. *Journal of Sports Sciences, 9* (special issue), 29–52.

Coyle, E. (1995). Substrate utilization during exercise in active people. *American Journal of Clinical Nutrition, 61* (suppl.), 968S–979S.

Cymerman, A. (1996). The physiology of high-altitude exposure. In B. M. Marriott & S. J. Carlson (Eds.), *Nutritional needs in cold and in high altitude environments* (pp. 295–317). Washington, DC: National Academy Press.

D'Eon, T. M., Sharoff, C., Chipkin, S. R., Grow, D., Ruby, B. C., & Braun, B. (2002). Regulation of exercise carbohydrate metabolism by estrogen and progesterone in women. *American Journal of Physiology: Endocrinology and Metabolism, 283*, E1046–E1055.

Doubt, T. (1991). Physiology of exercise in the cold. *Sports Medicine, 11*, 367–381.

Earnest, C., & Rudolph, C. (2001). Recovery. In J. Antonio & J. R. Stout (Eds.), *Sports supplements* (pp. 238–259). Philadelphia, PA: Lippincott Williams & Wilkins.

Ekblom, B. (1986). Applied physiology of football. *Sports Medicine, 3*, 50–60.

Essen, B. (1978). Studies on the regulation of metabolism in human skeletal muscle using intermittent exercise as an experimental model. *Acta Physiologica Scandinavica*, suppl. *454*, 1–32.

Fédération Internationale de Football Association (2004). *Regulations: Doping control for FIFA competitions and out of competitions*. Zurich, Switzerland: FIFA.

Ferretti, G. (1992). Cold and muscle performance. *International Journal of Sports Medicine, 13*, S185–S187.

Freund, B. J., & Sawka, M. N. (1996). Influence of cold stress on human fluid balance. In B. M. Marriott & S. J. Carlson (Eds.), *Nutritional needs in cold and in high altitude environments* (pp. 161–179). Washington, DC: National Academy Press.

Fulco, C. S., & Cymerman, A. (1988). Human performance and acute hypoxia. In K. B. Pandolf, M. N. Sawka, & R. R. Gonzalez (Eds.), *Human performance physiology and environmental medicine at terrestrial extremes* (pp. 467–496). Indianapolis, IN: Benchmark Press.

Fulco, C. S., Kambis, K. W., Friedlander, A. L., Rock, P. B., Muza, S. R., & Cymerman, A. (2005). Carbohydrate supplementation improves time-trial cycle performance during energy deficit at 4300 m altitude. *Journal of Applied Physiology, 99*, 867–876.

Fulco, C. S., Rock, P. B., Trad, L. A., Rose, M. R., Forte, V. A., Young, P. M. *et al.* (1989). *The effect of caffeine on endurance time to exhaustion.* Technical Report #T17-89. Natick, MA: US Army Research Institute of Environmental Medicine.

Galloway, S. D. R., & Maughan, R. J. (1997). Effects of ambient temperature on the capacity to perform prolonged cycle exercise in man. *Medicine and Science in Sports and Exercise, 29*, 1240–1249.

Galloway, S. D. R., & Maughan, R. J. (1998). The effects of substrate and fluid provision on thermoregulatory, cardiorespiratory and metabolic responses to prolonged exercise in a cold environment in man. *Experimental Physiology, 83*, 419–430.

Galloway, S. D. R., Wooten, S. A., Murphy, J. L., & Maughan, R. J. (2001). Exogenous carbohydrate oxidation from drinks ingested during prolonged exercise in a cold environment in humans. *Journal of Applied Physiology, 91*, 654–660.

Gill, M. B., & Pugh, L. G. C. E. (1964). Basal metabolism and respiration in men living at 5,800 m (19,000 ft). *Journal of Applied Physiology, 19*, 949–954.

Gleeson, M., & Bishop, N. C. (2000). Elite athlete immunology: Importance of nutrition. *International Journal of Sports Medicine, 21* (suppl. 1), S44–S50.

Gray, E. L., Consolazio, C. F., & Kark, R. M. (1951). Nutritional requirements for men at work in cold, temperate and hot environments. *Journal of Applied Physiology, 4*, 270–275.

Hawley, J. A., & Burke, L. M. (1997). Effect of meal frequency and timing on physical performance. *British Journal of Nutrition, 77*, S91–S103.

Hawley, J. A., Dennis, S. C., & Noakes, T. D. (1994). Carbohydrate, fluid, and electrolyte requirements of the football player: A review. *International Journal of Sports Nutrition, 4*, 221–236.

Hoyt, R. W., & Honig, A. (1996). Energy and macronutrient requirements for work at high altitudes. In B. M. Marriott & S. J. Carlson (Eds.), *Nutritional needs in cold and in high altitude environments* (pp. 379–391). Washington, DC: National Academy Press.

Hubbard, R. W., & Armstrong, L. E. (1988). The heat illnesses: Biochemical, ultrastructural and fluid-electrolyte considerations. In K. B. Pandolf, M. N. Sawka, & R. R. Gonzalez (Eds.), *Human performance physiology and environmental medicine at terrestrial extremes* (pp. 305–359). Indianapolis, IN: Benchmark Press.

Ivy, J. L. (1994). Food components that may optimize physical performance: An overview. In B. M. Marriott (Ed.), *Food components to enhance performance* (pp. 223–238). Washington, DC: National Academy Press.

Ivy, J. L., Res, P. T., Sprague, R. C., & Widzer, M. O. (2003). Effect of a carbohydrate-protein supplement on endurance performance during exercise of varying intensities. *International Journal of Sport Nutrition and Exercise Metabolism, 13*, 382–395.

Jehue, R., Street, D., & Huizenga, R. (1993). Effect of time zone and game time changes on team performance: National Football League. *Medicine and Science in Sports and Exercise, 25*, 127–131.

Kalman, D. (2002). Vitamins: Are athletes' needs different than the needs of sedentary people? In J. Antonio & J. R. Stout (Eds.), *Sports supplements* (pp. 137–159). Philadelphia, PA: Lippincott Williams & Wilkins.

Keller, U., Szinnai, G., Bilz, S., & Berneis, K. (2003). Effects of changes in hydration on protein, glucose and lipid metabolism in man: Impact on health. *European Journal of Clinical Nutrition*, 57 (suppl. 2), S69–S74.

Kenefick, R. W., Mahood, N. V., Hazzard, M. P., Quinn, T. J., & Castellani, J. W. (2004). Hypohydration effects on thermoregulation during moderate exercise in the cold. *European Journal of Applied Physiology*, 92, 565–570.

Kies, C. V. (1995). Sodium, potassium, and chloride status of college students: Competitive athletes, recreational athletes, and nonparticipants. In C. V. Kies & J. A. Driskell (Eds.), *Sports nutrition: Minerals and electrolytes* (pp. 206–214). Boca Raton, FL: CRC Press.

Kolka, M. A., & Stephenson, L. A. (1988). Exercise thermoregulation after prolonged wakefulness. *Journal of Applied Physiology*, 64, 1575–1579.

Kreider, R. B., Melton, C., Greenwood, M., Rasmussen, C., Lundberg, J., Earnest, C. et al. (2003). Effects of oral D-ribose supplementation on anaerobic capacity and selected metabolic markers in healthy males. *International Journal of Sport Nutrition and Exercise Metabolism*, 13, 76–86.

Kuzon, W. M., Rosenblatt, J. D., Huebel, S. C., Leatt, P., Plyley, M. J., McKee, N. H. et al. (1990). Skeletal muscle fiber type, fiber size, and capillary supply in elite football players. *International Journal of Sports Medicine*, 11, 99–102.

Latzka, W. A., & Sawka, M. N. (2000). Hyperhydration and glycerol: Thermoregulatory effects during exercise in hot climates. *Canadian Journal of Applied Physiology*, 25, 536–545.

Lieberman, H. R. (1994). Tyrosine and stress: Human and animal studies. In B. M. Marriott (Ed.), *Food components to enhance performance* (pp. 277–299). Washington, DC: National Academy Press.

Lieberman, H. R., & Shukitt-Hale, B. (1996). Food components and other treatments that may enhance mental performance at high altitudes and in the cold. In B. M. Marriott & S. J. Carlson (Eds.), *Nutritional needs in cold and in high altitude environments* (pp. 453–465). Washington, DC: National Academy Press.

Luce, G. G. (1970). *Biological rhythms in psychiatry and medicine*. Chevy Chase, MD: National Institutes of Mental Health.

Magkos, F., & Kavouras, S. A. (2005). Caffeine and ephedrine: Physiological, metabolic and performance-enhancing effects. *Sports Medicine (New Zealand)*, 34, 871–889.

Maughan, R. J. (2000). Water and electrolyte loss and replacement in exercise. In R. J. Maughan (Ed.), *Nutrition and sport* (pp. 226–240). Oxford: Blackwell Science.

Maughan, R. J. (2002). Plenary lecture. The athlete's diet: Nutritional goals and dietary strategies. *Proceedings of the Nutrition Society*, 61, 87–96.

Maughan, R. J. (2003a). Caffeine ingestion and fluid balance: A review. *Journal of Human Nutrition and Dietetics*, 16, 411–420.

Maughan, R. J. (2003b). Impact of mild dehydration on wellness and on exercise performance. *European Journal of Clinical Nutrition*, 57 (suppl. 2), S19–S23.

Maughan, R. J., & Leiper, J. B. (1994). Fluid replacement requirements in football. *Journal of Sports Sciences*, 12, S29–S34.

Maughan, R. J., Leiper, J. B., & Sherriffs, S. M. (1996). Restoration of fluid balance after exercise-induced dehydration: Effects of food and fluid intake. *European Journal of Applied Physiology*, 73, 317–325.

Maughan, R. J., Merson, S. J., Broad, N. P., & Shirreffs, S. M. (2004). Fluid and electrolyte intake and loss in elite football players during training. *International Journal of Sports Nutrition and Exercise Metabolism, 14,* 333–346.

Maughan, R. J., Shirreffs, S. M., Merson, S. J., & Horswill, C. A. (2005). Fluid and electrolyte balance in elite male football (soccer) players training in a cool environment. *Journal of Sports Sciences, 23,* 73–79.

Maxwell, N. S., Gardner, F., & Nimmo, M. A. (1999). Intermittent running: Muscle metabolism in the heat and effect of hypohydration. *Medicine and Science in Sports and Exercise, 31,* 675–683.

McConnel, G. K., Stephens, T. J., & Canny, B. J. (1999). Fluid ingestion does not influence intense 1-h exercise performance in a mild environment. *Medicine and Science in Sports and Exercise, 31,* 386–392.

Mefferd, R. B., Hale, H. B., & Martens, H. H. (1958). Nitrogen and electrolyte excretion of rats chronically exposed to adverse environments. *American Journal of Physiology, 192,* 209–218.

Miller, S. L., Maresh, C. M., Armstrong, L. E., Effeling, C. B., Lennon, S., & Rodriguez, N. R. (2002). Metabolic response to provision of mixed protein–carbohydrate supplementation during endurance exercise. *International Journal of Sport Nutrition and Exercise Metabolism, 12,* 384–397.

Mohr, M., Krustrup, P., & Bangsbø, J. (2003). Match performance of high-standard football players with special reference to development of fatigue. *Journal of Sports Sciences, 21,* 519–528.

Mustafa, K. Y., & Mahmoud, N. E. A. (1979). Evaporative water loss in African football players. *Journal of Sports Medicine and Physical Fitness, 19,* 181–183.

National Heart, Lung, and Blood Institute (1998). *Clinical guidelines on the identification, evaluation, and treatment of overweight and obesity in adults: The Evidence Report.* NIH Publication #98-4083. Washington, DC: National Institutes of Health.

Nehlig, A., & Debry, G. (1994). Caffeine and sports activity: A review. *International Journal of Sports Medicine, 15,* 215–223.

Newsholme, E. A., & Castell, L. M. (2000). Amino acids, fatigue, and immunodepression in exercise. In R. J. Maughan (Ed.), *Nutrition in sport* (pp. 153–170). Oxford: Blackwell Science.

Normand, H., Vargas, E., Bordachar, J., Benoit, O., & Raynaud, J. (1992). Sleep apneas in high altitude residents (3,800 m). *International Journal of Sports Medicine, 13* (suppl. 1), S40–S42.

Op't Eijnde, B., Van Leemputte, M., Brouns, F., Van Der Vusse, G. J., Labarque, V., Ramaekers, M. *et al.* (2001). No effects of oral ribose supplementation on repeated maximal exercise and *de novo* ATP resynthesis. *Journal of Applied Physiology, 91,* 2275–2281.

Pedersen, B. K., & Bruunsgaard, H. (1995). How physical exercise influences the establishment of infections. *Sports Medicine, 19,* 393–400.

Penetar, R. J. (1994). Effects of caffeine on cognitive performance, mood, and alertness in sleep-deprived humans. In B. M. Marriott (Ed.), *Food components to enhance performance* (pp. 407–431). Washington, DC: National Academy Press.

Phinney, S. D., Bistrian, B. R., Wolfe, R. R., & Blackburn, G. L. (1983). The human metabolic response to chronic ketosis without caloric restriction: Physical and biochemical adaptation. *Metabolism, 32,* 757–768.

Piérard, C., Beaumont, M., Enslen, M., Chauffard, F., Tan, D.-X., Reiter, R. J. *et al.* (2001). Resynchronization of hormonal rhythms after an eastbound flight in humans: Effects of slow-release caffeine and melatonin. *European Journal of Applied Physiology, 85,* 144–150.

Pozos, R. S., Roberts, D. E., Hackney, A. C., & Feith, S. J. (1996). Military schedules vs. biological clocks. In B. M. Marriott & S. J. Carlson (Eds.), *Nutritional needs in cold and in high altitude environments* (pp. 149–160). Washington, DC: National Academy Press.

Pugh, L. G. C. E. (1962). Physiological and medical aspects of the Himalayan scientific and mountaineering expedition, 1960–61. *British Medical Journal, 2,* 621–627.

Reilly, T., Atkinson, G., & Budgett, R. (1997a). Effects of temazepam on physiological and performance variables following a westerly flight across five time zones. *Journal of Sports Sciences, 15,* 62.

Reilly, T., Atkinson, G., & Waterhouse, J. (1997b). Travel fatigue and jet-lag. *Journal of Sports Sciences, 15,* 365–369.

Reynolds, R. D. (1996). Effects of cold and altitude on vitamin and mineral requirements. In B. M. Marriott & S. J. Carlson (Eds.), *Nutritional needs in cold and in high altitude environments* (pp. 215–244). Washington, DC: National Academy Press.

Ritz, P., Salle, A., Simard, G., Dumas, J. F., Foussard, F., & Malthiery, Y. (2003). Effects of changes in water compartments on physiology and metabolism. *European Journal of Clinical Nutrition, 57* (suppl. 2), S2–S5.

Roberts, A. C., Butterfield, G. E., Cymerman, C., Reeves, J. T., Wolfel, E. E., & Brooks, G. A. (1996). Acclimatization to 4,300-m altitude decreases reliance on fat as a substrate. *Journal of Applied Physiology, 81,* 1762–1771.

Rose, M. S., Houston, C. S., Fulco, C. S., Coates, G., Sutton, J. R., & Cymerman, A. (1988). Operation Everest II: Nutrition and body composition. *Journal of Applied Physiology, 65,* 2545–2551.

Saltin, B. (1973). Metabolic fundamentals in exercise. *Medicine and Science in Sports, 5,* 137–146.

Sawka, M. N., Gonzalez, R. R., & Pondolf, K. B. (1984). Effects of sleep deprivation on thermoregulation during exercise. *American Journal of Physiology, 246,* R72–R77.

Sawka, M. N., & Pandolf, K. B. (1990). Effects of body water loss on physiological function and exercise performance. In C. V. Gisolfi & D. R. Lamb (Eds.), *Perspectives in exercise science and sports medicine, Vol. 3: Fluid homeostasis during exercise* (pp. 1–38). Carmel, IN: Benchmark Press.

Sawka, M. N., & Wenger, C. B. (1988). Physiological responses to acute exercise-heat stress. In K. B. Pandolf, M. N. Sawka, & R. R. Gonzalez (Eds.), *Human performance physiology and environmental medicine at terrestrial extremes* (pp. 97–152). Indianapolis, IN: Benchmark Press.

Schmidt, M. C., Askew, E. W., Roberts, D. E., Prior, R. L., Ensign, W. Y., & Hesslink, R. E. (2002). Oxidative stress in humans training in a cold, moderate altitude environment and their response to a phytochemical antioxidant supplement. *Wilderness and Environmental Medicine, 13,* 94–105.

Shephard, R. J. (1993). Metabolic adaptations to exercise in the cold: An update. *Sports Medicine (New Zealand), 16,* 266–289.

Shephard, R. J. (1999). Biology and medicine of football: An update. *Journal of Sports Sciences, 17,* 757–786.

Sherman, W. M. (1992). Recovery from endurance exercise. *Medicine and Science in Sports and Exercise, 24,* S336–S339.

Sherman, W. M., & Wimer, G. S. (1991). Insufficient dietary carbohydrate during training: Does it impair athletic performance? *International Journal of Sports Nutrition, 1*, 28–44.

Shirreffs, S. M. (2005). The importance of good hydration for work and exercise performance. *Nutrition Reviews, 63*, S14–S21.

Shirreffs, S. M., Aragon-Vargas, L. F., Chamorro, M., Maughan, R. J., Serratosa, L., & Zachwieja, J. J. (2005). The sweating response of elite professional football players to training in the heat. *International Journal of Sports Medicine, 26*, 90–95.

Shirreffs, S. M., Armstrong, L. E., & Cheuvront, S. N. (2004). Fluid and electrolyte needs for preparation and recovery from training and competition. *Journal of Sports Sciences, 22*, 57–63.

Shirreffs, S. M., Taylor, A. J., Leiper, J. B., & Maughan, R. J. (1996). Post-exercise rehydration in man: Effects of volume consumed and drink sodium content. *Medicine and Science in Sports and Exercise, 28*, 1260–1271.

Simon-Schnass, I. M. (1992). Nutrition at high altitude. *Journal of Nutrition, 122*, 778–781.

Simon-Schnass, I. (1996). Oxidative stress at high altitudes and effects of vitamin E. In B. M. Marriott & S. J. Carlson (Eds.), *Nutritional needs in cold and in high altitude environments* (pp. 393–418). Washington, DC: National Academy Press.

Spriet, L. L. (2002). Caffeine. In M. S. Bahrke & C. E. Yesalis (Eds.), *Performance-enhancing substances in sport and exercise* (pp. 267–278). Champaign, IL: Human Kinetics.

Srivastava, K. K., & Kumar, R. (1992). Human nutrition in cold and high terrestrial altitudes. *International Journal of Biometerology, 36*, 10–13.

Stephenson, L. A., & Kolka, M. A. (1988). Effect of gender, circadian period and sleep loss on thermal responses during exercise. In K. B. Pandolf, M. N. Sawka, & R. R. Gonzalez (Eds), *Human performance physiology and environmental medicine at terrestrial extremes* (pp. 267–304). Indianapolis, IN: Benchmark Press.

Strydom, N. B., Kotze, H. F., Van der Walt, W. H., & Rogers, G. G. (1976). Effect of ascorbic acid on rate of heat acclimatization. *Journal of Applied Physiology, 2*, 202–205.

Tiedt, H. J., Grimm, M., & Unger, K. D. (1991). Research progress on iron, copper, zinc, calcium, magnesium, ferritin and transferrin as well as haemoglobin and hematocrit in the blood of high-performance athletes: Part 2. *Medizin und Sport, 31*, 161–165.

Tipton, M. J., Franks, G. M., Meneilly, G. S., & Mekjavic, I. B. (1997). Substrate utilization during exercise and shivering. *European Journal of Applied Physiology, 76*, 103–108.

Toner, M. M., & McArdle, W. D. (1988). Physiological adjustments of man to the cold. In K. B. Pandolf, M. N. Sawka, & R. R. Gonzalez (Eds.), *Human performance physiology and environmental medicine at terrestrial extremes* (pp. 361–400). Indianapolis, IN: Benchmark Press.

Tullson, P. C., & Terjung, R. L. (1991). Adenine nucleotide synthesis in exercising and endurance-trained skeletal muscle. *American Journal of Physiology, 261*, C342–C347.

Van Erp-Baart, A. M. J., Saris, W. H. M., Binkhorst, R. A., Vos, J. A., & Elvers, W. H. (1989). Nationwide survey on nutritional habits in elite athletes: Part II. Mineral and vitamin intake. *International Journal of Sports Medicine, 10* (suppl. I), S11–S16.

Wagenmakers, A. J. M. (1999). Supplementation with branched-chain amino acids, glutamine, and protein hydrolysates: Rationale for effects on metabolism and performance. In *The role of protein and amino acids in sustaining and enhancing performance* (pp. 309–329). Washington, DC: National Academy Press.

Waterhouse, J., Kao, S., Edwards, B., Weinert, D., Atkinson, G., & Reilly, T. (2005). Transient changes in the pattern of food intake following a simulated time zone transition to the east across eight time zones. *Chronobiology International, 22,* 299–319.

Watson, G., Judelson, D. A., Armstrong, L. E., Yeargin, S. W., Casa, D. J., & Maresh, C. M. (2005). Influence of diuretic-induced dehydration on competitive sprint and power performance. *Medicine and Science in Sports and Exercise, 37,* 1168–1174.

Webster, M. J. (2002). Sodium bicarbonate. In M. S. Bahrke & C. E. Yesalis (Eds.), *Performance-enhancing substances in sport and exercise* (pp. 197–208). Champaign, IL: Human Kinetics.

Welch, B. E., Buskirk, E. R., & Iampietro, P. F. (1958). Relation of climate and temperature to food and water intake in men. *Metabolism, 7,* 141–148.

Wenger, C. B. (1988). Human heat acclimatization. In K. B. Pandolf, M. N. Sawka, & R. R. Gonzalez (Eds.), *Human performance physiology and environmental medicine at terrestrial extremes* (pp. 153–197). Indianapolis, IN: Benchmark Press.

Westerterp, K. R., Kayser, B., Brouns, F., Herry, J. P., & Saris, W. H. (1992). Energy expenditure climbing Mt. Everest. *Journal of Applied Physiology, 73,* 1815–1819.

Westerterp-Plantenga, M. S., Westerterp, K. R., Rubbens, M., Verwegen, C. R. T., Richelet, J. P., & Gardette, B. (1999). Appetite at "high altitude" [Operation Everest III (Comex-'97)]: a simulated ascent of Mount Everest. *Journal of Applied Physiology, 87,* 391–399.

Wilbur, R. L. (2004). *Altitude training and athletic performance.* Champaign, IL: Human Kinetics.

Williams, C. (1995). Macronutrients and performance. *Journal of Sport Sciences, 13,* S1–S10.

Williams, C., & Serratosa, L. (2006). Nutrition on match day. *Journal of Sports Sciences, 24,* 687–607.

Wilson, W. M., & Maughan, R. J. (1992). A role for serotonin in the genesis of fatigue in man: Administration of a 5-hydroxytryptamine reuptake inhibitor (Paroxetine) reduces the capacity to perform prolonged exercise. *Experimental Physiology, 77,* 921–924.

Winget, C. M., DeRoshia, C. W., & Holley, D. C. (1985). Circadian rhythms and athletic performance. *Medicine and Science in Sports and Exercise, 17,* 498–516.

Wright, V. P., Klawitter, P. F., Iscru, D. F., Merola, A. J., & Clanton, T. L. (2005). Superoxide scavengers augment contractile but not energetic responses to hypoxia in rat diaphragm. *Journal of Applied Physiology, 98,* 1753–1760.

Wurtman, R. J. (1994). Effects of nutrients on neurotransmitter release. In B. M. Marriott (Ed.), *Food components to enhance performance* (pp. 239–261). Washington, DC: National Academy Press.

Young, A. J. (1988). Human adaptation to cold. In K. B. Pandolf, M. N. Sawka, & R. R. Gonzalez (Eds.), *Human performance physiology and environmental medicine at terrestrial extremes* (pp. 401–434). Indianapolis, IN: Benchmark Press.

Youngstedt, S. D., & Buxton, O. M. (2003). Jet lag and athletic performance. *American Journal of Medicine and Sports, 5,* 219–226.

Zeisel, S. H. (1994). Choline: Human requirements and effects on human performance. In B. M. Marriott (Ed.), *Food components to enhance performance* (pp. 381–406). Washington, DC: National Academy Press.

126   *Armstrong*

Zuo, L., Christofi, F. L., Wright, V. P., Liu, C. Y., Merola, A. J., Berliner, L. J. *et al.* (2000). Intra- and extracellular measurement of reactive oxygen species produced during heat stress in diaphragm muscle. *American Journal of Physiology: Cell Physiology, 279,* C1058–C1066.

Zuo, L., & Clanton, T. L. (2005). Reactive oxygen species formation in the transition to hypoxia in skeletal muscle. *American Journal of Physiology: Cell Physiology, 289,* C207–C216.

7   Alcohol and football

R. J. MAUGHAN

The use of alcohol is often intimately associated with sport, and the association is particularly strong in football. As well as providing a source of energy, alcohol (ethanol) has metabolic, cardiovascular, thermoregulatory, and neuromuscular actions that may affect exercise performance. Its actions on the central nervous system, however, result in decrements in skill and behavioural changes that may have adverse effects on performance. There is also evidence of dose-dependent decrements in aerobic capacity. Although the mechanisms are not well understood, the aftermath of alcohol use (hangover) may also adversely affect performance for many hours after intoxication. Alcohol intoxication may adversely affect the player's dietary choices by displacing carbohydrate from the diet at a time when restoration of glycogen stores should be a priority.

Keywords: Ethanol, intoxication, exercise, sport, soccer

Introduction

Alcohol is an energy-supplying nutrient that forms a small but important part of the normal dietary intake of a large part of the world's population. Unlike the other macronutrients, however, alcohol is not an essential part of the human diet, and is absent from the diets of a significant portion of the population. Alcohol intake may be measured in grams or millilitres of ethanol, or in units of alcohol: each unit of alcohol in the UK contains approximately 8 g (10 ml) of ethanol. The UK Department of Health recommends that adult men should not consume more than 3–4 units of alcohol per day and women should not consume more than 2–3 units daily. In the USA, however, a standard drink delivers about 12–14 g of alcohol, and the US Department of Agriculture recommends that men should not drink more than one or two drinks per day and that women should not exceed one drink per day.

Alcohol intake and drinking behaviours vary widely between countries and cultures, and data from the UK will be used here for illustrative purposes. The National Diet and Nutrition Survey (NDNS) of adults aged 19–64 years living in private households in Great Britain, carried out between July 2000 and June 2001, found that, among men and women who drank alcoholic beverages, alcohol contributed on average 8.1% and 5.7% respectively of their total energy intake (National Diet and Nutrition Survey, 2003). Mean daily alcohol intake was 21.9 g for men and 9.3 g for women: if those who consumed no alcohol were excluded, the figures were 27.2 g for men and 13.5 g for women. Data from the NDNS suggest that, on average, men were consuming 21.1 units per week and women were consuming 9.0 units per week. The NDNS also high-lighted that a number of men and women were drinking more than the UK Department of Health recommended guidelines for safe drinking. Among those people who consumed alcohol, 38% of men and 24% of women had more than the maximum, with younger age groups consuming more units per week than older age groups. It was estimated that 5% of adult men and 10% of adult women in the UK consume no alcohol (National Diet and Nutrition Survey, 2003). About one in 13 adults in the UK, however, is dependent on alcohol (Ibrahim & Gilvarry, 2005).

Alcohol-containing foods – most of which are in liquid form – have a rela-tively high energy content (29 kJ [7 kcal] per gram of alcohol), but are generally poor in other nutrients. As with other components of the diet, intake of alcohol has implications for health and for sports performance, and both acute and chronic alcohol intake in large amounts can be a reason for concern. There is compelling evidence that regular ingestion of moderate amounts of alcohol may confer some health benefits; in particular, there seems to be a 25–40% reduction in the risk of adverse cardiovascular events (Goldberg, Mosca, Piano, & Fisher, 2001). The mechanisms by which alcohol may reduce the inci-dence of mortality of cardiovascular diseases are the subject of much debate, but there is certainly an increased level of high-density lipoprotein cholesterol in regular moderate consumers (El-Sayed, Ali, & El-Sayed, 2005). Available evidence also suggests that moderate alcohol consumption may have favourable effects on blood coagulation and fibrinolysis. Excessive intake is associated with several negative health outcomes, including an increased risk of various liver disorders, some cancers, and suicide. There are a number of unique features associated with the consumption of alcohol, including its psychological and behavioural effects, its effects on physiological and metabolic functions, and the social connotations of alcohol intake.

There is a long history of association between alcohol and sport (Collins & Vamplew, 2002). Sponsorship by alcohol companies remains an important source for many football clubs, further emphasizing the association. Alcohol consumption is associated in particular with celebration, but consumption can also be used as a shield to escape from the realization of failure. In this regard, sport is not different from most other social contexts, but the actions of intoxi-cated high-profile sportsmen and women are likely to attract attention from the media. Excessive alcohol intake is also likely to have a negative effect on a foot-baller's ability to perform the tasks for which he or she is employed.

Alcohol use in football and in sport

It is not entirely clear whether the prevalence of alcohol use is different in foot-ball players or other athletes from that of the general population, and the contradictory information in the literature reflects the variability in alcohol use in different population groups. It may also reflect the social connotations associated with alcohol use, and questionnaire-derived data on alcohol use may be even more prone to misrepresentation than those relating to use of other food groups. Reports from American school populations suggest a greater prevalence of alcohol use in team sports participants than in non-participants (Garry & Morrissey, 2000), and data from a New Zealand student population show higher rates of hazardous drinking behaviours in elite sportspeople (O'Brien, Blackie, & Hunter, 2005). In contrast, it seems that sports participation delays drinking andintoxication debut in Norwegian youngsters (Hellandsjo Bu *et al.*, 2002). Data from Spain (Pastor, Balaguer, Pons, & Garcia-Merita, 2003) suggest that alcohol use in athletic students is less than in their non-athletic peers. There are data from France that show a lower prevalence of alcohol use in athletic students (Lorente, Peretti-Watel, Griffet, & Grelot, 2003) but also data that show a greater prevalence of use (Lorente, Souville, Griffet, & Grelot, 2004). Moore and Werch (2004) have highlighted some of the complexities that influence analyses of the relationship between sports participation and substance use. In their survey, school-sponsored, male-dominated sports were associated with increased alcohol use, but out-of-school, mixed-gender sports participation was associated with greater use among females.

There are few surveys of the prevalence of alcohol use in senior football players and in those playing in professional leagues, and the reliability of these surveys is unknown. Maughan (1997) reported an average intake of about 10–12 g · day^{-1}, representing about 2–3% of total energy intake in the first team squads of two Scottish Premier League teams. There was, however, an individual value in excess of 10% of energy intake, as well as several players who consumed no alcohol. Burke and Read (1988) reported that alcohol accounted for about 4% of total energy intake in elite Australian Rules football players, about the same as in the general population. In a somewhat alarming report, Ama, Betnga, Ama Moor and Kamga (2003) found that 25% of amateur football players surveyed in Yaounde, Cameroon, admitted drinking methylated spirits, and that 16% drank alcohol before matches (including 12% of "elite" players).

Care is needed in the interpretation of alcohol intake figures. "Moderate drinking", usually defined as the ingestion of about 10–40 g of ethanol per day for men and 10–20 g · day^{-1} for women, is not generally considered to be harmful to health. Indeed, those who drink alcohol in moderation have lower overall mortality rates than those who drink more heavily or those who do not drink at all (Macdonald, 1999). Problems arise, however, when intake at these levels is episodic – that is, when the average intake for a week is compressed into a short space of time. Unfortunately, binge drinking is commonly found in football, and the culture of the game is such that many players will abstain from alcohol in training but will drink copious amounts after a game (Burke & Maughan, 2000). This pattern was demonstrated in a dietary survey of Australian Rules football players whose mean daily intake of alcohol was reported to be a modest 20 g or two standard drinks (Burke & Read, 1988).

However, almost all this intake occurred on match day, when the mean intake was 120 g (range = 27–368 g); alcohol provided a mean contribution of 19% to total energy intake on match day (range = 3–43%). These self-reports of excessive alcohol intake after the game were confirmed when blood alcohol levels were estimated at a training session on the morning after a game: 34% of players registered a positive blood alcohol level with 10% of players showing a level above the legal limit for driving a motor vehicle.

Metabolism of ethanol

Alcohol (ethanol) is readily absorbed from the gastrointestinal tract and quickly becomes distributed throughout all body tissues. It is absorbed faster than it can be metabolized, so blood (and tissue) concentration increases, but there is no storage depot for alcohol, so it must be removed by oxidation. After a single drink, the blood alcohol concentration usually reaches a peak after about 40 min, but this time will vary with prior exercise, the co-ingestion of other nutrients, and habitual alcohol intake. A small amount (less than 10% of an ingested dose) may be lost in the urine and via the lungs.

Metabolism of alcohol occurs primarily in the liver, and it can be oxidized at a rate of about 100 mg per kilogram of body mass per hour. The first step in the metabolism of alcohol is the oxidation of ethanol to acetaldehyde ($CH_3CH=O$), a reaction catalysed by alcohol dehydrogenase (Reaction 1 below), with conversion of the coenzyme NAD^+ to NADH in the process. The acetaldehyde is further oxidized to acetate in a reaction catalysed by aldehyde dehydrogenase (Reaction 2 below), and the acetate so formed can then enter the citric acid cycle, where it is converted to carbon dioxide and water. A number of the metabolic effects of alcohol are directly linked to the production of an excess of both NADH and acetaldehyde. Acetaldehyde is thought to be responsible for many of the adverse effects of alcohol.

$$CH_3CH_2OH + NAD^+ \rightarrow CH_3CH=O + NADH + H^+ \qquad (1)$$

$$CH_3CH=O + NAD^+ + H_2O \rightarrow CH_3COO^- + NADH + 2H^+ \qquad (2)$$

Alcohol also can be metabolized by the microsomal ethanol-oxidizing system (MEOS) within the liver. The MEOS plays a minor role in alcohol metabolism when alcohol intake is small or absent, but its activity is upregulated by chronic intake of alcohol in high doses. Once the pathway is activated, MEOS greatly enhances the rate of conversion of alcohol to acetaldehyde: in doing so, it can disrupt the oxidation-reduction status of the cell by reducing the available pool of the reduced cofactor NADPH. The rate at which ethanol is cleared by the liver varies between individuals, and the response of the individual will depend on a number of factors, including the amount of ethanol consumed in relation to their habitual intake. There is conflicting information about whether the rate of metabolism of alcohol is increased by exercise.

Alcohol and performance

It is generally assumed that performance is impaired in individuals who are intoxicated, but there is a substantial body of anecdotal evidence to suggest that alcohol intake before exercise will not have an adverse effect on performance. Because of the understandable reluctance of institutional ethics committees to approve studies involving the administration of alcohol, there is limited experimental evidence relating to the effects of alcohol on exercise performance. There are reasons to believe that acute alcohol intake may impair performance of endurance exercise because of effects on metabolic, cardiovascular, or thermoregulatory function, and that it may affect performance of skilled tasks because of effects on reaction time, fine motor control, levels of arousal, and judgement.

There generally seem to be no effects of alcohol ingestion, at least in moderate amounts, on muscle strength and power (Reilly, 2003). An exception, however, is an early study by Hebbelinck (1963) that showed no effect of alcohol ($0.6\,\text{ml}$ of 94% ethanol $\cdot$ kg body mass^{-1}) on isometric strength, but a 6% reduction in vertical jump height and a 10% decrease in performance in an $80\,\text{m}$ sprint. In a study of the effects of alcohol on sprinting and middle-distance running performance, McNaughton and Preece (1986) showed a progressive impairment in performance at distances of 200, 400, 800, and $1500\,\text{m}$ with increasing doses of alcohol in amounts that resulted in blood alcohol concentrations between 0.01 and 0.1% (i.e. $10\text{–}100\,\text{mg} \cdot 100\,\text{ml}^{-1}$); performance in the $100\,\text{m}$ sprint was not affected. In a study by Houmard, Lagenfield and Wiley (1987), performance time in a 5 mile ($8\,\text{km}$) treadmill run was $28\,\text{s}$ slower after low-dose alcohol ingestion (blood alcohol count below $0.05\,\text{g} \cdot 100\,\text{ml}^{-1}$): this effect was not statistically significant, but is nonetheless meaningful to the athlete. Kendrick, Affrime and Lowenthal (1993) reported that runners who drank alcohol before a treadmill run had higher heart rates, lower blood sugar levels, and more trouble finishing their runs compared with runners who had non-alcoholic drinks. Performance in events that require skill, accuracy, judgement, and information processing are more obviously affected than are tasks that do not require these attributes.

Acute effects of alcohol that may influence performance

Metabolic effects

It is widely recognized that ethanol has a variety of effects on carbohydrate metabolism in skeletal muscle and in liver. Much of the available evidence comes from animal models, showing that synthesis of glycogen in both liver (Cook et al., 1988) and oxidative skeletal muscle (Xu, Heng, & Palmer, 1993) is impaired in the presence of even relatively low levels of ethanol, though there seems to be no effects on Type II muscle fibres. Alcohol also delays gastric emptying, delaying the delivery of co-ingested glucose to the small intestine, and also appears to impair intestinal glucose absorption (Cook et al., 1988).

Ingestion of alcohol will increase the risk of hypoglycaemia due to the suppression of glucose production by the liver (Jorfeldt & Juhlin-Dannfelt, 1978). This may be of particular concern during prolonged, moderate-intensity exercise when glucose output from the liver is an important source of energy.

The animal data on impairment of glycogen storage in liver and muscle are often used as a reason for athletes to avoid alcohol during the recovery period after exercise, but it is not entirely clear that these data can be extrapolated to post-exercise recovery in humans. One of the key priorities during recovery between training sessions or games is the replacement of the limited carbohydrate stores, and this is achieved by ensuring an adequate intake of carbohydrate from the diet during the recovery period. Burke *et al.* (2003) reported the effects of alcohol intake on muscle glycogen storage in humans over 8 h and 24 h of recovery from a prolonged cycling bout that resulted in a substantial reduction of carbohydrate stores. The athletes who participated in this study undertook three different diets following their glycogen-depleting exercise: a high-carbohydrate diet intended to optimize recovery, an alcohol displacement diet (reduced carbohydrate, in which about 210 g of dietary carbohydrate was replaced by about 120 g alcohol), and an alcohol + carbohydrate diet (about 120 g alcohol added to the high-carbohydrate diet). Muscle glycogen storage was significantly reduced (by almost 50% at 8 h and about 16% at 24 h) on the alcohol displacement diet when the amount of carbohydrate provided by the diet was less than adequate (Figure 1). On the other hand, when the high-carbohydrate diet was eaten, there was no clear evidence that alcohol intake caused a reduction in muscle glycogen storage: there was a small, not statistically significant reduction at 8 h and no effect at all at 24 h. There was, however, a large variability of the responses of different participants, and it may well be that some individuals are unable to effectively replenish their glycogen reserves between daily training sessions if substantial amounts of alcohol are consumed.

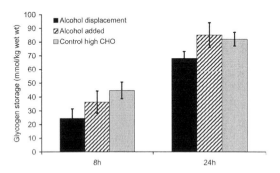

Figure 1. Effects of alcohol on post-exercise muscle glycogen storage. After glycogen-depleting exercise, participants were fed a control high-carbohydrate diet, an isoenergetic diet with 1.5 g alcohol $\cdot$ kg^{-1} displacing carbohydrate, or the high-carbohydrate diet with 1.5 g alcohol $\cdot$ kg^{-1} added. Displacing carbohydrate reduced glycogen storage at 8 h and 24 h; adding alcohol tended to reduce glycogen storage at 8 h, but there was no effect at 24 h. Drawn from the data of Burke *et al.* (2003).

Even if there is no direct metabolic effect of ethanol on glycogen storage when dietary carbohydrate intake is high, it is likely that players who consume large amounts of alcohol during the recovery period after training or a match will have a reduced carbohydrate intake, either as a result of a decreased total (non-alcohol) energy intake or because of a failure to follow the recommended eating strategies at this time.

Aerobic function

Acute ingestion of moderate doses of alcohol appears to have little effect on cardiorespiratory function and exercise performance (ACSM, 1982). In a study by Bond, Franks and Howley (1984), 12 males (six moderate drinkers and six abstainers) undertook three separate maximal exercise tests consisting of progressive workloads on a bicycle ergometer. Before each work bout, the participants consumed a placebo ($0.0\,ml \cdot kg^{-1}$), a small ($0.44\,ml \cdot kg^{-1}$), or a moderate ($0.88\,ml \cdot kg^{-1}$) dose of a 95% ethanol solution. Neither amount of alcohol had any significant effect on heart rate, blood pressure, ventilation, oxygen uptake, or work performance. Other studies, however, have suggested a decreased performance in events demanding a high aerobic capacity, such as middle-distance running (see Reilly, 2003).

Hydration effects

The diuretic action of ethanol is well recognized, and Eggleton (1942) estimated an excess urine production of about 10 ml for each gram of ethanol ingested. Alcohol acts via suppression of the release of anti-diuretic hormone from the pituitary (Roberts, 1963). Alcohol has a negligible diuretic effect when consumed in dilute solution following a moderate level of hypohydration induced by exercise in the heat (Shirreffs & Maughan, 1997). There appears to be no difference in recovery from dehydration whether the rehydration beverage is alcohol-free or contains up to 2% alcohol, but drinks containing 4% alcohol tend to delay the recovery process by promoting urine loss. Based on the data of Eggleton (1942), however, it is apparent that concentrated alcohol solutions will result in net negative fluid balance: a 25 ml measure of spirits (40% ethanol) contains 10 ml of alcohol and 15 ml of water, resulting in a urine output of about 100 ml and net negative water balance of 85 ml. Ingestion of large volumes of dilute alcohol will result in a water diuresis, but should promote restoration of fluid balance provided that there is also an intake of sodium. The alcohol content of some standard drinks is shown in Table 1.

Effects on thermoregulatory function

The 1982 ACSM Position Stand on the use of alcohol in sports identified perturbations of thermoregulatory mechanisms, especially in the cold, as one of the reasons to abstain from alcohol prior to exercise. Small doses of ethanol,

Table 1. A standard drink contains approximately
10 g of alcohol

Drink	Volume
Standard beer (4% alcohol)	250 ml
Low-alcohol beer (2% alcohol)	500 ml
Cider, wine coolers, alcoholic soft drinks	250 ml
Wine	100 ml
Champagne	100 ml
Fortified wines, sherry, port	60 ml
Spirit	30 ml

given to human volunteers at rest in the absence of a thermal stress, have very little effect on body temperature, but large doses administered before exercise at low ambient temperatures result in increased peripheral vasodilatation and a marked fall in core temperature. In combination with the concomitant fall in blood glucose concentration that is normally observed in this situation, there is clearly potential for an adverse effect on performance. Graham (1981) showed that ingestion of alcohol ($2.5\,\text{ml} \cdot \text{kg}^{-1}$) before prolonged (3 h) exercise in the cold resulted in increased heat loss, though this effect was somewhat attenuated by co-ingestion of glucose. In animal studies, the administration of alcohol to animals exposed to ambient temperatures both above and below the thermoneutral zone has shown that alcohol acts to impair adaptation to both heat and cold (Kalant & Lê, 1983).

In another animal study, rats were given 0, 4, 8, 12, or 16% ethanol as the sole source of drinking water for 14 days. Time to fatigue in treadmill running in the heat (35°C) of rats drinking 4% ethanol was similar to that of rats consuming water (32 and 32.9 min respectively), but the running time of rats drinking 16% ethanol was reduced (Francesconi & Mager, 1981). There appear to be no further recent studies in this important area.

Psychomotor and behavioural effects

Alcohol has a number of direct effects – rather than via any of its metabolites – on central neurotransmitter synthesis and release. These actions have been reviewed by Reilly (2003). It is not surprising, therefore, that ingestion of large doses of alcohol will affect some or all of the actions of the central nervous system. The American College of Sports Medicine published a position stand on the use of alcohol in sports (ACSM, 1982) in which it was concluded that small to moderate amounts of alcohol – that is, less than the amount necessary to cause intoxication – result in impaired reaction time, hand–eye coordination, accuracy, balance, and gross motor skills. The evidence that has accumulated since then has confirmed these findings. The same mechanisms may operate to increase the risks associated with driving while under the influence of alcohol: about a half of all fatal road traffic accidents involve drivers who are intoxicated (National Institute on Alcohol Abuse and Alcoholism, 2000). An initial response to ingestion of small doses of alcohol is an enhanced sense of well-being, but even low doses (sufficient to elevate the blood alcohol concentration to about $30 \, \text{ml} \cdot \text{dl}^{-1}$) will impair hand–eye coordination. Progressively increasing the dose leads to loss of social inhibition, loss of fine motor control, erratic behaviour, increased aggression, and finally loss of control of voluntary activity.

The aftermath of alcohol use

According to O'Brien and Lyons (2000), 74% of a population of football players reported that they drank alcohol, and 65% reported drinking the day before training or a match. There is limited and conflicting evidence on the effects of post-alcohol/hangover effects on functional capacity, but there is sufficient evidence of adverse effects the day after a heavy drinking session for such activities to be discouraged (Barker, 2004). O'Brien (1993) showed reductions in aerobic exercise performance of rugby players the day after an evening bout of drinking involving an intake of 1–38 units of alcohol, though anaerobic performance was unaffected. The negative effect on aerobic performance was apparent at even the smallest dose of alcohol. For obvious reasons, there are few studies of the effects of high alcohol intakes on soccer-specific performance, and there appear to be no studies on well-trained footballers. Symptoms of hangover are thought to be due to dehydration, acid–base disturbances, disruption of cytokine and prostaglandin pathways, and alterations in glucose metabolism via effects on circulating insulin and glucagon levels (Wiese, Shlipak, & Browner, 2000). There are also cardiovascular effects during the hangover phase, including increased heart rate, decreased left ventricular performance, and increased blood pressure (Kupari, 1983).

Chronic effects of alcohol

Alcoholism is a complex disorder, with a strong genetic predisposition that interacts with precipitating factors in the environment (Macdonald, 1999). Some alcoholics consume alcohol in relatively moderate amounts on a regular basis while others engage in episodes of binge drinking that may vary in their frequency. Chronic intake of large amounts of ethanol is usually associated with multiple nutritional deficiencies as well as various muscle, liver, and cardiac pathologies. Animal studies show muscle atrophy, primarily in Type II fibres, in response to chronic alcohol exposure (Preedy, Duane, & Peters, 1988). It is unclear whether the habitual intake of small amounts of alcohol may adversely affect the metabolic adaptations in muscle that result from training. Although the management of the nutritional deficiencies is clinically relevant in the treatment of alcoholism, it has little practical relevance to the athlete. Impairment of performance because of the other effects of alcohol abuse is likely to be apparent long before nutrient deficiencies begin to be a concern.

Effects of alcohol on injury and incapacity

The ingestion of alcohol is likely to have a number of behavioural and other effects that may influence the risk of injury and the recovery process after injury. The history of the game of football contains many instances of players taking part in games while under the influence of alcohol. Prior alcohol consumption appears to increase the risk of sports-related injury, with an injury prevalence of 55% in drinkers compared with 24% in non-drinkers ($P < 0.005$) (O'Brien & Lyons, 2000). The mechanisms by which this association may be mediated are not entirely clear, but the increased risk of injury, and the increased severity of injuries that do occur, may be a consequence of increased risk-taking behaviours, as alcohol removes some of the restraints that normally operate (O'Brien, 1993). This may also account for the increased aggression often displayed by young men while under the influence of alcohol.

Intoxication during match-play is fortunately rather rare, at least at the higher levels of the game, though it is not completely absent. It is perhaps not so unusual, though, for players training the morning after a high alcohol intake the previous night to be still under the influence of alcohol, and several high-profile players have publicly admitted to alcohol addiction.

Some degree of muscle damage, either of intrinsic or extrinsic origin, is commonplace in both training and competition. This may often be in the form of minor damage that results in efflux of muscle-specific proteins into the vascular space, accompanied by some degree of pain and disability that may persist for hours or days (Clarkson & Hubal, 2002). This damage results in turn in an inflammatory response that involves an increase in local blood flow and macrophage infiltration of the damaged area. Recommended treatments include application of ice, compression, and elevation of the limb to reduce blood flow. Because alcohol can act as a peripheral vasodilator, it is often stated that alcohol intake should be avoided after any exercise that may have resulted in muscle damage. There appears, however, to be no experimental evidence to support these anecdotal observations. Clarkson and Reichsman (1990) investigated the effects of alcohol ingestion on muscle damage induced by eccentric exercise of the upper arm muscles. Female participants exercised one arm on two separate occasions, with alcohol ($0.8\,g \cdot kg^{-1}$) ingested 35 min before exercise on one occasion and a non-alcoholic drink on the other. Muscle damage was assessed by leakage of muscle-specific enzymes into the circulation, function was assessed by force generation, and subjective soreness and stiffness were also assessed. The exercise resulted in muscle damage, pain, loss of strength, and decreased range of motion, but there was no effect of alcohol on any of these responses. Nonetheless, intoxication is likely to result in inappropriate behaviours that may exacerbate existing muscle damage and delay the recovery process, and is unwise.

As more serious injury or surgical intervention results in longer-term inability to train or play, footballers may face some special problems. There may be a temptation to drink more, perhaps because of the absence of a requirement to prepare for upcoming games or because of depression at being absent from the game and from the routine of training. This may result in unwanted weight gain, apart from the potential for negative effects on the repair process in muscle and other tissues.

Alcohol and the spectator

Alcohol consumption affects not only those on the field but also those spectators on the terraces and those watching at home on television. One consequence of a ban on alcohol sales at an (American) university football stadium was a decrease in security problems: decreases in arrests, assaults, ejections from the stadium, and student disciplinary hearings were reported after implementation of the ban (Bormann & Stone, 2001). These positive outcomes were not associated with any reduction in season ticket renewals in spite of a generally negative perception from spectators. An earlier study (Spaite *et al.*, 1990) had shown no effect on the overall incidence of medical incidents among spectators after a ban on bringing alcohol into a college football stadium; there were, however, some changes in the nature of the medical emergencies treated.

Alcohol was banned from football grounds in the UK in the mid-1980s, but this has not prevented intoxication among supporters attending games. A review of medical consultations with stadium medical staff at a major Scottish football ground in a single season revealed a total of 127 casualties seen at 26 games (Crawford *et al.*, 2001). "Alcohol excess" was identified as a major contributing factor in 26 (20%) cases.

The 1998 World Cup in Paris had effects on supporters and television spectators around the world. A total of 151 patients attended the Accident and Emergency Department of Edinburgh Royal Infirmary, Scotland, over a 5 week period with conditions that were identified as being related to the World Cup (Mattick, 1999). The majority of patients were suffering from alcohol-related trauma. During the 2002 World Cup held in Korea and Japan, 47 patients attended the Emergency Department of the University College Hospital, Galway, Ireland (Mattick, Mehta, Hanrahan, & O'Donnell, 2003); more than half of all cases were alcohol-related.

References

Ama, P. F. M., Betnga, B., Ama Moor, V. J., & Kamga, J. P. (2003). Football and doping: Study of African amateur footballers. *British Journal of Sports Medicine, 37,* 301–310.

American College of Sports Medicine (ACSM) (1982). The use of alcohol in sports. *Medicine and Science in Sports and Exercise, 14,* ix–xi.

Barker, C. T. (2004). The alcohol hangover and its potential impact on the UK armed forces: A review of the literature on post-alcohol impairment. *Journal of the Royal Army Medical Corps, 150,* 168–174.

Bond, V., Franks, B. D., & Howley, E. T. (1984). Alcohol, cardiorespiratory function and work performance. *British Journal of Sports Medicine, 18,* 203–206.

Bormann, C. A., & Stone, M. H. (2001). The effects of eliminating alcohol in a college stadium: The Folsom Field beer ban. *Journal of the American College of Health, 50,* 81–88.

Burke, L. M., Collier, G. R., Broad, E. M., Davis, P. G., Martin, D. T., Sanigorski, M. A. J. *et al.* (2003). Effect of alcohol intake on muscle glycogen storage after prolonged exercise. *Journal of Applied Physiology, 95,* 983–990.

Burke, L. M., & Maughan, R. J. (2000). Alcohol in sport. In R. J. Maughan (Ed.), *Nutrition in sport* (pp. 405–416). Oxford: Blackwell.

Burke, L. M., & Read, R. S. (1988). A study of dietary patterns of elite Australian football players. *Canadian Journal of Sports Science, 13,* 15–19.

Clarkson, P. M., & Hubal, M. J. (2002). Exercise-induced muscle damage in humans. *American Journal of Physical Medicine and Rehabilitation, 81,* S52–S59.

Clarkson, P. M., & Reichsman, F. (1990). The effect of ethanol on exercise-induced muscle damage. *Journal of Studies on Alcohol, 51,* 19–23.

Collins, T., & Vamplew, W. (2002). *Mud, sweat and beers.* Oxford: Berg.

Cook, E. B., Preece, J. A., Tobin, S. D., Sugden, M. C., Cox, D. J., & Palmer, T. N. (1988). Acute inhibition by ethanol of intestinal absorption of glucose and hepatic glycogen synthesis on glycogen refeeding after starvation in the rat. *Biochemical Journal, 254,* 59–65.

Crawford, M., Donnelly, J., Gordon, J., MacCallum, R., MacDonald, I., McNeill, N. *et al.* (2001). An analysis of consultations with the crowd doctors at Glasgow Celtic football club, season 1999–2000. *British Journal of Sports Medicine, 35,* 245–249.

Eggleton, M. G. (1942). The diuretic action of alcohol in man. *Journal of Physiology, 101,* 172–191.

El-Sayed, M. S., Ali, N., & El-Sayed, A. Z. (2005). Interactions between alcohol and exercise: Physiological and haematological implications. *Sports Medicine, 35,* 257–269.

Francesconi, R., & Mager, M. (1981). Alcohol consumption in rats: Effects on work capacity in the heat. *Journal of Applied Physiology, 50,* 1006–1010.

Garry, J. P., & Morrissey, S. L. (2000). Team sports participation and risk-taking behaviours among a biracial middle school population. *Clinical Journal of Sports Medicine, 10,* 185–190.

Goldberg, I. J., Mosca, L., Piano, M. R., & Fisher, E. A. (2001). AHA science advisory: Wine and your heart. *Circulation, 103,* 472–475.

Graham, T. (1981). Alcohol ingestion and man's ability to adapt to exercise in a cold environment. *Canadian Journal of Applied Sport Science, 6,* 27–31.

Hebbelinck, M. (1963). The effects of a small dose of ethyl alcohol on certain basic components of human physical performance. *Archives in Pharmacodynamics, 143,* 247–257.

Hellandsjø, Bu, E. T., Watten, R. G., Foxcroft, D. R., Ingebrigtsen, J. E., & Relling, G. (2002). Teenage alcohol and intoxication debut: The impact of family socialization factors, living area and participation in organised sports. *Alcohol and Alcoholism, 37,* 74–80.

Houmard, J. A., Lagenfield, M. E., & Wiley, R. L. (1987). Effects of the acute ingestion of small amounts of alcohol upon 5-mile run times. *Journal of Sports Medicine and Physical Fitness*, *27*, 253–257.

Ibrahim, F., & Gilvarry, E. (2005). Alcohol dependence and treatment strategies. *British Journal of Hospital Medicine*, *66*, 462–465.

Jorfeldt, L., & Juhlin-Dannfelt, A. (1978). The influence of ethanol on splanchnic and skeletal muscle metabolism in man. *Metabolism*, *27*, 97–106.

Kalant, H., & Lê, A. D. (1983). Effects of ethanol on thermoregulation. *Pharmacological Therapy*, *23*, 313–364.

Kendrick Z. V., Affrime, M. B., & Lowenthal, D. T. (1993). Effect of ethanol on metabolic responses to treadmill running in well-trained men. *Journal of Clinical Pharmacology*, *33*, 136–139.

Kupari, M. (1983). Drunkenness, hangover, and the heart. *Acta Medica Scandinavica*, *213*, 84–90.

Lorente, F. O., Peretti-Watel, P., Griffet, J., & Grelot, L. (2003). Alcohol use and intoxication in sport university students. *Alcohol and Alcoholism*, *38*, 427–430.

Lorente, F. O., Souville, M., Griffet, J., & Grelot, L. (2004). Participation in sports and alcohol consumption among French adolescents. *Addiction and Behaviour*, *29*, 941–946.

Macdonald, I. (1999). *Health issues related to alcohol consumption* (2nd edn.). Oxford: Blackwell Science.

Mattick, A. P. (1999). The Football World Cup 1998: An analysis of related attendances to an accident and emergency department. *Scottish Medical Journal*, *44*, 75–76.

Mattick, A. P., Mehta, R., Hanrahan, H., & O'Donnell, J. J. (2003). The Football World Cup 2002 – analysis of related attendances to an Irish Emergency Department. *Irish Medical Journal*, *96*, 90–91.

Maughan, R. J. (1997). Energy and macronutrient intakes of professional football (soccer) players. *British Journal of Sports Medicine*, *31*, 45–47.

McNaughton, L., & Preece, D. (1986). Alcohol and its effects on sprint and middle distance running. *British Journal of Sports Medicine*, *20*, 56–59.

Moore, M. J., & Werch, C. E. (2004). Sport and physical activity participation and substance use among adolescents. *Journal of Adolescent Health*, *36*, 486–493.

National Diet and Nutrition Survey (2003). http://www.food.gov.uk/multimedia/pdfs/ndnsv2 (accessed 18 July 2005).

National Institute on Alcohol Abuse and Alcoholism (2000). *Tenth annual report to the US Congress on alcohol and health*. Washington, DC: National Institute on Alcohol Abuse and Alcoholism.

O'Brien, C. P. (1993). Alcohol and sport: Impact of social drinking on recreational and competitive sports. *Sports Medicine*, *15*, 71–77.

O'Brien, C. P., & Lyons, F. (2000). Alcohol and the athlete. *Sports Medicine*, *29*, 295–300.

O'Brien, K. S., Blackie, J. M., & Hunter, J. A. (2005). Hazardous drinking in elite New Zealand sportspeople. *Alcohol and Alcoholism*, *40*, 239–241.

Pastor, Y., Balaguer, I., Pons, D., & Garcia-Merita, M. (2003). Testing direct and indirect effects of sports participation on perceived health in Spanish adolescents between 15 and 18 years of age. *Journal of Adolescence*, *26*, 717–730.

Preedy, V. R., Duane, P., & Peters, T. J. (1988). Comparison of the acute effects of ethanol on liver and skeletal muscle protein synthesis in the rat. *Alcohol and Alcoholism, 23*, 155–162.

Reilly, T. (2003). Alcohol, anti-anxiety drugs and sport. In D. R. Mottram (Ed.), *Drugs in sport* (3rd edn., pp 256–285). London: Routledge.

Roberts, K. E. (1963). Mechanism of dehydration following alcohol ingestion. *Archives of Internal Medicine, 112*, 154–157.

Shirreffs, S. M., & Maughan, R. J. (1997). Restoration of fluid balance after exercise-induced dehydration: Effects of alcohol consumption. *Journal of Applied Physiology, 83*, 1152–1158.

Spaite, D. W., Meislin, H. W., Valenzuela, T. D., Criss, E. A., Smith, R., & Nelson, A. (1990). Banning alcohol in a major college stadium: Impact on the incidence and patterns of injury and illness. *Journal of the American College of Health, 39*, 125–128.

Wiese, J. G., Shlipak, M. G., & Browner, W. S. (2000). The alcohol hangover. *Annals of Internal Medicine, 132*, 897–902.

Xu, D., Heng, J. K., & Palmer, T. N. (1993). The mechanism(s) of the alcohol-induced impairment in glycogen synthesis in oxidative skeletal muscles. *Biochemistry and Molecular Biology International, 30*, 169–176.

8 Dietary supplements for football

P. HESPEL, R. J. MAUGHAN AND
P. L. GREENHAFF

Physical training and competition in football markedly increase the need for macro- and micronutrient intake. This requirement can generally be met by dietary management without the need for dietary supplements. In fact, the efficacy of most supplements available on the market is unproven. In addition, players must be cautious of inadequate product labelling and supplement impurities that may cause a positive drug test. Nonetheless, a number of dietary supplements may beneficially affect football performance. A high endurance capacity is a prerequisite for optimal match performance, particularly if extra time is played. In this context, the potential of low-dose caffeine ingestion (2–5 mg·kg body mass^{-1}) to enhance endurance performance is well established. However, in the case of football, care must be taken not to overdose because visual information processing might be impaired. Scoring and preventing goals as a rule requires production of high power output. Dietary creatine supplementation (loading dose: 15–20 g·day^{-1}, 4–5 days; maintenance dose: 2–5 g g·day^{-1}) has been found to increase muscle power output, especially during intermittent sprint exercises. Furthermore, creatine intake can augment muscle adaptations to resistance training. Team success and performance also depend on player availability, and thus injury prevention and health maintenance. Glucosamine or chondroitin may be useful in the treatment of joint pain and osteoarthritis, but there is no evidence to support the view that the administration of these supplements will be preventative. Ephedra-containing weight-loss cocktails should certainly be avoided due to reported adverse health effects and positive doping outcomes. Finally, the efficacy of antioxidant or vitamin C intake in excess of the normal recommended dietary dose is equivocal. Responses to dietary supplements can vary substantially between individuals, and therefore the ingestion of any supplement must be assessed in training before being used in competition. It is recommended that dietary supplements are only used based on the advice of a qualified sports nutrition professional.

Keywords: Soccer, exercise, muscle, nutrition

Introduction

The marketing pressure by the sports nutrition industry on athletic populations and sports nutrition professionals has engendered the widely held belief that the intake of dietary supplements is an essential part of participation in sports and physical activity. Many sports organizations and federations, as well as teams or individual athletes, also obtain substantial sponsorship from supplement companies. In the case of football, the administration of sports supplements has become a more or less standard procedure, often promoted by team physicians, coaches, and even the parents of young players. In this review, the relevance of supplement intake in football is discussed from a scientific perspective, together with some ethical concerns associated with supplement intake and sports education.

It is important to recognize that adequate intake of fluid and carbohydrate is crucial to endurance capacity and thus also to match performance in football, but these supplements are excluded from this review as they are covered elsewhere. In contrast to all supplements discussed in this review, the ingestion of supplements/drinks containing only water, electrolytes, and carbohydrates (so-called "fluid replenishers" and "energy drinks/gels/bars") can be seen as essential to adequate energy supply and rehydration during football at any level of competition (Burke, Loucks, & Broad, 2006; Shirreffs, Sawka, & Stone, 2006). Supplementation of water and carbohydrates in football not only serves ergogenic purposes but is also important for the prevention of adverse effects that could be associated with carbohydrate depletion and/or dehydration. Secondly, evidence is increasing to indicate that the ingestion of carbohydrate/protein-amino acid mixtures during the early phase of recovery from high-intensity exercise could facilitate post-exercise muscle glycogen storage as well as muscle protein synthesis, and thereby may enhance recovery and long-term adaptations to training (Hawley, Tipton, & Millard-Stafford, 2006).

Is there a need for supplements in football?

Training for and playing football can markedly increase the need for macro- and micronutrients. At a professional level, with often sustained periods of two matches per week, interspersed with training sessions, this increase can be substantial. However, this need can be covered adequately by dietary management, and establishing good eating practices to achieve the consistent intake of a well-balanced and healthy diet should be the primary nutritional strategy to support optimum performance in football (Burke *et al.*, 2006). Such practices include manipulation of the quantity and type of foods to meet fluctuating energy needs, the selection of food sources to provide adequate carbohydrate, protein, and micronutrients and, last but not least, the specific timing of intake of nutrients to facilitate recovery between exercise and promote adaptations to training (Hawley *et al.*, 2006; Williams & Serratosa, 2006). Therefore, coaches, physicians, parents, and others who are engaged in the training and education process of footballers must pay particular attention to developing adequate eating habits in players, rather than promoting the use of dietary supplements to compensate for presumed dietary shortcomings. This is particularly true for young players, who should be able to develop their football talent by the optimum combination of training and diet. It is most doubtful that the addition of dietary supplements could facilitate the expression of football talent.

Nevertheless, appropriate ingestion of some specific supplements in conjunction with appropriate training can contribute to enhanced performance in football. At its most basic, the most important measure of performance in football is the number of goals scored versus the number of goals conceded, but there are no research data to show that nutritional supplements can improve this balance. But there is sound scientific evidence that some supplements can affect factors that determine football performance. The so-called "ergogenic" effects of these supplements, however, are generally small, and thus probably relevant only in top-class footballers where extremely small differences in performance can make the difference between loss and victory, with potentially major financial and career implications. To counterbalance the strong marketing pressures generated by the supplement industry, it is important that players are well educated about effective procedures for supplement intake. It is also important to recognize that responses to supplements vary among players, and supplements that work for one player may not necessarily work for another. Furthermore, the use of supplements must always be tested in training before being applied in competition, to avoid unexpected side-effects. Each individual player must consider whether the small benefit obtained from supplement ingestion outweighs the associated risks (see below).

Risks associated with the use of dietary supplements

The market for nutritional supplements has become a multi-billion dollar business, spreading supplements worldwide. Unfortunately, in many cases, the labelling of products does not correspond with the actual content of the product. Some products contain less active ingredients than indicated on the label, or no active substance at all (Green, Catlin, & Starcevic, 2001). A typical example of such malpractice is the so-called "creatine-serum", which after several years of aggressive marketing and sales was recently demonstrated by several independent laboratories to contain no creatine (Harris, Almada, Harris, Dunnett, & Hespel, 2004). On the other hand, products have been found to contain substances not included on the label or much more active ingredients than indicated on the label (Gurley, Gardner, & Hubbard, 2000; Parasrampuria, Schwartz, & Petesch, 1998). Most alarming is the finding from recent field surveys that apparently innocent over-the-counter products that, according to the label, were supposed to contain only harmless compounds, contained pharmacological quantities of the anabolic steroid metadienone (De Cock *et al.*, 2001; Geyer *et al.*, 2004; Parr, Geyer, Reinhart, & Schanzer, 2004). This indicates that some companies will not hesitate to potentiate the purported actions of their sports supplements by the addition of dangerous prescription drugs, a practice that is criminal. Besides conceivable adverse health effects, the intake of such supplements could result in a positive doping test. For example, a substantial fraction (10–25%) of a variety of "off-the-shelf" supplements was found to be contaminated by androgenic prohormones, including compounds related to testosterone and nandrolone (Geyer *et al.*, 2004; www.dopinginfo.de). Ingestion of some androgenic prohormones (19-noradrostenedione and 19-norandrostenediol) can produce a positive doping test for nandrolone (Delbeke, Van

Eenoo, Van Thuyne, & Desmet, 2002; Geyer *et al.*, 2004), as has occurred on many occasions in football and in other sports. Some supplements produced from plant extracts may contain substances that are on the banned substances list, primarily ephedrine (=ephedra) and morphine (Van Thuyne, Van Eenoo, & Delbeke, 2003). Typically, the product label would identify the plant of origin, such as "Ma Huang", but not the illegal compound, ephedra. It is important to emphasize that players at the higher levels of the game must expect to be tested for substance abuse, and must accept the consequences, irrespective of whether the doping regulations have been violated on purpose or by accident, for instance by the ingestion of a contaminated supplement. Furthermore, many dietary supplements have been found to contain micro- and macro-contaminants resulting from poor production and packaging practices in often unhygienic conditions. Last but not least, it is important to note that adequate long-term safety data are lacking for most sports supplements. The absence of reported side-effects in small-scale or short-term studies does not therefore prove that the supplement *is* safe. In addition, even if the active ingredient appears to be safe, the real risk may lie with the impurity of the product. Thus, consistent caution is warranted.

Selection of supplements that are relevant to football

Thousands of supplements, mostly pseudo-supplements, are available for purchase. To recognize supplements that are potentially effective and relevant to football, three requirements have been identified:

1. The supplement must work, which means that it must influence physical/ physiological, mental, or health factors that determine performance in football.
2. The supplement must not cause any adverse health effects.
3. The supplement must be legal – that is, it must not contain any substance named in the banned substance list, or alternatively a substance that could result in a positive doping test.

It is reasonable to state that athletes should not ingest supplements that simply have no effect. Thus, supplements must have measurable effects on performance or on performance-related factors that go beyond the placebo effect that may result from the psychological effect of supplement intake. Still, football coaches and physicians should probably also appreciate that dietary supplements can serve as excellent placebos, provided they have no detrimental effects on either health or performance. If used as a placebo, it must be done for a small selection of important matches only.

It is probably correct to conclude that the acute ingestion of some dietary supplements could produce an ergogenic effect in football by directly enhancing match performance. Similarly, it is probably correct to state that some supplements could improve performance over the longer term by having a beneficial

Table 1. Supplements that work in some exercise situations

Supplement	Ergogenic or health effects	Physiological mechanisms linked to the observed effects
Amino acids/ protein hydrolysate/ protein[a]	Increases muscle volume/ fat-free mass Stimulates recovery from exercise	Stimulates muscle amino acid uptake Stimulates muscle protein synthesis Stimulates insulin release Stimulates muscle glycogen resynthesis
Caffeine	Enhances endurance performance Stimulates reaction time, mental alertness, and visual information processing	Stimulates lipolysis and muscle fat oxidation rate Stimulates exogenous carbohydrate oxidation Increases heart rate Psychostimulatory action
Carbohydrates[b]	Enhance endurance performance Stimulates recovery from exercise	Stimulates and maintains muscle carbohydrate oxidation Prevents hypoglycaemia Stimulates muscle glycogen resynthesis Stimulates insulin release Increases endurance training workload Inhibits muscle protein degradation
Creatine	Stimulates muscle strength and power Increases muscle volume/ fat-free mass Stimulates recovery from exercise	Increases muscle creatine content Facilitates muscle phosphocreatine resynthesis Shortens muscle relaxation time Increases resistance training workload Stimulates muscle glycogen resynthesis
Ephedra[c]	Facilitates short-term weight loss	Stimulates sympathetic nervous system Enhances resting energy expenditure

[a] For details on this category of supplements, see Hawley *et al.* (2006).
[b] For details on this category of supplements, see Burke *et al.* (2006), Shirreffs *et al.* (2006), and Williams and Serratosa (2006).
[c] This supplement is on the list of substances banned by WADA.

effect on health and injury prevention. Table 1 lists a number of supplements that work, and from a scientific perspective appear to be relevant to football. For most of these supplements, one or more physiological mechanisms have been elucidated to explain its purported performance or health effect. Table 2, on the other hand, contains a number of supplements that *may* work. Scientific evidence to support these supplements is at present inconclusive, yet there are some valid data to suggest that these compounds might have some potential in aiding performance. However, further research is needed to justify any recommendation to use these products (see Table 2). Scrutiny of Tables 1 and 2 will demonstrate that most commercially available supplements are not listed. This means that scientific support for an ergogenic or health effect is currently lacking, or more frequently that available research data indicate that

Table 2. Supplements that may work in some exercise situations*

Supplement	Ergogenic or health effects claimed	Proposed physiological mechanisms linked to the effects claimed
Antioxidants	Prevents muscle damage	Enhances defence against formation of reactive oxygen species in contracting muscles
Beta-hydroxy-β-methylbutyrate	Stimulates muscle strength and power Increases muscle volume/fat-free mass	Inhibits contraction-induced muscle cell degradation
Glucosamine	Alleviates joint pain Reduces symptoms of osteoarthritis	Stimulates the formation of bone cartilage
Vitamin C	Stimulates the immune system	Stimulates the activity of neutrophils, monocytes, and lymphocytes

* The available literature is inconclusive in supporting a possible "ergogenic" action in healthy individuals. Further studies are warranted.

these supplements do not work in healthy individuals and athletes. Some of the most popular sports supplements, such as l-carnitine, co-enzyme Q10, ginseng and other so-called "adaptogens", glutamine, and ribose fall within this category of pseudo-sports supplements. Therefore, they will not be considered further.

Supplements for endurance

Aerobic endurance is a pivotal determinant of performance in football. Match duration in football is 90 min and can increase to 120 min when extra time is played. During this period, players on average perform between 9 and 12 km of intermittent running exercise, of which about 10% is sprinting (Reilly, 2005). There is no doubt that adequate pre-match and half-time carbohydrate intake can substantially improve endurance capacity as well as intermittent sprint power in the final stages of a match (Williams & Serratosa, 2006). Furthermore, bicarbonate and other alkalinizing agents like sodium citrate are also frequently considered as ergogenic supplements in all-out anaerobic exercise (Horswill, 1995; Matson & Tran, 1993). Bicarbonate intake (200–300 mg · kg body mass^{-1}) increases buffer capacity, and can significantly enhance performance during short maximal exercise bouts lasting from about 20 s to about 5 min. However, gastrointestinal distress, mostly cramping, diarrhoea or vomiting, associated with bicarbonate intake can be substantial. It is unlikely that the small beneficial effect possibly obtained from bicarbonate intake during the initial stage of a football match could outweigh the risk for gastrointestinal distress in a later stage, usually starting about 1 h after ingestion. Therefore, bicarbonate is not considered to be a sensible supplement in the context of football. Other supplements to be considered are caffeine and creatine.

Caffeine

Caffeine is a popular stimulant used by most individuals, including athletes. Caffeine is contained in coffee, tea, chocolate, and many other caffeinated food sources like cola. The physiological mechanisms of action of caffeine are only partially understood. Caffeine has been shown to stimulate fat utilization, leading to a reduced rate of muscle glycogen breakdown, but this does not appear to explain changes in performance. More likely, caffeine beneficially affects performance by reducing perception of fatigue, enhancing central drive, and/or improving muscle fibre recruitment (Graham, 2001; Magkos & Kavouras, 2004). The stimulatory action of caffeine on the brain is probably mediated by adenosine receptor blockade (Davis *et al.*, 2003).

The ergogenic effect of caffeine in endurance exercise performance is well established (for recent reviews, see Doherty & Smith, 2005; Graham, 2001; Magkos & Kavouras, 2004), which explains its extensive use by endurance athletes. Early studies demonstrated that the ingestion of caffeine doses of between 5 and 13 mg · kg body mass^{-1} caused a substantial improvement in endurance exercise capacity (Graham & Spriet, 1991; Pasman, Van Baak, Jeukendrup, & de Haan, 1995). However, more recent studies have shown that caffeine can be equally as effective at lower doses in the range of 2–6 mg · kg body mass^{-1} (Graham & Spriet, 1995; Kovacs, Stegen, & Brouns, 1998). In a study that used a sensitive exercise performance model and that employed well-trained cyclists as participants, it was shown that the ingestion of as little as about 90 mg of caffeine during a 2 h exercise test could result in significant performance improvements in a subsequent time-trial (Cox *et al.*, 2002b). Caffeine is rapidly absorbed and if ingested during the pre-match warm-up, the performance effects will be maintained for the entire match, even if extra time is played (Bell & McLellan, 2002). For example, when ingested on an empty stomach, peak plasma levels are usually reached within 1 h. However, the ergogenic effect is maintained for at least 3 h after ingestion. Intake of a caffeine in the form of coffee yields smaller effects than intake of a similar dose of pure caffeine (Graham, Hibbert, & Sathasivam, 1998), and there may be some gastrointestinal distress associated with drinking strong coffee (Tarnopolsky, 1994).

Responses to caffeine intake and withdrawal can vary greatly among individuals depending on the degree of habituation (Bangsbo, Jacobsen, Nordberg, Christensen, & Graham, 1992; Bell & McLellan, 2002; Fisher, McMurray, Berry, Mar, & Forsythe, 1986; Graham, 2001; Hetzler, Warhaftig-Glynn, Thompson, Dowling, & Weltman, 1994; Magkos & Kavouras, 2004; Van Soeren & Graham, 1998; Van Soeren, Sathasivam, Spriet, & Graham, 1993). Therefore, individual tuning of the dosage in the context of training is very important. Frequent high-dose caffeine intake results in rapid desensitization.

This in turn establishes the need to use even higher doses. Hence a rational use of caffeine in football probably ideally includes moderate daily caffeine use, with acute caffeine spikes on match days (3–6 mg · kg body mass^{-1} during warming up). It is sometimes suggested that habitual caffeine users should consider withdrawing from caffeine for about 4 days to enhance the beneficial effects of an acute pre-match caffeine dose, but the evidence for performance benefits when this is done is not entirely convincing. In addition, the participants in the study of Cox et al. (2002b) were habitual caffeine users and yet a positive effect on performance was seen with only 90 mg of caffeine. Besides its effect on endurance, small doses of caffeine (1–2 mg · kg body mass^{-1}) can also beneficially influence reaction time, alertness, and visual information processing, which are crucial to success in goalkeeping and outfield play (Haskell, Kennedy, Wesnes, & Scholey, 2005). However, overdosing will negatively affect reaction time and alertness, which might counterbalance the stimulatory effect of caffeine on endurance performance (Figure 1). Similarly, it could be argued that the metabolic effects of high-dose caffeine intake could induce insulin resistance in skeletal muscle and tachycardia. For the goalkeeper the lower dose (1–2 mg · kg body mass^{-1}) is obvious, while the outfield players should

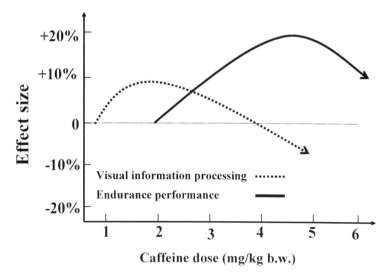

Figure 1. Caffeine affects both visual information processing and endurance capacity. However, the dose needed to yield an optimal effect on visual information processing is substantially lower than that required to yield an optimal effect on endurance capacity. If too high a dose of caffeine is ingested, caffeine can impair visual information processing. Therefore, outfield players should seek a dose to enhance endurance capacity, without negatively affecting visual information processing, whereas goalkeepers should stick to the lower dose. Depending on the degree of habituation, responses to a given caffeine dose can vary greatly between individuals, with habitual caffeine users needing higher doses. Therefore, the doses indicated on the x-axis, as well as the effect-size on the y-axis, are indicative.

rather seek a dosage to enhance endurance without causing mental over-arousal and gross metabolic and heart rate perturbations.

The common use of caffeine as a social stimulant in society probably proves that low-dose caffeine intake can be considered safe. However, high-dose caffeine intake is widely thought to be associated with adverse health effects, in particular at the level of the cardiovascular system (Tarnopolsky, 1994). The diuretic effect of caffeine at the doses recommended here is negligible, which means that there is no reason to avoid caffeine intake or withdraw from caffeine-containing beverages in the approach to matches to be played in hot environmental conditions (Armstrong *et al.*, 2005; Maughan & Griffin, 2003).

Caffeine use in competition was formerly considered as doping by the International Olympic Committee in cases where the intake produced urinary caffeine concentrations higher than $12\,\mu g \cdot ml^{-1}$. However, in early 2004 the World Anti-Doping Agency (WADA) removed caffeine from the list of banned substances, although its use is being monitored. Still, the discussion does not seem to be closed and the regulations might change again.

Creatine

Dietary creatine supplementation is popular in athletic populations, and it has been reported on numerous occasions to increase muscle strength and power (see next section for further details on this topic). However, co-ingestion of creatine with a carbohydrate-rich diet can enhance post-exercise glycogen repletion in humans (Robinson, Sewell, Hultman, Greenhaff, 1999; van Loon *et al.*, 2004). There is no direct evidence for a beneficial effect on endurance performance (Terjung *et al.*, 2000), but this latter effect might facilitate the restoration of muscle glycogen stores following exercise, especially when recovery time between matches is limited.

Supplements for strength and power

In addition to the requirement for a high endurance capacity to maintain running ability throughout a match, footballers must also be able to produce high power outputs. It is unquestionable that the ability to suddenly accelerate, perform short maximal intermittent sprints, jump higher than the opponent, or generate high kicking and tackling forces is a prerequisite of high-level football performance (Reilly, 2005). Muscle strength is an important determinant of maximal power output in all athletes. Therefore, supplements that have the potential to enhance muscle strength and power are important to football. Issues pertaining to the stimulation of resistance training adaptations as a result of the ingestion of amino acid-protein-carbohydrate supplements are addressed in detail elsewhere (Hawley *et al.*, 2006). In the context of this review, however, two additional supplements need to be considered, creatine and to a lesser extent 3-hydroxymethylbutyrate.

Creatine

Creatine is a natural guanidine compound occurring in meat and fish in concentrations of between 3 and $7 \, g \cdot kg^{-1}$ (Walker, 1979). Synthetic creatine supplements exist as creatine monohydrate or various creatine salts, such as creatine citrate or creatine pyruvate. There is no evidence that so-called "special" creatine formulations are better than simple (and cheaper!) creatine monohydrate powder. However, creatine salts, in contrast with creatine monohydrate, are easily soluble and stable in solution and thus could be included in sports drinks or gels. On the other hand, creatine monohydrate must be consumed soon after it is brought in to solution. It is well established that creatine supplementation can enhance power output during short maximal sprints (Terjung *et al.*, 2000), in particular during intermittent exercise modes (Casey, Constantin-Teodosiu, Howell, Hultman, & Greenhaff, 1996; Greenhaff, Casey, Short, Harris, & Söderlund, 1993; Hespel *et al.*, 2001; Van Leemputte, Vandenberghe, & Hespel, 1999; Vandenberghe *et al.*, 1996, 1997), even when contained in an endurance exercise event like football (Cox, Mujika, Tumilty, & Burke, 2002a; Mujika, Padilla, Ibañez, Izquierdo, & Gorostiaga, 2000; Vandebuerie, Vanden Eynde, Vandenberghe, & Hespel, 1998). Furthermore, several studies have shown that creatine supplementation can potentiate the gains in fat-free mass and muscle force and power output that accompany resistance training (Hespel *et al.*, 2001; Kreider *et al.*, 1998; Maganaris & Maughan, 1998; Volek *et al.*, 1999).

A classical creatine loading regimen consists of an initial loading phase ($15-20 \, g \cdot day^{-1}$ for 4–7 days) followed by a maintenance dose ($2-5 \, g \cdot day^{-1}$) (Terjung *et al.*, 2000). However, there are some data to indicate that the effects of creatine supplementation may fade after 2 months (Derave, Eijnde, & Hespel, 2003). Although research data in this regard are still lacking, it is probably sensible to interrupt periods of creatine supplementation (8–10 weeks) with wash-out periods of at least 4 weeks. Individuals with a low initial muscle creatine content, like vegetarians (Burke *et al.*, 2003; Delanghe *et al.*, 1989; Watt, Garnham, & Snow, 2004), respond better to creatine supplementation than others with a high natural muscle creatine content. Ingesting creatine in conjunction with training sessions can stimulate muscle creatine uptake, as exercise is known to facilitate the disposal of ingested creatine into musculature (Harris, Söderlund, & Hultman, 1992; Robinson *et al.*, 1999). Ingesting creatine supplements in combination with post-exercise carbohydrate-amino acid-protein supplements can enhance muscle creatine retention by virtue of elevated circulating insulin concentrations (Green, Hultman, Macdonald, Sewell, & Greenhaff, 1996; Steenge, Simpson, & Greenhaff, 2000).

Creatine is not on the doping list and creatine intake in healthy adults, following the aforementioned guidelines, has been found to be generally safe (Terjung *et al.*, 2000). Initial concern with regard to the potential adverse effects of creatine on renal function has been dampened by studies showing intact renal function after acute and prolonged dietary creatine intake (Poortmans *et al.*,

1997; Poortmans & Francaux, 1999). Creatine loading is often accompanied by a rapid increase in body mass (1–3 kg within 3–4 days is not uncommon), which probably results mainly from intracellular water and/or glycogen accumulation driven by muscle creatine uptake. This increase in muscle water content may increase intramuscular pressure, which in some few individuals may predispose to development of a compartment syndrome (Schroeder *et al.*, 2001).

The physiological mechanisms underlying the effects of creatine supplementation are only partly understood. There are data to indicate that the increased muscle creatine content due to creatine intake can facilitate flux through the creatine kinase reaction and thereby prevent net ATP degradation during high-intensity muscle contractions (Casey *et al.*, 1996). This could also explain the shortening of muscle relaxation time seen after creatine loading (Van Leemputte *et al.*, 1999). Furthermore, stimulation of muscle phosphocreatine resynthesis probably contributes to enhanced recovery between intermittent bouts of short maximal exercise (Greenhaff, Bodin, Söderlund, & Hultman, 1994). The mechanisms underlying the potential of creatine to stimulate muscle anabolism during resistance training are unclear. One study has found creatine intake to stimulate satellite cell proliferation (Dangott, Schultz, & Mozdziak, 1999). Others have observed creatine to impinge on intracellular signalling pathways involved in regulation of muscle protein metabolism (Deldicque *et al.*, 2005; Louis, Van Beneden, Dehoux, Theisen, & Francaux, 2004). However, direct evidence that creatine can stimulate net protein synthesis in human muscle is missing (Louis *et al.*, 2003a, 2003b). Alternatively, changes in muscle protein accretion can occur as a consequence of individuals performing more work during high-intensity training programmes while consuming creatine (Kreider *et al.*, 1998). At least part of the increase in body mass due to creatine intake does not reflect protein accretion but intracellular water accumulation (Ziegenfuss, Lowery, & Lemon, 1998).

Beta-hydroxy-β-methylbutyrate (HMB)

HMB is a naturally occurring metabolite of the branched-chain amino acid leucine. Based on observations in animals (Chua, Siehl, & Morgan, 1979; Tischler, Desautels, & Goldberg, 1982), it was hypothesized that this compound could contribute to muscle anabolism by mediating the action of leucine to inhibit muscle protein breakdown (Gallagher, Carrithers, Godard, Schulze, & Trappe, 2000a; Nissen *et al.*, 1996). Over the past 10 years, a small number of studies have looked at the potential of oral HMB to stimulate muscle hypertrophy (for a recent review, see Nissen & Sharp, 2003). Published results are equivocal, yet a recent meta-analysis of available data suggested that HMB intake at a rate of 1.5–$3.0 \, \mathrm{g \cdot day^{-1}}$ could result in larger gains in fat-free mass and muscle power output associated with resistance training. This effect may be due to inhibition of contraction-induced proteolysis (Nissen *et al.*, 1996). Short-term HMB intake (1–8 weeks) does not appear to induce any detrimental side-effects (Gallagher, Carrithers, Godard, Schulze, & Trappe, 2000b; Nissen *et al.*, 1996; Nissen & Sharp, 2003), but there are no data on its long-term (>8 weeks) effects and side-effects. HMB is not on the doping list. In summary, overall evidence in favour of an ergogenic action of HMB is weak and more data from independent laboratories are needed.

Supplements for health

Long-term team performance in football depends to a large extent on the degree of match participation by the better players. In this respect, some supplements might contribute to injury prevention or rehabilitation from injury, health maintenance, or prevention of fatigue and overtraining.

Antioxidants

Oxygen utilization in contracting muscles results in the formation of reactive oxygen species (ROS), which, if produced in excess of the muscle antioxidant defence system, may result in muscle cell damage (Sen, 2001). However, one should also consider that the formation of ROS probably also contributes to promoting training adaptations by impinging on intracellular signalling pathways during exercise (Sen, 2001). Still, using only the former argument, a number of antioxidant nutritional supplements are marketed to prevent muscle tissue damage in athletes. This primarily includes beta carotene, vitamins C and E, selenium, ubiquinone, and several phytochemicals (Clarkson & Thompson, 2000; Ji & Peterson, 2004; Sen, 2001; Urso & Clarkson, 2003). Available research on the potential ergogenic effects of antioxidant supplements is equivocal, and there is no consensus as to whether strenuous exercise training increases the need for antioxidants in the diet. Numerous studies have looked at the potential of single or combined antioxidant supplements on indices of exercise-induced muscle damage. Some studies have found small beneficial effects, but others have found no effect, while one study even reported antioxidant intake to exaggerate tissue damage (Barr & Rideout, 2004; Clarkson & Thompson, 2000; Sen, 2001; Urso & Clarkson, 2003). Against this background, and awaiting further scientific evidence, there is probably no sound scientific rationale to recommend antioxidant supplementation in footballers. It definitely is a better option to include a selection of foods with a high content of antioxidants in the daily diet (Kris-Etherton, Lichtenstein, Howard, Steinberg, & Witztum, 2004; and see www.americanheart.org).

Creatine

Creatine can enhance the gain of fat-free mass produced by a given amount of resistance training. It also has been demonstrated that creatine supplementation can facilitate the recovery of muscle volume and muscular functional capacity during rehabilitation training following an episode of muscle atrophy due to leg immobilization (Hespel *et al.*, 2001). Given the high incidence of leg injuries and concomitant muscle disuse atrophy in football, creatine supplementation may be a worthwhile option to enhance post-injury rehabilitation and thereby speed up return to training and competition.

Glucosamine

The incidence of knee- and ankle-joint injuries is conceivably higher in football than in any other sport and frequently prevents players from participating in training and competition. Glucosamine and chondroitin are two popular substances being promoted for maintenance of joint health (Gorsline & Kaeding, 2005). In Europe these substances are sold only in the form of prescription drugs, while in the USA they are available as over-the-counter dietary supplements. It is believed that both glucosamine and chondroitin can help to enhance the structural integrity and resilience of bone cartilage. Discordant findings with regard to the effects of glucosamine and chondroitin have been reported (McAlindon, LaValley, Gulin, & Felson, 2000). However, it is probably correct to conclude from some well-controlled studies that glucosamine can retard the progression of osteoarthritis, at least in older people (Pavelka *et al.*, 2002; Reginster *et al.*, 2001). Furthermore, observations in older individuals with chronic knee pain indicate that glucosamine can yield an analgesic effect and serve as an alternative or adjuvant treatment to non-steroid anti-inflammatory drugs (Braham, Dawson, & Goodman, 2003). A recent safety review of glucosamine concluded that glucosamine supplementation in accordance with current indications and dosage regimens (20–25 mg · kg body mass^{-1}) is probably safe. Bloating or diarrhoea may occur, and individuals with shellfish allergies should refrain from glucosamine intake (Anderson, Nicolosi, & Borzelleca, 2005).

Footballers could also consider using glucosamine or chondroitin supplementation as a strategy to prevent knee pain or osteoarthritis. However, this practice is certainly premature because there is currently no evidence to indicate that glucosamine or chondroitin could serve to prevent osteoarthritis and/or joint pain in healthy athletes. It is also important to note that most data with regard to the effects of glucosamine and chondroitin have been obtained from studies involving older individuals, and thus it is unclear whether these findings can be readily extrapolated to young footballers afflicted by knee pain or osteoarthritis.

Vitamin C

It is well established that strenuous exercise training, including the repetition of football games, can have an immunosuppressive effect (Gleeson & Bishop, 2000; Gleeson, Lancaster, & Bishop, 2001; Gleeson, Nieman, & Pedersen, 2004; Gleeson & Pyne, 2000; Hiscock & Pedersen, 2002; Lakier, 2003; Malm, Ekblom, Ekblom, 2004; Nieman, 2001, Nieman *et al.*, 2003; Nieman *et al.*, 2002; Pedersen & Toft, 2000). Because vitamin C has been suggested to be implicated in immunoregulation (Bhaskaram, 2002), it could play a role in reducing the incidence of infectious disease, which is important for keeping players fit and available to play. Research findings on the effect of vitamin C on infectious disease or on markers of immune function are equivocal. Recent reviews of available studies concluded that vitamin C supplementation does not beneficially affect the risk of developing a cold, yet could slightly (~8%) reduce the duration of a cold (Douglas, Hemila, D'Souza, Chalker, & Treacy, 2004; Hemila, 1996, 2004). However, such an effect requires a vitamin C dose of only about $200 \text{ mg} \cdot \text{day}^{-1}$, which is very easy to obtain from a well-balanced diet (see Table 3).

Supplements for weight reduction

Body weight gains can be a problem for some athletes, including footballers. Excess body fat can impair endurance capacity and power output during football. The logical strategy to reduce body weight is to shift the balance of dietary energy intake relative to energy expenditure towards a net deficit, primarily by reducing energy intake. However, not all players can achieve the expected body fat goal in this way. Therefore, players often seek the assistance of "fat-burning supplements" to facilitate body weight reduction. Ephedra is a popular supplement in this regard. As mentioned earlier, L-carnitine is not an effective dietary supplement. Although carnitine plays an essential role in fat oxidation in skeletal muscle, dietary supplementation with L-carnitine does not increase

Table 3. Some foods with a very high content ($>50 \text{ mg} \cdot 100 \text{ g}^{-1}$) of vitamin C

Food product*	Typical amount of food product needed to obtain a vitamin C intake of ~200 mg
Blackberries	130 g
Breakfast cereals	300 g
Broccoli	180 g
Cauliflower	250 g
Cress	400 g
Guava	75 g
Fennel (root)	220 g
Kiwi	280 g
Mango	400 g
Orange	400 g
Papaya	250 g
Pepper (green or red)	130 g
Parsley	130 g
Red cabbage	330 g
Sprouts	130 g
Strawberries	330 g

* Vitamin C content refers to fresh products. Similar canned or deep-frozen food products contain substantially less vitamin C.

the muscle store of carnitine and therefore it cannot serve to reduce body weight by increasing fat oxidation rates.

Ephedra

Ephedra is a herbal equivalent of ephedrine and is contained in Ma Huang (Pittler & Ernst, 2005; Saper, Eisenberg, & Phillips, 2004). Ephedra can act as a beta-adrenoceptor agonist, which means it can increase resting energy expenditure by virtue of activation of the sympathetic nervous system, which also results in increased heart rate. Research data indicate that dietary intake of ephedra can be effective in facilitating short-term weight loss (Dwyer, Allison, & Coates, 2005; Shekelle *et al.*, 2003a, 2003b). Furthermore, the effects of ephedra on body weight reduction can be exaggerated by the simultaneous ingestion of caffeine and aspirin (Daly, Krieger, Dulloo, Young, & Landsberg, 1993; Dulloo, 2002; Dwyer *et al.*, 2005). The herbals guarana and white willow bark may be valid alternatives for caffeine and aspirin, respectively (Daly *et al.*, 1993). Other supplements that are believed to enhance the effects of ephedra are green tea and yohimbine. However, there is also substantial evidence that the adverse effects to health associated with the intake of these "weight-loss cocktails" are substantial (Andraws, Chawla, & Brown, 2005; Haller, Benowitz, & Jacob, 2005; Pittler, Schmidt, & Ernst, 2005; Shekelle *et al.*, 2003a). Adverse events documented include nausea, vomiting, psychiatric symptoms, autonomic hyperactivity, and cardiac arrhythmias. Moreover, cases of myocardial infarction, cerebrovascular accident, serious psychiatric pathology, and even death have been reported. In addition, ephedrine and ephedra are included on the list of banned substances issued by WADA. Intake of ephedra can result in a positive doping test, and from a health perspective the use of ephedra and ephedra-containing mixtures is dangerous, so its use must be strongly discouraged at any level of competition.

Combination of supplements and timing of supplement intake

A prevailing view of athletes is "if a little is good, then more is better", and therefore it is not uncommon for them to ingest excessive amounts of various supplements. This is an expensive practice and is unlikely to facilitate the ergogenic effects of the respective supplements. In addition, such practice raises a safety concern because on the one hand the side effects of supplement overdosing are unknown, and on the other hand overdosing also increases the intake rate of contaminants possibly contained in the supplements. Furthermore, athletes as a rule use multiple supplements. From a theoretical point of view, supplements acting via different physiological mechanisms could act additively or even in a synergistic way. However, the physiological mechanisms of action of the various supplements discussed in this section are incompletely understood. Moreover, very few studies have looked at combinations of supplements, which render it difficult to make specific recommendations. However, available data and field experience taken together indicate that there is no significant interaction between the supplements discussed in this review. There is one exception: caffeine has been found to negate at least the short-term effects of creatine supplementation, which suggests that co-ingestion of these substances should probably be avoided (Hespel, Op't, & Van Leemputte, 2002; Van Leemputte et al., 1999). It is well established that exercise can enhance the responses of muscle to creatine and protein/amino acid intake (Harris et al., 1992; Robinson et al., 1999; Tipton & Wolfe, 2004; Wolfe, 2000). Furthermore, co-ingestion of an insulinogenic carbohydrate/amino acid mixture and creatine could conceivably facilitate muscle creatine retention, when the mixture is consumed in sufficient quantities to stimulate marked insulin release (Green et al., 1996; Steenge, Lambourne, Casey, Macdonald, & Greenhaff, 1998; Steenge et al., 2000). Also, from a practical point of view it is probably a sensible idea to time the intake of the above-mentioned supplements to coincide with strength and power exercise sessions, including early recovery (1–3 h). There are no specific recommendations with regard to the timing of intake of the other supplements addressed here.

References

Anderson, J. W., Nicolosi, R. J., & Borzelleca, J. F. (2005). Glucosamine effects in humans: A review of effects on glucose metabolism, side effects, safety considerations and efficacy. *Food and Chemical Toxicology, 43,* 187–201.

Andraws, R., Chawla, P., & Brown, D. L. (2005). Cardiovascular effects of ephedra alkaloids: A comprehensive review. *Progress in Cardiovascular Diseases, 47,* 217–225.

Armstrong, L. E., Pumerantz, A. C., Roti, M. W., Judelson, D. A., Watson, G., Dias, J. C. et al. (2005). Fluid, electrolyte, and renal indices of hydration during 11 days of controlled caffeine consumption. *International Journal of Sports Nutrition and Exercise Metabolism, 15,* 252–265.

Bangsbo, J., Jacobsen, K., Nordberg, N., Christensen, N. J., & Graham, T. (1992) Acute and habitual caffeine ingestion and metabolic responses to steady-state exercise. *Journal of Applied Physiology, 72,* 1297–1303.

Barr, S. I., & Rideout, C. A. (2004). Nutritional considerations for vegetarian athletes. *Nutrition, 20,* 696–703.

Bell, D. G., & McLellan, T. M. (2002). Exercise endurance 1, 3, and 6 h after caffeine ingestion in caffeine users and nonusers. *Journal of Applied Physiology, 93,* 1227–1234.

Bhaskaram, P. (2002). Micronutrient malnutrition, infection, and immunity: An overview. *Nutrition Reviews, 60,* S40–S45.

Braham, R., Dawson, B., & Goodman, C. (2003). The effect of glucosamine supplementation on people experiencing regular knee pain. *British Journal of Sports Medicine, 37,* 45–49.

Burke, D. G., Chilibeck, P. D., Parise, G., Candow, D. G., Mahoney, D., & Tarnopolsky, M. (2003). Effect of creatine and weight training on muscle creatine and performance in vegetarians. *Medicine and Science in Sports and Exercise, 35,* 1946–1955.

Burke, L. M., Loucks, A., & Broad, N. (2006). Energy and carbohydrate for training and recovery. *Journal of Sports Sciences, 24*, 675–685.

Casey, A., Constantin-Teodosiu, D., Howell, S., Hultman, E., & Greenhaff, P. L. (1996). Creatine ingestion favorably affects performance and muscle metabolism during maximal exercise in humans. *American Journal of Physiology: Endocrinology and Metabolism, 271*, E31–E37.

Chua, B., Siehl, D. L., & Morgan, H. E. (1979). Effect of leucine and metabolites of branched chain amino acids on protein turnover in heart. *Journal of Biological Chemistry, 254*, 8358–8362.

Clarkson, P. M., & Thompson, H. S. (2000). Antioxidants: What role do they play in physical activity and health? *American Journal of Clinical Nutrition, 72*, 637S–646S.

Cox, G. R., Desbrow, B., Montgomery, P. G., Anderson, M. E., Bruce, C. R., Macrides, T. A. et al. (2002b). Effect of different protocols of caffeine intake on metabolism and endurance performance. *Journal of Applied Physiology, 93*, 990–999.

Cox, G., Mujika, I., Tumilty, D., & Burke, L. (2002a). Acute creatine supplementation and performance during a field test simulating match play in elite female football players. *International Journal of Sports Nutrition and Exercise Metabolism, 12*, 33–46.

Daly, P. A., Krieger, D. R., Dulloo, A. G., Young, J. B., & Landsberg, L. (1993). Ephedrine, caffeine and aspirin: Safety and efficacy for treatment of human obesity. *International Journal of Obesity and Related Metabolic Disorders, 17* (suppl. 1), S73–S78.

Dangott, B., Schultz, E., & Mozdziak, P. E. (1999). Dietary creatine monohydrate supplementation increases satellite cell mitotic activity during compensatory hypertrophy. *International Journal of Sports Medicine, 20*, 13–16.

Davis, J. M., Zhao, Z., Stock, H. S., Mehl, K. A., Buggy, J., & Hand, G. A. (2003). Central nervous system effects of caffeine and adenosine on fatigue. *American Journal of Physiology: Regulatory and Integrative Comparative Physiology, 284*, R399–R404.

De Cock, K. J., Delbeke, F. T., Van Eenoo, P., Desmet, N., Roels, K., & De Backer, P. (2001). Detection and determination of anabolic steroids in nutritional supplements. *Journal of Pharmaceutical and Biomedical Analysis, 25*, 843–852.

Delanghe, J., De Slypere, J. P., De Buyzere, M., Robbrecht, J., Wieme, R., & Vermeulen, A. (1989). Normal reference values for creatine, creatinine, and carnitine are lower in vegetarians. *Clinical Chemistry, 35*, 1802–1803.

Delbeke, F. T., Van Eenoo, P., Van Thuyne, W., & Desmet, N. (2002). Prohormones and sport. *Journal of Steroid Biochemistry and Molecular Biology, 83*, 245–251.

Deldicque, L., Louis, M., Theisen, D., Nielens, H., Dehoux, M., Thissen, J. P. et al. (2005). Increased IGF mRNA in human skeletal muscle after creatine supplementation. *Medicine and Science in Sports and Exercise, 37*, 731–736.

Derave, W., Eijnde, B. O., & Hespel, P. (2003). Creatine supplementation in health and disease: What is the evidence for long-term efficacy? *Molecular and Cellular Biochemistry, 244*, 49–55.

Doherty, M., & Smith, P. M. (2005). Effects of caffeine ingestion on rating of perceived exertion during and after exercise: A meta-analysis. *Scandinavian Journal of Medicine and Science in Sports, 15*, 69–78.

Douglas, R. M., Hemila, H., D'Souza, R., Chalker, E. B., & Treacy, B. (2004). Vitamin C for preventing and treating the common cold. *Cochrane Database of Systemic Review*, CD000980.

Dulloo, A. G. (2002). Herbal simulation of ephedrine and caffeine in treatment of obesity. *International Journal of Obesity and Related Metabolic Disorders, 26,* 590–592.

Dwyer, J. T., Allison, D. B., & Coates, P. M. (2005). Dietary supplements in weight reduction. *Journal of the American Dietetic Association, 105,* S80–S86.

Fisher, S. M., McMurray, R. G., Berry, M., Mar, M. H., & Forsythe, W. A. (1986). Influence of caffeine on exercise performance in habitual caffeine users. *International Journal of Sports Medicine, 7,* 276–280.

Gallagher, P. M., Carrithers, J. A., Godard, M. P., Schulze, K. E., & Trappe, S. W. (2000a). β-Hydroxy- β-methylbutyrate ingestion. Part I: Effects on strength and fat free mass. *Medicine and Science in Sports and Exercise, 32,* 2109–2115.

Gallagher, P. M., Carrithers, J. A., Godard, M. P., Schulze, K. E., & Trappe, S. W. (2000b). β-Hydroxy- β-methylbutyrate ingestion. Part II: Effects on hematology, hepatic and renal function. *Medicine and Science in Sports and Exercise, 32,* 2116–2119.

Geyer, H., Parr, M. K., Mareck, U., Reinhart, U., Schrader, Y., & Schanzer, W. (2004). Analysis of non-hormonal nutritional supplements for anabolic-androgenic steroids – results of an international study. *International Journal of Sports Medicine, 25,* 124–129.

Gleeson, M., & Bishop, N. C. (2000). Special feature for the Olympics. Effects of exercise on the immune system: Modification of immune responses to exercise by carbohydrate, glutamine and anti-oxidant supplements. *Immunology and Cell Biology, 78,* 554–561.

Gleeson, M., Lancaster, G. I., & Bishop, N. C. (2001). Nutritional strategies to minimise exercise-induced immunosuppression in athletes. *Canadian Journal of Applied Physiology, 26* (suppl.), S23–S35.

Gleeson, M., Nieman, D. C., & Pedersen, B. K. (2004). Exercise, nutrition and immune function. *Journal of Sports Sciences, 22,* 115–125.

Gleeson, M., & Pyne, D. B. (2000). Special feature for the Olympics. Effects of exercise on the immune system: Exercise effects on mucosal immunity. *Immunology and Cell Biology, 78,* 536–544.

Gorsline, R. T., & Kaeding, C. C. (2005). The use of NSAIDs and nutritional supplements in athletes with osteoarthritis: Prevalence, benefits, and consequences. *Clinical Sports Medicine, 24,* 71–82.

Graham, T. E. (2001). Caffeine and exercise: Metabolism, endurance and performance. *Sports Medicine, 31,* 785–807.

Graham, T. E., Hibbert, E., & Sathasivam, P. (1998). Metabolic and exercise endurance effects of coffee and caffeine ingestion. *Journal of Applied Physiology, 85,* 883–889.

Graham, T. E., & Spriet, L. L. (1991). Performance and metabolic responses to a high caffeine dose during prolonged exercise. *Journal of Applied Physiology, 71,* 2292–2298.

Graham, T. E., & Spriet, L. L. (1995). Metabolic, catecholamine, and exercise performance responses to various doses of caffeine. *Journal of Applied Physiology, 78,* 867–874.

Green, A. L., Hultman, E., Macdonald, I. A., Sewell, D. A., & Greenhaff, P. L. (1996). Carbohydrate ingestion augments skeletal muscle creatine accumulation during creatine supplementation in humans. *American Journal of Physiology: Endocrinology and Metabolism, 271,* E821–E826.

Green, G. A., Catlin, D. H., & Starcevic, B. (2001). Analysis of over-the-counter dietary supplements. *Clinical Journal of Sport Medicine, 11*, 254–259.

Greenhaff, P. L., Bodin, K., Söderlund, K., & Hultman, E. (1994). Effect of oral creatine supplementation on skeletal muscle phosphocreatine resynthesis. *American Journal of Physiology: Endocrinology and Metabolism, 266*, E725–E730.

Greenhaff, P. L., Casey, A., Short, A. H., Harris, R., & Söderlund, K. (1993). Influence of oral creatine supplementation on muscle torque during repeated bouts of maximal voluntary exercise in man. *Clinical Science, 84*, 565–571.

Gurley, B. J., Gardner, S. F., & Hubbard, M. A. (2000). Content versus label claims in ephedra-containing dietary supplements. *American Journal of Health: System Pharmacy, 57*, 963–969.

Haller, C. A., Benowitz, N. L., & Jacob, P., III (2005). Hemodynamic effects of ephedra-free weight-loss supplements in humans. *American Journal of Medicine, 118*, 998–1003.

Harris, R. C., Almada, A. L., Harris, D. B., Dunnett, M., & Hespel, P. (2004). The creatine content of creatine serum and the change in the plasma concentration with ingestion of a single dose. *Journal of Sports Sciences, 22*, 851–857.

Harris, R. C., Söderlund, K., & Hultman, E. (1992). Elevation of creatine in resting and exercised muscle of normal subjects by creatine supplementation. *Clinical Science, 83*, 367–374.

Haskell, C. F., Kennedy, D. O., Wesnes, K. A., & Scholey, A. B. (2005). Cognitive and mood improvements of caffeine in habitual consumers and habitual non-consumers of caffeine. *Psychopharmacology (Berlin), 179*, 813–825.

Hawley, J. A., Tipton, K. D., & Millard-Stafford, M. L. (2006). Promoting training adaptations through nutritional interventions. *Journal of Sports Sciences, 24*, 709–721.

Hemila, H. (1996). Vitamin C and common cold incidence: A review of studies with subjects under heavy physical stress. *International Journal of Sports Medicine, 17*, 379–383.

Hemila, H. (2004). Vitamin C supplementation and respiratory infections: A systematic review. *Military Medicine, 169*, 920–925.

Hespel, P., Op't, E. B., & Van Leemputte, M. (2002). Opposite actions of caffeine and creatine on muscle relaxation time in humans. *Journal of Applied Physiology, 92*, 513–518.

Hespel, P., Op't Eijnde, B., Van Leemputte, M., Ursø, B., Greenhaff, P., Labarque, V. *et al.* (2001). Oral creatine supplementation facilitates the rehabilitation of disuse atrophy and alters the expression of muscle myogenic factors in humans. *Journal of Physiology, 536*, 625–633.

Hetzler, R. K., Warhaftig-Glynn, N., Thompson, D. L., Dowling, E., & Weltman, A. (1994). Effects of acute caffeine withdrawal on habituated male runners. *Journal of Applied Physiology, 76*, 1043–1048.

Hiscock, N., & Pedersen, B. K. (2002). Exercise-induced immunodepression – plasma glutamine is not the link. *Journal of Applied Physiology, 93*, 813–822.

Horswill, C. A. (1995). Effects of bicarbonate, citrate, and phosphate loading on performance. *International Journal of Sport Nutrition, 5* (suppl.), S111–S119.

Ji, L. L., & Peterson, D. M. (2004). Aging, exercise, and phytochemicals: Promises and pitfalls. *Annals of the New York Academy of Sciences, 1019*, 453–461.

Kovacs, E. M. R., Stegen, J. H. C. H., & Brouns, F. (1998). Effect of caffeinated drinks on substrate metabolism, caffeine excretion, and performance. *Journal of Applied Physiology, 85,* 709–715.

Kreider, R. B., Ferreira, M., Wilson, M., Grinstaff, P., Plisk, S., Reinardy, J. *et al.* (1998). Effects of creatine supplementation on body composition, strength, and sprint performance. *Medicine and Science in Sports and Exercise, 30,* 73–82.

Kris-Etherton, P. M., Lichtenstein, A. H., Howard, B. V., Steinberg, D., & Witztum, J. L. (2004). Antioxidant vitamin supplements and cardiovascular disease. *Circulation, 110,* 637–641.

Lakier, S. L. (2003). Overtraining, excessive exercise, and altered immunity: Is this a T helper-1 versus T helper-2 lymphocyte response? *Sports Medicine, 33,* 347–364.

Louis, M., Poortmans, J. R., Francaux, M., Berre, J., Boisseau, N., Brassine, E. *et al.* (2003a). No effect of creatine supplementation on human myofibrillar and sarcoplasmic protein synthesis after resistance exercise. *American Journal of Physiology: Endocrinology and Metabolism, 285,* E1089–E1094.

Louis, M., Poortmans, J. R., Francaux, M., Hultman, E., Berre, J., Boisseau, N. *et al.* (2003b). Creatine supplementation has no effect on human muscle protein turnover at rest in the postabsorptive or fed states. *American Journal of Physiology: Endocrinology and Metabolism, 284,* E764–E770.

Louis, M., Van Beneden, R., Dehoux, M., Thissen, J. P., & Francaux, M. (2004). Creatine increases IGF-I and myogenic regulatory factor mRNA in C(2)C(12) cells. *FEBS Letters, 557,* 243–247.

Maganaris, C. N., & Maughan, R. J. (1998). Creatine supplementation enhances maximum voluntary isometric force and endurance capacity in resistance trained men. *Acta Physiologica Scandinavica, 163,* 279–287.

Magkos, F., & Kavouras, S. A. (2004). Caffeine and ephedrine: Physiological, metabolic and performance-enhancing effects. *Sports Medicine, 34,* 871–889.

Malm, C., Ekblom, O., & Ekblom, B. (2004). Immune system alteration in response to two consecutive football games. *Acta Physiologica Scandinavica, 180,* 143–155.

Matson, L. G., & Tran, Z. V. (1993). Effects of sodium bicarbonate ingestion on anaerobic performance: A meta-analytic review. *International Journal of Sports Nutrition, 3,* 2–28.

Maughan, R. J., & Griffin, J. (2003). Caffeine ingestion and fluid balance: A review. *Journal of Human Nutrition and Dietetics, 16,* 411–420.

McAlindon, T. E., LaValley, M. P., Gulin, J. P., & Felson, D. T. (2000). Glucosamine and chondroitin for treatment of osteoarthritis: A systematic quality assessment and meta-analysis. *Journal of the American Medical Association, 283,* 1469–1475.

Mujika, I., Padilla, S., Ibañez, J., Izquierdo, M., & Gorostiaga, E. (2000). Creatine supplementation and sprint performance in football players. *Medicine and Science in Sports and Exercise, 32,* 518–525.

Nieman, D. C. (2001). Exercise immunology: Nutritional countermeasures. *Canadian Journal of Applied Physiology, 26* (suppl.), S45–S55.

Nieman, D. C., Dumke, C. L., Henson, D. A., McAnulty, S. R., McAnulty, L. S., Lind, R. H., & Morrow, J. D. (2003). Immune and oxidative changes during and following the Western States Endurance Run. *International Journal of Sports Medicine, 24,* 541–547.

Nieman, D. C., Henson, D. A., McAnulty, S. R., McAnulty, L., Swick, N. S., Utter, A. C., Vinci, D. M., Opiela, S. J., & Morrow, J. D. (2002). Influence of vitamin C supplementation on oxidative and immune changes following an ultra-marathon. *Journal of Applied Physiology*, 92, 1970–1977.

Nissen, S. L., & Sharp, R. L. (2003). Effect of dietary supplements on lean mass and strength gains with resistance exercise: A meta-analysis. *Journal of Applied Physiology*, 94, 651–659.

Nissen, S., Sharp, R., Ray, M., Rathmacher, J. A., Rice, D., Fuller, J. C., Jr. *et al.* (1996). Effect of leucine metabolite beta-hydroxy-beta-methylbutyrate on muscle metabolism during resistance-exercise training. *Journal of Applied Physiology*, 81, 2095–2104.

Parasrampuria, J., Schwartz, K., & Petesch, R. (1998). Quality control of dehydro-epiandrosterone dietary supplement products. *Journal of the American Medical Association*, 280, 1565.

Parr, M. K., Geyer, H., Reinhart, U., & Schanzer, W. (2004). Analytical strategies for the detection of non-labelled anabolic androgenic steroids in nutritional supplements. *Food Additives and Contaminants*, 21, 632–640.

Pasman, W. J., Van Baak, M. A., Jeukendrup, A. E., & de Haan, A. (1995). The effect of different dosages of caffeine on endurance performance time. *International Journal of Sports Medicine*, 16, 225–230.

Pavelka, K., Gatterova, J., Olejarova, M., Machacek, S., Giacovelli, G., & Rovati, L. C. (2002). Glucosamine sulfate use and delay of progression of knee osteoarthritis: A 3-year, randomized, placebo-controlled, double-blind study. *Archives of Internal Medicine*, 162, 2113–2123.

Pedersen, B. K., & Toft, A. D. (2000). Effects of exercise on lymphocytes and cytokines. *British Journal of Sports Medicine*, 34, 246–251.

Pittler, M. H., & Ernst, E. (2005). Complementary therapies for reducing body weight: A systematic review. *International Journal of Obesity and Related Metabolic Disorders*, 29, 1030–1038.

Pittler, M. H., Schmidt, K., & Ernst, E. (2005). Adverse events of herbal food supplements for body weight reduction: Systematic review. *Obesity Reviews*, 6, 93–111.

Poortmans, J. R., Auquier, H., Renaut, V., Durussel, A., Saugy, M., & Brisson, G. R. (1997). Effect of short-term creatine supplementation on renal responses in men. *European Journal of Applied Physiology*, 76, 566–567.

Poortmans, J. R., & Francaux, M. (1999). Long-term oral creatine supplementation does not impair renal function in healthy athletes. *Medicine and Science in Sports and Exercise*, 31, 1108–1110.

Reginster, J. Y., Deroisy, R., Rovati, L. C., Lee, R. L., Lejeune, E., Bruyere, O. *et al.* (2001). Long-term effects of glucosamine sulphate on osteoarthritis progression: A randomised, placebo-controlled clinical trial. *Lancet*, 357, 251–256.

Reilly, T. (2005). An ergonomics model of the football training process. *Journal of Sports Sciences*, 23, 561–572.

Robinson, T. M., Sewell, D. A., Hultman, E., & Greenhaff, P. L. (1999). Role of sub-maximal exercise in promoting creatine and glycogen accumulation in human skeletal muscle. *Journal of Applied Physiology*, 87, 598–604.

Saper, R. B., Eisenberg, D. M., & Phillips, R. S. (2004). Common dietary supplements for weight loss. *American Family Physician*, 70, 1731–1738.

Schroeder, C., Potteiger, J., Randall, J., Jacobsen, D., Magee, L., Benedict, S. *et al.* (2001). The effects of creatine dietary supplementation on anterior compartment pressure in the lower leg during rest and following exercise. *Clinical Journal of Sports Medicine*, 11, 87–95.

Sen, C. K. (2001). Antioxidants in exercise nutrition. *Sports Medicine, 31,* 891–908.

Shekelle, P., Hardy, M. L., Morton, S. C., Maglione, M., Suttorp, M., Roth, E. *et al.* (2003a). Ephedra and ephedrine for weight loss and athletic performance enhancement: Clinical efficacy and side effects. *Evidence Report Technological Assessment* (Summ.), 1–4.

Shekelle, P. G., Hardy, M. L., Morton, S. C., Maglione, M., Mojica, W. A., Suttorp, M. J. *et al.* (2003b). Efficacy and safety of ephedra and ephedrine for weight loss and athletic performance: A meta-analysis. *Journal of the American Medical Association, 289,* 1537–1545.

Shirreffs, S. M., Sawka, M. N., & Stone, M. (2006). Water and electrolyte needs for soccer training and match-play. *Journal of Sports Sciences, 24,* 699–707.

Steenge, G. R., Lambourne, J., Casey, A., Macdonald, I. A., & Greenhaff, P. L. (1998). Stimulatory effect of insulin on creatine accumulation in human skeletal muscle. *American Journal of Physiology: Endocrinology and Metabolism, 275,* E974–E979.

Steenge, G. R., Simpson, E. J., & Greenhaff, P. L. (2000). Protein- and carbohydrate-induced augmentation of whole body creatine retention in humans. *Journal of Applied Physiology, 89,* 1165–1171.

Tarnopolsky, M. (1994). Caffeine and endurance performance. *Sports Medicine, 18,* 109–125.

Terjung, R. L., Clarkson, P. M., Eichner, E. R., Greenhaff, P. L., Hespel, P., Israel, R. G. *et al.* (2000). The physiological and health effects of oral creatine supplementation. *Medicine and Science in Sports and Exercise, 32,* 706–717.

Tipton, K. D., & Wolfe, R. R. (2004). Protein and amino acids for athletes. *Journal of Sports Sciences, 22,* 65–79.

Tischler, M. E., Desautels, M., & Goldberg, A. L. (1982). Does leucine, leucyl-tRNA, or some metabolite of leucine regulate protein synthesis and degradation in skeletal and cardiac muscle? *Journal of Biological Chemistry, 257,* 1613–1621.

Urso, M. L., & Clarkson, P. M. (2003). Oxidative stress, exercise, and antioxidant supplementation. *Toxicology, 189,* 41–54.

Vandebuerie, F., Vanden Eynde, B., Vandenberghe, K., & Hespel, P. (1998). Effect of creatine loading on endurance capacity and sprint power in cyclists. *International Journal of Sports Medicine, 83,* 2055–2063.

Vandenberghe, K., Gillis, N., Van Leemputte, M., Van Hecke, P., Vanstapel, F., & Hespel, P. (1996). Caffeine counteracts the ergogenic action of muscle creatine loading. *Journal of Applied Physiology, 80,* 452–457.

Vandenberghe, K., Goris, M., Van Hecke, P., Van Leemputte, M., Vangerven, L., & Hespel, P. (1997). Long-term creatine intake is beneficial to muscle performance during resistance training. *Journal of Applied Physiology, 83,* 2055–2063.

Van Leemputte, M., Vandenberghe, K., & Hespel, P. (1999). Shortening of muscle relaxation time after creatine loading. *Journal of Applied Physiology, 86,* 840–844.

van Loon, L. J., Murphy, R., Oosterlaar, A. M., Cameron-Smith, D., Hargreaves, M., Wagenmakers, A. J. *et al.* (2004). Creatine supplementation increases glycogen storage but not GLUT-4 expression in human skeletal muscle. *Clinical Science (London), 106,* 99–106.

Van Soeren, M. H., & Graham, T. E. (1998). Effect of caffeine on metabolism, exercise endurance and catecholamine responses after withdrawal. *Journal of Applied Physiology, 85,* 1493–1501.

Van Soeren, M. H., Sathasivam, P., Spriet, L. L., & Graham, T. E. (1993). Caffeine metabolism and epinephrine responses during exercise in users and nonusers. *Journal of Applied Physiology, 75*, 805–812.

Van Thuyne, W., Van Eenoo, P., & Delbeke, F. T. (2003). Urinary concentrations of morphine after the administration of herbal teas containing *Papaveris fructus* in relation to doping analysis. *Journal of Chromatography B: Analytical Technologies in the Biomedical and Life Sciences, 785*, 245–251.

Volek, J. S., Duncan, N. D., Mazzetti, S. A., Staron, R. S., Putukian, M., Gómez, A. L. et al. (1999). Performance and muscle fiber adaptations to creatine supplementation and heavy resistance training. *Medicine and Science in Sports and Exercise, 31*, 1147–1156.

Walker, J. B. (1979). Creatine: biosynthesis, regulation, and function. *Advances in Enzymology, 50*, 177–242.

Watt, K. K., Garnham, A. P., & Snow, R. J. (2004). Skeletal muscle total creatine content and creatine transporter gene expression in vegetarians prior to and following creatine supplementation. *International Journal of Sports Nutrition and Exercise Metabolism, 14*, 517–531.

Williams, C., & Serratosa, L. (2006). Nutrition on match day. *Journal of Sports Sciences, 24*, 687–697.

Wolfe, R. R. (2000). Protein supplements and exercise. *American Journal of Clinical Nutrition, 72*, 551S–557S.

Ziegenfuss, T. M., Lowery, L. M., & Lemon, P. W. R. (1998). Acute fluid volume changes in men during three days of creatine supplementation. *Journal of Exercise Physiology, 1*, 1–9.

9 Nutritional strategies to counter stress to the immune system in athletes, with special reference to football

DAVID C. NIEMAN AND NICOLETTE C. BISHOP

Although epidemiological data indicate that athletes are at increased risk of upper respiratory tract infection during periods of heavy training and the 1–2 week period following endurance race events, there is very limited information on the responses to football training and match-play. For several hours after heavy exertion, components of both the innate (e.g. natural killer cell activity and neutrophil oxidative burst activity) and adaptive (e.g. T and B cell function) immune system exhibit suppressed function. Although such responses to football training and competition do not appear to be as pronounced, variations in immune cell numbers and function are reported in professional footballers over the course of a season. Attempts have been made through nutritional means (e.g. glutamine, vitamins C and E, and carbohydrate supplementation) to attenuate immune changes following intensive exercise and thus lower the risk of upper respiratory tract infection. Carbohydrate supplementation during heavy exercise has emerged as a partial countermeasure and attenuates increases in blood neutrophil counts, stress hormones, and inflammatory cytokines, but has little effect on decrements in salivary IgA output or natural killer cell function. Animal research indicates that other nutritional components such as beta-glucan, quercetin, and curcumin warrant human investigations to determine if they are effective countermeasures to exercise-induced immune dysfunction.

Keywords: Exercise, lymphocytes, neutrophils, cytokines, antioxidants, carbohydrate

Introduction

Mounting evidence indicates that physical activity influences immune function and risk of certain types of infection, such as upper respiratory tract infections (URTI). In contrast to moderate physical activity, prolonged and intensive exertion causes numerous negative changes in immunity and an increased risk of URTI. Footballers, as elite athletes, must train intensively to compete at the highest levels and therefore may also be at increased risk of URTI and suppressed immune function. There is a growing interest in potential nutritional countermeasures to exercise-induced immune dysfunction. This article is a current review of these nutritional countermeasures. To date, only a few studies have observed susceptibility for URTI and immunological changes in professional footballers (with fewer still examining nutritional countermeasures); most studies in this area have been conducted on endurance athletes. However, wherever possible data will be highlighted from footballers collected over a season or in response to a match, or from studies employing football-specific protocols. Where this is not possible, any extrapolation of findings from endurance athletes to football play should be made with caution, since the physiological demands of football training and play are not necessarily the same as those of endurance training and competition. This highlights the need for further football-specific research in this area.

Exercise, immunity, and URTI risk

Although the relationship between exercise and URTI and other types of infections has been explored since early in the twentieth century (Baetjer, 1932), the number of well-designed epidemiological and exercise training experimental trials on humans is still small, limiting our understanding of this important topic (Nieman, 1997a, 2003).

There is a common belief among fitness enthusiasts that regular exercise confers resistance against URTI. A survey of 750 masters athletes (ranging in age from 40 to 81 years) showed that 76% perceived themselves as less vulnerable to viral illnesses than their sedentary peers (Shephard, Kavanagh, Mertens, Qureshi, & Clark, 1995). Three epidemiological studies (Kostka, Berthouze, Lacour, & Bonnefoy, 2000; Matthews *et al.*, 2002; Strasner, Barlow, Kampert, & Dunn, 2001) and three randomized experimental trials (Nieman *et al.*, 1990b, 1993, 1998a) have provided important data in support of the value of frequent and moderate physical activity in reducing URTI risk. Other studies indicate that during moderate exercise or vigorous exercise that incorporate rest intervals, several positive changes occur in the immune system (Nehlsen-Cannarella *et al.*, 1991; Nieman, 2000; Nieman & Nehlsen-Cannarella, 1994; Nieman, Henson, Austin, & Brown, 2005b).

In contrast to the benefits of moderate physical activity, a common perception among elite athletes and their coaches is that heavy exertion and overtraining lead to immune dysfunction and an elevated risk of URTI. A growing number of epidemiological investigations support this belief and will be reviewed in the next section. Data from animal studies have been difficult to apply to the human condition, but in general have supported the finding that one or two periods of exhaustive exercise following inoculation leads to a more frequent appearance of infection and a higher fatality rate (but results differ depending on the pathogen, with some more affected by exercise than others) (Davis *et al.*, 1997; Pedersen & Bruunsgaard, 1995).

Heavy exertion and URTI: Epidemiological evidence

The relationship between exercise and URTI may be modelled in the form of a "J" curve (Nieman, 1997a). This model suggests that although the risk of URTI may decrease below that of a sedentary individual when one engages in moderate exercise training, risk may rise above average during periods of excessive amounts of high-intensity exercise.

The "J" curve model also suggests that immunosurveillance mirrors the relationship between infection risk and exercise workload. In other words, it makes sense that if regular moderate exercise lowers infection risk, it should be accompanied by enhanced immunosurveillance. On the other hand, when an athlete engages in unusually heavy exercise workloads (e.g. overtraining, a competitive endurance race event, or even heavy match schedules), infection risk should be related to diminished immunosurveillance.

Much more research using larger pools of participants and improved research designs is necessary before this model can be wholly accepted or rejected. The epidemiological studies used self-reported URTI data (primarily retrospective, with two studies using one-year daily logs). Few have attempted to verify symptomatology using viral identification or verification by physicians. There is some concern that the symptoms reported by endurance athletes following competitive race events may reflect those associated with an inflammatory response rather than URTI (Castell *et al.*, 1997; Drenth *et al.*, 1995; Nehlsen-Cannarella *et al.*, 1997).

With these limitations in mind, several epidemiological reports suggest that athletes who engage in marathon-type events and/or very heavy training are at increased risk of URTI. Nieman, Johanssen, Lee, Cermal and Arabatzis (1990a) reported that 12.9% of marathon runners reported URTI during the week following the Los Angeles Marathon compared with 2.2% of control marathon runners (odds ratio = 5.9). Forty percent of the runners reported at least one URTI episode during the 2 month winter period before the marathon race. Controlling for various confounding factors, it was determined that runners training more than 96 km · week^{-1} doubled their odds for sickness compared with those training less than 32 km · week^{-1}. Similar results have been reported by Heath *et al.* (1991), Linde (1987), Nieman *et al.* (2002a, 2003b, in press), and Peters and colleagues (Peters, 1990; Peters & Bateman, 1983; Peters, Goetzsche, Grobbelaar, & Noakes, 1993; Peters, Goetzsche, Joseph, & Noakes, 1996; Peters-Futre, 1997). Risk of URTI following a race event may depend on the distance, with an increased incidence conspicuous only following a marathon or ultramarathon (Nieman, Johanssen, & Lee, 1989). With this is mind, the question arises of how relevant these findings are to football training and match-play. Unfortunately, research to assess this is limited. Nevertheless, one small study of 15 top league professional Belgian footballers over a season showed a higher incidence of URTI compared with untrained controls (Bury, Marechal, Mahieu, & Pirnay, 1998). Over a year (July to July), 22 episodes of URTI were diagnosed by a respiratory physician in the footballers, with only 9 episodes diagnosed in the control group. The majority of the infections in players were diagnosed during the winter months, which is in line with usual seasonal variations in URTI rates. Interestingly, this period also coincided with the main part of the competitive season, when it may be speculated that physiological demands on players were increased (although no training or match data were reported by the authors).

Together, these epidemiological studies imply that heavy acute or chronic exercise is associated with an increased risk of URTI. Thus it makes sense that URTI risk may be increased when an athlete goes through repeated cycles of unusually heavy exertion, has been exposed to novel pathogens, and experienced other stressors to the immune system including lack of sleep, severe mental stress, malnutrition, or weight loss. A one-year retrospective study of 852 German athletes showed that risk of URTI was highest in endurance athletes who also reported significant stress and sleep deprivation (Konig, Grathwohl, Weinstock, Northoff, & Berg, 2000). In other words, URTI risk is related to many factors, and when brought together during travel to important competitive events, the athlete may be unusually susceptible. This could be of equal relevance to professional footballers, particularly during periods of fixture congestion with domestic, regional, and international competitions taking place. Furthermore, other factors also play an important role in a player's susceptibility for URTI. Being in close proximity with other players who may have or be incubating a cold-causing virus through shared accommodation, changing facilities, and the practice of sharing drinking bottles during training and matches will increase exposure to the viruses that cause URTI.

Most endurance athletes, however, do not report URTI after competitive race events. For example, only one in seven marathon runners reported an episode of URTI during the week following the March 1987 Los Angeles Marathon, compared to two in 100 who did not compete (Nieman *et al.*, 1990a). When athletes train hard, but avoid overreaching and overtraining, URTI risk is typically unaltered. For example, during a $2\frac{1}{2}$ month period (winter/spring) in which elite female rowers trained $2\text{--}3\,\text{h}\cdot\text{day}^{-1}$ (rowing drills, resistance training), the incidence of URTI did not vary significantly from that of non-athletic controls (Nieman *et al.*, 2000a).

Exercise-induced changes in immune function

Together, these data imply that there is a relationship between exercise and infection, and that heavy exertion may suppress various components of immunity. Research data on the resting immunity of athletes and non-athletes, however, are limited and present a confusing picture at present (Nieman, 1997b). For example, the few studies available suggest that the innate immune system responds differentially to the chronic stress of intensive exercise, with natural killer cell activity tending to be enhanced while neutrophil function is suppressed (Nieman *et al.*, 1995b, 1999; Pyne, Baker, Fricker, McDonald, & Nelson, 1995; Smith & Pyne, 1997). The adaptive immune system (resting state) in general seems to be largely unaffected by athletic endeavour.

Each acute bout of cardiorespiratory endurance exercise leads to transient but significant changes in immunity and host defence (Gabriel & Kindermann,

1997; Hoffman-Goetz and Pedersen, 1994; Nieman *et al.*, 1997b, 2002a, 2003a, 2004; Pedersen & Brunsgaard, 1995; Petersen & Pedersen, 2005). Natural killer cell activity, various measures of T and B cell function, upper airway neutrophil function, and salivary IgA concentration have all been reported to be suppressed for at least several hours during recovery from prolonged, intense endurance exercise (Bruunsgaard *et al.*, 1997; Gabriel & Kindermann, 1997; Mackinnon & Hooper, 1994; Müns 1993; Nieman *et al.*, 1995a, 1995c, 2001, 2003b; Shinkai *et al.*, 1993).

Compared with endurance events, only a few papers have examined immunological changes in professional footballers. Bury *et al.* (1998) found no effect of a competitive season on total numbers of leukocytes, but did observe an increase in numbers of circulating neutrophils and a decrease in the numbers of total lymphocytes (accounted for by a decrease in CD$^+$ T lymphocytes and resulting in a decrease in the CD4/CD8 ratio) over the course of the season. Furthermore, significant falls in both neutrophil chemotaxis and phagocytosis and in PHA-stimulated T lymphocyte proliferation were reported. However, there was little change in NK cell number or cytotoxity during the season. Rebelo *et al.* (1998) also observed increases in neutrophil numbers and a fall in the CD4/CD8 ratio in 13 professional Portuguese players at the end of a competitive season compared with pre-season values. More recently, Gleeson (2004) monitored immune changes of 18 members of the first team squad of an English Premier League team that was involved in the European Champions League in addition to domestic competition. In this study, no changes in neutrophils, lymphocytes, or CD4/CD8 ratio were found yet a decrease in NK cell numbers was observed, in contrast to the findings of Bury *et al.* (1998) and Rebelo *et al.* (1998). Furthermore, during the season, the numbers of CD45RO$^+$ T lymphocytes (a mixture of memory cells, important in long-term recognition of antigens and in generating the adaptive response to recall antigens, and short-term activated T cells) fell significantly, with very low levels recorded by the end of the season. The numbers of CD45RA$^+$ T lymphocytes (nave cells that have not yet encountered antigen) increased. The fall in CD45RO$^+$ cells and NK cells can be viewed as potentially disadvantageous to the body's defence against viral pathogens, such as URTI (Gleeson, 2004). Interestingly, salivary IgA concentration and MHCII expression on monocytes were also lowest at the time when form (wins/losses ratio and league position) was at its lowest. Finally, Malm, Ekblom and Ekblom (2004a) found that a 5 day football training camp for Swedish elite junior footballers resulted in decreases in T and B lymphocytes, but no change in total leukocytes and NK cells compared with values before the camp.

A few studies have investigated the acute effects of football play following matches (Malm, Ekblom, & Ekblom, 2004b) or in response to field or laboratory-based tests designed to simulate the activity patterns and physiological demands of football (Bishop, Blannin, Robson, Walsh, & Gleeson, 1999; Bishop, Gleeson, Nicholas, & Ali, 2002; Bishop *et al.*, 2005). In these studies, increases in numbers of circulating neutrophils, lymphocytes and lymphocyte subsets, leukocyte adhesion molecules, and plasma levels of IL-6 have been observed after exercise, in addition to decreases in neutrophil function. However, the magnitude of these alterations is not as great as that observed following endurance-type events, even when exercise was performed following an overnight fast (Bishop *et al.*, 1999, 2002, 2005). Two of these studies have looked at the effect of match or simulated play on consecutive days on immunological measures: Bishop *et al.* (2005) found that lymphocyte proliferation responses following exposure to influenza were unaffected by the exercise on the first day but were significantly lower before exercise on the second day compared with the same time on day 1. On both days, exercise was performed at the same time of day. Malm *et al.* (2004b) reported reduced expression of lymphocyte adhesion and signalling molecules 6 h after the second of two games played 20 h apart. Unfortunately, this study did not take any measurements after the first game or immediately before the second game, making it difficult to assess the extent of any "carry-over" from the first game. Furthermore, the games were held at different times of day and thus it could be argued that diurnal changes may have had some influence on the results.

It is suggested that alterations in immune measures observed following intensive exercise create an "open window" of decreased host protection, during which viruses and bacteria may gain a foothold, increasing the risk of subclinical and clinical infection (Figure 1). Although this is an attractive hypothesis, no one has yet demonstrated conclusively that athletes showing the most extreme immunosuppression are those that contract an infection (Lee, Meehan, Robinson, Mabry, & Smith, 1992; Mackinnon, Ginn, & Seymour, 1993). In one study, salivary IgA secretion rate decreased by nearly half in a group of 155 ultramarathon runners following a 160 km race (Nieman *et al.*, 2005c). Nearly

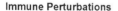

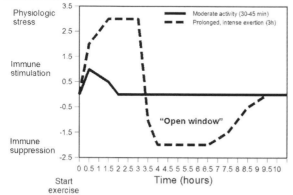

Figure 1. The "open window theory". Moderate exercise causes mild immune changes; in contrast, prolonged, intensive exercise (90 min or longer) leads to a downturn in immunosurveillance that increases the likelihood for opportunistic upper respiratory tract infections.

one in four runners reported an URTI episode during the 2 weeks following the race, and the decrease in sIgA secretion rate was significantly greater in these runners (54%) than in those not reporting URTI (31%). It is doubtful, however, that sIgA output alone can be used to predict URTI at the individual athlete level. In this study, the overall predictive value for URTI was 55%, indicating that sIgA output was more useful at the group than the individual level, and that other factors need to be discovered and combined with sIgA before URTI risk can be predicted for individual athletes.

Nutritional countermeasure strategies

Nutrition impacts the development of the immune system, both in the growing fetus and in the early months of life. Nutrients are also necessary for the immune response to pathogens so that cells can divide and produce antibodies and cytokines. Many enzymes in immune cells require the presence of micronutrients, and critical roles have been defined for zinc, iron, copper, selenium, vitamins A, B6, C, and E in the maintenance of optimum immune function.

Nutritional immunology is a rapidly growing area of scientific scrutiny, and four key principles have emerged:

1. Almost all nutrients in the diet play a crucial role in maintaining an "optimal" immune response (Calder & Kew, 2002). A varied, healthy diet provides all the nutrients needed for good immune function in most healthy adults, and vitamin/mineral supplements do not "boost" immunity above normal levels.
2. Deficient intakes of energy and nutrients can have negative consequences on immune status and susceptibility to pathogens. Protein-energy-malnutrition (PEM) causes a downturn in most aspects of immune function and strongly increases the risk of various types of infection (Keusch, 2003).
3. Some nutrients (i.e. glutamine, arginine, fatty acids, vitamin E) provide additional benefits to immunocompromised persons (i.e. the frail elderly) or patients who suffer from various infections, and is now called "immuno-nutrition" (Calder, 2004; Grimble, 2005).
4. Advanced supplements may prove useful in countering immune suppression for healthy adults during unusual mental and physical stress (Hamer, Wolvers, & Albers, 2004). For example, dietary beta-glucans shift inflammatory profiles to a Th1 type and thus enhance resistance against bacterial and parasitic infections, n-3 fatty acids from fish oils (eicosapentaenoic acid and docosahexaenoic acid) dampen inflammatory responses, and Gingko biloba lowers NFκB and activator protein 1 activation, possibly due to its high content of polyphenols (Plat & Mensink, 2005).

The influence of nutritional supplements on the immune and infection response to intense and prolonged exercise is an active area of research by multiple investigators (Gleeson, Nieman, & Pedersen, 2004). Supplements studied thus far in humans include zinc, dietary fat, plant sterols, antioxidants (e.g. vitamins C and E, beta-carotene, N-acetylcysteine, and butylated hydroxyanisole), glutamine, and carbohydrate. Except for carbohydrate beverages, none of these supplements has emerged as an effective countermeasure to exercise-induced immune suppression (Gleeson *et al.*, 2004; Nieman, 2001; Nieman & Pedersen, 2000). Antioxidants and glutamine have received much attention, but the data thus far do not support their role in negating immune changes after heavy exertion.

Carbohydrate supplements

Research during the 1980s and early 1990s established that a reduction in blood glucose was linked to hypothalamic-pituitary-adrenal activation, an increased release of adrenocorticotrophic hormone and cortisol, increased plasma growth hormone, and increased plasma epinephrine concentrations (Murray, Paul, Seifert, & Eddy, 1991). Stress hormones have an intimate link with some aspects of immune function.

Several studies with runners and cyclists have shown that carbohydrate beverage ingestion plays a role in attenuating changes in immunity when the athlete experiences physiologic stress and depletion of carbohydrate stores in response to high-intensity ($\sim$75–80% $\dot{V}O_{2max}$) exercise bouts lasting more than 90 min (Nehlsen-Cannarella *et al.*, 1997; Nieman *et al.*, 1997a, 1997c, 1998b, 2001, 2003a). In particular, carbohydrate ingestion (about one litre per hour of a typical sports drink) compared to a placebo has been linked to reduced change in blood immune cell counts, and lower pro- and anti-inflammatory cytokines. However, carbohydrate ingestion during intense and prolonged exercise is largely ineffective in countering post-exercise decrements in natural killer and salivary IgA output.

The average intensity of a football match is in the region of 70% $\dot{V}O_{2max}$ and laboratory-based protocols that closely simulate the activity patterns and physiological demands of football match-play have shown that carbohydrate ingestion compared to placebo can negate some of the immune responses associated with placebo ingestion (Bishop *et al.*, 2005). In response to a validated football-specific intermittent running protocol performed at the same time of day on consecutive days, carbohydrate ingestion was associated with lower post-exercise $CD3^+$ counts on both days. Furthermore, before exercise on the second day T lymphocyte proliferative responses to influenza were 80% higher with carbohydrate ingestion than placebo. Interestingly, these responses occurred despite no significant fall in plasma glucose concentration immediately after exercise with placebo ingestion and no effect of carbohydrate ingestion on cortisol responses to the exercise. This perhaps suggests that the role of cortisol is not as crucial as was originally thought. One note of caution to consider when extrapolating these findings to a true training session or match is that the exercise was performed following an overnight fast and so the magnitude of the alterations observed may be greater than might be seen had a pre-match meal been consumed.

These effects appear to be dependent on the average intensity of the exercise. Protocols in which the average intensity has been lower than that typically observed in competitive matches have found smaller changes in immune measures and little effect of carbohydrate ingestion on these (Bishop *et al.*, 1999). With this in mind, it is likely that immune responses to match-play could depend on an individual's playing position.

Overall, these data indicate that physiological stress to some aspects of the immune system is reduced when athletes use carbohydrate during intense exertion lasting 90 min or more. Does this mean that athletes using carbohydrate beverages during competitive events will lower their risk of sickness afterwards? One study in endurance athletes suggests this is so, but more research is needed (Nieman *et al.*, 2002a).

Antioxidants

Heavy exertion increases the generation of free radicals and reactive oxygen species (ROS) through several pathways, including oxidative phosphorylation, an increase in catecholamines, prostanoid metabolism, xanthine oxidase, and NAD(P)H oxidase (Urso & Clarkson, 2003). Neutrophils and macrophages migrate to the site of contraction-induced muscle damage, infiltrate the muscle tissue, activate the release of cytokines, and produce additional ROS. Most ROS are neutralized by a sophisticated antioxidant defence system consisting of a variety of enzymes and non-enzymatic antioxidants including vitamin A, E, and C, glutathione, ubiquinone, and flavonoids. Intensive and sustained exercise, however, can create an imbalance between ROS and antioxidants, leading to oxidative stress that not only causes lipid peroxidation and protein oxidation, but may also impact immune function. A recent study of professional Polish footballers reported the presence of elevated levels of specific antibodies against oxidized low-density lipoproteins in 7 of the 11 players studied (Klapcińska *et al.*, 2005). This reflects enhanced oxidative stress, suggested by the authors to be induced by these players' regular participation in intensive physical training. Interestingly, this oxidative stress was evident despite their apparently normal blood antioxidant status.

Can taking additional antioxidant supplements attenuate exercise-induced changes in immune function and infection risk? Unfortunately, no studies in footballers have attempted to answer this question. However, several double-blind placebo studies of South African ultramarathon runners did demonstrate that vitamin C (but not E or beta-carotene) supplementation (about 600 mg · day^{-1} for 3 weeks) was related to fewer reports of URTI symptoms (Peters 1990; Peters & Bateman, 1983; Peters *et al.*, 1993, 1996; Peters-Futre, 1997). This has not been replicated, however, by other research teams. Himmelstein, Robergs, Koehler, Lewis and Qualls (1998), for example, reported no alteration in URTI incidence among 44 marathon runners and 48 sedentary individuals randomly assigned to a 2 month regimen of $1000\,mg \cdot day^{-1}$ of vitamin C or placebo. Most randomized, placebo-controlled studies have been unable to demonstrate that vitamin C supplements modulate immune responses following heavy exertion (Nieman *et al.*, 1997b, 2002b; Nieman, Peters, Henson, Nevines, & Thompson, 2000b).

Vitamin E functions primarily as a non-specific, chain-breaking antioxidant that prevents the propagation of lipid peroxidation. The vitamin is a peroxyl radical scavenger and protects polyunsaturated fatty acids within membrane phospholipids and in plasma lipoproteins. The effect of vitamin E supplementation on the inflammatory and immune response to intensive and prolonged exercise is largely unstudied and equivocal. Cannon *et al.* (1991) found that vitamin E supplementation of $800\,IU \cdot day^{-1}$ for 48 days attenuated endotoxin-induced IL-6 secretion from mononuclear cells for 12 days after running downhill on an inclined treadmill. Singh *et al.* (1999) showed no effect of vitamin E supplementation (4 days, $800\,IU \cdot day^{-1}$) on the increase in plasma IL-6 following a 98 min treadmill run at 65–70% $\dot{V}O_{2max}$ to exhaustion. Petersen *et al.* (2002) reported no influence of vitamin E and C supplementation (500 mg and 400 mg, respectively, for 14 days before and 7 days after) on the plasma cytokine response to a 5% downhill 90 min treadmill run at 75% $\dot{V}O_{2max}$.

Two months of vitamin E supplementation at a dose of $800\,IU/ \cdot day^{-1}$ α-tocopherol did not affect increases in plasma cytokines, perturbations in other measures of immunity, or oxidative stress in triathletes competing in the Kona Triathlon World Championship race event (Nieman *et al.*, 2004). On the contrary, athletes in the vitamin E group experienced greater lipid peroxidation and increases in plasma levels of several cytokines than members of the placebo group following the triathlon. Despite these indications that vitamin E exerted pro-oxidant and pro-inflammatory effects, race performance did not differ between athletes in the vitamin E and placebo groups. In general, vitamin E supplementation to counter immune suppression and oxidative stress in endurance athletes cannot be recommended.

Glutamine

Glutamine, a non-essential amino acid, has attracted much attention by investigators (Mackinnon & Hooper, 1996; Rohde *et al.*, 1995; Rohde, MacLean, & Pedersen, 1998). Glutamine is the most abundant amino acid in the body, and is synthesized by skeletal muscle and other tissues. Glutamine is an important fuel for lymphocytes and monocytes, and decreased amounts *in vitro* have a direct effect in lowering proliferation rates of lymphocytes.

Reduced plasma glutamine has been observed in response to various stressors, including prolonged exercise. Since skeletal muscle is the major tissue involved in glutamine production and is known to release glutamine into the blood compartment at a high rate, it has been hypothesized that muscle activity may directly influence the immune system by altering the availability of this immune cell fuel substrate. A reduction in URTI incidence rates has been reported following marathon race events in runners consuming beverages containing glutamine (Castell, Poortmans, & Newsholme, 1996; Castell *et al.*, 1997).

Whether exercise-induced reductions in plasma glutamine are linked to impaired immunity and host protection against viruses in athletes is still unclear, but the majority of studies have not favoured such a relationship (Nieman & Pedersen, 2000). For example, in a crossover, placebo-controlled study of eight males, glutamine supplementation abolished the post-exercise decrease in plasma glutamine concentration but still had no influence relative to placebo on exercise-induced decreases in T and natural killer cell function (Rohde *et al.*, 1998).

One problem with the glutamine hypothesis is that plasma concentrations following exercise do not decrease below threshold values that are detrimental to lymphocyte function as demarcated by *in vitro* experiments. In other words, even marathon-type exertion does not deplete the large body stores of glutamine enough to diminish lymphocyte function.

Nutritional components requiring further study in athletes

There are many nutritional components that have the potential to serve as countermeasures to immune dysfunction in athletes. Data from cellular and animal studies indicate that quercetin, beta-glucan, and curcumin warrant further testing in human athletes, and many other advanced supplements will be added to this list over the next decade.

Polyphenolic compounds are abundant throughout the plant kingdom and are found in a wide variety of human foods. The effects of dietary polyphenols are of great current interest due to their antioxidative, anti-inflammatory, and possible anti-carcinogenic activities (Gee & Johnson, 2001). The flavonoids, which are the best defined group of polyphenols in the human diet, comprise a large and complex group, all of which contain a three-ring structure with two aromatic centres and a central oxygenated heterocycle. Flavonoids provide much of the flavour and colour to fruits and vegetables. More than 5000 different flavonoids have been described (Ross & Kasum, 2002). There are six major subclasses of flavonoids, including flavonols, the subclass that includes quercetin. Epidemiological studies have shown flavonoid intake (mostly quercetin) to be inversely associated with mortality from cardiac heart disease. Quercetin is a potent antioxidant *in vitro*, and protection against the oxidative damage to LDL implicated in atherogenesis has been suggested as a possible mechanism (Wiseman, 1999). There is consistent evidence that quercetin may reduce the risk of lung cancer, and this may be due to its effects on cell cycle control and apoptosis (Neuhouser, 2004). Humans can absorb significant amounts of quercetin (particularly in the glucoside form) and it would appear to be sufficiently bioavailable to act as an antioxidant *in vivo* (Wiseman, 1999).

Quercetin regulates the expression of some genes including transcription factor nuclear factor-kappaB (NFκB) (Moskaug, Carlsen, Myhrstad, & Blomhoff, 2004). In one study, quercetin inhibited NFκB activation and diminished the induction of both pro-inflammatory cytokine transcription for IL-1beta, TNF-alpha, monocytes chemoattractant protein-1, and macrophage inflammatory protein-1 (Rangan, Wang, Tay, & Harris, 1999). In another study, rats fed 100 mg quercetin per kilogram of body mass daily for 7 weeks had significantly enhanced natural killer cell activity (NKCA) compared with controls (Exon, Magnuson, South, & Hendrix, 1998). Quercetin as a potent antioxidant may reduce free radical damage to tissues during exercise, and thus reduce NFκB activation of gene expression for IL-1beta and TNF-alpha. Thus there is some biologic plausibility that quercetin could influence immune function changes, inflammation, and oxidative stress in exercising humans, and studies have been initiated to determine if quercetin is an effective countermeasure.

Beta-glucan, a polysaccharide derived from the cell wall of yeast, fungi, algae, and oats, has well-documented immunostimulant properties. Beta-glucan can enhance the activities of both innate and specific immune function and has been shown to enhance the resistance to various viral, bacterial, protozoan, and fungal diseases, as well as to promote anti-tumour activity. A series of studies have shown that oral feedings of oat beta-glucan can offset exercise-induced immune suppression and decrease susceptibility to URTI and tumour metastasis in a mouse model of exhaustive exercise and short-term heavy training (Davis *et al.*, 2004; Murphy *et al.*, 2004). In one study, oat beta-glucan blocked the increase in morbidity and mortality after intranasal inoculation of herpes simplex virus type 1 (HSV-1) combined with treadmill running to fatigue for three consecutive days (Davis *et al.*, 2004). This protective effect was linked to an increase in macrophage antiviral resistance to HSV-1 but not NK cytotoxicity. Studies have been initiated to determine if this effect also occurs in human athletes.

Curcumin is the major curcuminoid in the Indian spice turmeric, and has potent anti-inflammatory activity. Ingestion of curcumin for 3 days prior to muscle-damaging downhill running attenuated muscle damage and hastened recovery of endurance performance in mice (J. M. Davis, personal communication). Curcumin may serve as a more effective anti-inflammatory than ibuprofen during and following heavy exertion, but research in human athletes is needed. Use of ibuprofen during ultramarathon race events has been linked to elevated plasma cytokine and endotoxaemia (Nieman *et al.*, 2005a).

Conclusions

The risk of upper respiratory tract infection can increase when athletes push beyond normal limits. The infection risk is amplified when other factors related to immune function are present, including exposure to novel pathogens during travel, lack of sleep, severe mental stress, malnutrition, or weight loss.

Many components of the immune system exhibit adverse change after prolonged, heavy exertion lasting more than 90 min. These immune changes occur in several compartments of the immune system and body (e.g. the skin, upper respiratory tract mucosal tissue, lung, blood, and muscle). During this "open window" of impaired immunity (which may last between 3 and 72 h, depending on the immune measure), viruses and bacteria may gain a foothold, increasing the risk of subclinical and clinical infection. Of the various nutritional countermeasures that have been evaluated thus far, ingestion of carbohydrate beverages during intense and prolonged exercise has emerged as the most effective. However, carbohydrate supplementation during exercise decreases exercise-induced increases in plasma cytokines and stress hormones, but is largely ineffective against other immune components including natural killer cell function and salivary IgA. Ongoing research will determine the value of other nutritional components in countering immune dysfunction in heavily exercising athletes.

References

Baetjer, A. M. (1932). The effect of muscular fatigue upon resistance. *Physiological Reviews, 12*, 453–468.

Bishop, N. C., Blannin, A. K., Robson, P. J. Walsh, N. P., & Gleeson, M. (1999). The effects of carbohydrate supplementation on immune responses to a football-specific exercise protocol. *Journal of Sports Sciences, 17*, 787–796.

Bishop, N. C., Gleeson, M., Nicholas, C. W., & Ali, A. (2002). Influence of carbohydrate supplementation on plasma cytokine and neutrophil degranulation responses to high intensity intermittent exercise. *International Journal of Sport Nutrition and Exercise Metabolism, 12*, 145–156.

Bishop, N. C., Walker, G. J., Bowley, L. A., Evans, K. F., Molyneux, K., Wallace, F. A. et al. (2005). Lymphocyte responses to influenza and tetanus toxoid in vitro following intensive exercise and carbohydrate ingestion on consecutive days. *Journal of Applied Physiology, 99*, 1327–1335.

Bruunsgaard, H., Hartkopp, A., Mohr, T., Konradsen, H., Heron, I., Mordhorst, C. H. et al. (1997). In vivo cell-mediated immunity and vaccination response following prolonged, intense exercise. *Medicine and Science in Sports and Exercise, 29*, 1176–1181.

Bury, T., Marechal, R., Mahieu, P., & Pirnay, F. (1998). Immunological status of competitive football players during the training season. *International Journal of Sports Medicine, 19*, 364–368.

Calder, P. C. (2004). N-3 fatty acids, inflammation, and immunity – relevance to post-surgical and critically ill patients. *Lipids, 39*, 1147–1161.

Calder, P. C., & Kew, S. (2002). The immune system: A target for functional foods? *British Journal of Nutrition, 88* (suppl. 2), S165–S177.

Cannon, J. G., Meydani, S. N., Fiedling, R. A., Fiatarone, M. A., Meydani, M., Farhangmehr, M. et al. (1991). Acute phase response to exercise. II. Associations between vitamin E, cytokines, and muscle proteolysis. *American Journal of Physiology, 260*, R1235–R1240.

Castell, L. M., Poortmans, J. R., Leclercq, R., Brasseur, M., Duchateau, J., & Newsholme, E. A. (1997). Some aspects of the acute phase response after a marathon race, and the effects of glutamine supplementation. *European Journal of Applied Physiology*, 75, 47–53.

Castell, L. M., Poortmans, J. R., & Newsholme, E. A. (1996). Does glutamine have a role in reducing infections in athletes? *European Journal of Applied Physiology*, 73, 488–490.

Davis, J. M., Kohut, M. L., Colbert, L. H., Jackson, D. A., Ghaffar, A., & Mayer, E. P. (1997). Exercise, alveolar macrophage function, and susceptibility to respiratory infection. *Journal of Applied Physiology*, 83, 1461–1466.

Davis, J. M., Murphy, E. A., Brown, A. S., Carmichael, M. D., Ghaffar, A., & Mayer, E. P. (2004). Effects of oat beta-glucan on innate immunity and infection after exercise stress. *Medicine and Science in Sports and Exercise*, 36, 1321–1327.

Drenth, J. P., Van Uum, S. H. M., Van Deuren, M., Pesman, G. J., Van Der VenJongekrijg, J., & Van Der Meer, J. W. M. (1995). Endurance run increases circulating IL-6 and IL-1ra but down regulates *ex vivo* TNF-α and IL-1β production. *Journal of Applied Physiology*, 79, 1497–1503.

Exon, J. H., Magnuson, B. A., South, E. H., & Hendrix, K. (1998). Dietary quercetin, immune functions and colonic carcinogenesis in rats. *Immunopharmacology and Immunotoxicology*, 20, 173–190.

Gabriel, H., & Kindermann, W. (1997). The acute immune response to exercise: What does it mean? *International Journal of Sports Medicine*, 18 (suppl. 1), S28–S45.

Gee, J. M., & Johnson, I. T. (2001). Polyphenolic compounds: Interactions with the gut and implications for human health. *Current Medicinal Chemistry*, 8, 1245–1255.

Gleeson, M. (2004). Exercise and immune function. *European Journal of Sports Sciences*, 4, 52–66.

Gleeson, M., Nieman, D. C., & Pedersen, B. K. (2004). Exercise, nutrition and immune function. *Journal of Sports Sciences*, 22, 115–125.

Grimble, R. F. (2005). Immunonutrition. *Current Opinion in Gastroenterology*, 21, 216–222.

Hamer, M., Wolvers, D., & Albers, R. (2004). Using stress models to evaluate immuno-modulating effects of nutritional intervention in healthy individuals. *Journal of the American College of Nutrition*, 23, 637–646.

Heath, G. W., Ford, E. S., Craven, T. E., Macera, C. A., Jackson, K. L., & Pate, R. R. (1991). Exercise and the incidence of upper respiratory tract infections. *Medicine and Science in Sports and Exercise*, 23, 152–157.

Himmelstein, S. A., Robergs, R. A., Koehler, K. M., Lewis, S. L., & Qualls, C. R. (1998). Vitamin C supplementation and upper respiratory tract infections in marathon runners. *Journal of Exercise Physiolology (Online)*, 1, 1–17.

Hoffman-Goetz, L., & Pedersen, B. K. (1994). Exercise and the immune system: A model of the stress response? *Immunology Today*, 15, 382–387.

Keusch, G. T. (2003). The history of nutrition: Malnutrition, infection and immunity. *Journal of Nutrition*, 133, 336S–3340S.

Klapcińska, B., Kempa, K., Sobczak, A., Sadowska-Krepa, E., Jagsz, S., & Szoltysek, I. (2005). Evaluation of autoantibodies against oxidized LDL (oLAB) and blood anti-oxidant status in professional football players. *International Journal of Sports Medicine*, 26, 71–78.

Konig, D., Grathwohl, D., Weinstock, C., Northoff, H., & Berg, A. (2000). Upper respiratory tract infection in athletes: Influence of lifestyle, type of sport, training effort, and immunostimulant intake. *Exercise Immunology Reviews*, 6, 102–120.

Kostka, T., Berthouze, S. E., Lacour, J., & Bonnefoy, M. (2000). The symptomatology of upper respiratory tract infections and exercise in elderly people. *Medicine and Science in Sports and Exercise, 32,* 46–51.

Lee, D. J., Meehan, R. T., Robinson, C., Mabry, T. R., & Smith, M. L. (1992). Immune responsiveness and risk of illness in U.S. Air Force Academy cadets during basic cadet training. *Aviation, Space and Environmental Medicine, 63,* 517–523.

Linde, F. (1987). Running and upper respiratory tract infections. *Scandinavian Journal of Sports Sciences, 9,* 21–23.

Mackinnon, L. T., Ginn, E. M., & Seymour, G. J. (1993). Temporal relationship between decreased salivary IgA and upper respiratory tract infection in elite athletes. *Australian Journal of Science and Medicine in Sport, 25,* 94–99.

Mackinnon, L. T., & Hooper, S. (1994). Mucosal (secretory) immune system responses to exercise of varying intensity and during overtraining. *International Journal of Sports Medicine, 15,* S179–S183.

Mackinnon, L. T., & Hooper, S. L. (1996). Plasma glutamine and upper respiratory tract infection during intensified training in swimmers. *Medicine and Science in Sports and Exercise, 28,* 285–290.

Malm, C., Ekblom, Ö., & Ekblom E. (2004a). Immune system alteration in response to increased physical training during a five day football training camp. *International Journal of Sports Medicine, 25,* 471–476.

Malm, C., Ekblom, Ö., & Ekblom, E. (2004b). Immune system alteration in response to two consecutive football games. *Acta Physiologica Scandinavica, 180,* 143–155.

Matthews, C. E., Ockene, I. S., Freedson, P. S., Rosal, M. C., Merriam, P. A., & Hebert, J. R. (2002). Moderate to vigorous physical activity and risk of upper-respiratory tract infection. *Medicine and Science in Sports and Exercise, 34,* 1242–1248.

Moskaug, J. O., Carlsen, H., Myhrstad, M., & Blomhoff, R. (2004). Molecular imaging of the biological effects of quercetin and quercetin-rich foods. *Mech Ageing and Development., 125,* 315–324.

Müns, G. (1993). Effect of long-distance running on polymorphonuclear neutrophil phagocytic function of the upper airways. *International Journal of Sports Medicine, 15,* 96–99.

Murphy, E. A., Davis, J. M., Brown, A. S., Carmichael, M. D., Mayer, E. P., & Ghaffar, A. (2004). Effects of moderate exercise and oat beta-glucan on lung tumor metastases and macrophage antitumor cytotoxicity. *Journal of Applied Physiology, 97,* 955–959.

Murray, R., Paul, G. L., Seifert, G. J., & Eddy, D. E. (1991). Responses to varying rates of carbohydrate ingestion during exercise. *Medicine and Science in Sports and Exercise, 23,* 713–718.

Nehlsen-Cannarella, S. L., Fagoaga, O. R., Nieman, D. C., Henson, D. A., Butterworth, D. E., Schmitt, R. L. *et al.* (1997). Carbohydrate and the cytokine response to 2.5 hours of running. *Journal of Applied Physiology, 82,* 1662–1667.

Nehlsen-Cannarella, S. L., Nieman, D. C., Jessen, J., Chang, L., Gusewitch, G., Blix, G. G. *et al.* (1991). The effects of acute moderate exercise on lymphocyte function and serum immunoglobulins. *International Journal of Sports Medicine, 12,* 391–398.

Neuhouser, M. L. (2004). Dietary flavonoids and cancer risk: Evidence from human population studies. *Nutrition and Cancer, 50,* 1–7.

Nieman, D. C. (1997a). Exercise immunology: Practical applications. *International Journal of Sports Medicine, 18* (suppl. 1), S91–S100.

Nieman, D. C. (1997b). Immune response to heavy exertion. *Journal of Applied Physiology*, 82, 1385–1394.

Nieman, D. C. (2000). Exercise effects on systemic immunity. *Immunology and Cell Biology*, 78, 496–501.

Nieman, D. C. (2001). Exercise immunology: Nutritional countermeasures. *Canadian Journal of Applied Physiology*, 26 (suppl.), S45–S55.

Nieman, D. C. (2003). Current perspective on exercise immunology. *Current Sports Medicine Reports*, 2, 239–242.

Nieman, D. C., Ahle, J. C., Henson, D. A., Warren, B. J., Suttles, J., Davis, J. M. *et al.* (1995a). Indomethacin does not alter the natural killer cell response to 2.5 hours of running. *Journal of Applied Physiology*, 79, 748–755.

Nieman, D. C., Buckley, K. S., Henson, D. A., Warren, B. J., Suttles, J., Ahle, J. C. *et al.* (1995b). Immune function in marathon runners versus sedentary controls. *Medicine and Science in Sports and Exercise*, 27, 986–992.

Nieman, D. C., Davis, J. M., Henson, D. A., Walberg-Rankin, J., Shute, M., Dumke, C. L. *et al.* (2003a). Carbohydrate ingestion influences skeletal muscle cytokine mRNA and plasma cytokine levels after a 3-h run. *Journal of Applied Physiology*, 94, 1917–1925.

Nieman, D. C., Dumke, C. L., Henson, D. A., McAnulty, S. R., Gross, S. J., & Lind, R. H. (2005a). Muscle damage is linked to cytokine changes following a 160-km race. *Brain and Behavioural Immunity*, 19, 298–403.

Nieman, D. C., Dumke, C. L., Henson, D. A., McAnulty, S. R., McAnulty, L. S., Lind, R. H. *et al.* (2003b). Immune and oxidative changes during and following the Western States Endurance Run. *International Journal of Sports Medicine*, 24, 541–547.

Nieman, D. C., Fagoaga, O. R., Butterworth, D. E., Warren, B. J., Utter, A., Davis, J. M. *et al.* (1997a). Carbohydrate supplementation affects blood granulocyte and monocyte trafficking but not function following 2.5 hours of running. *American Journal of Clinical Nutrition*, 66, 153–159.

Nieman, D. C., Henson, D. A., Austin, M. D., & Brown, V. A. (2005b). The immune response to a 30-minute walk. *Medicine and Science in Sports and Exercise*, 37, 57–62.

Nieman, D. C., Henson, D. A., Butterworth, D. E., Warren, B. J., Davis, J. M., Fagoaga, O. R. *et al.* (1997b). Vitamin C supplementation does not alter the immune response to 2.5 hours of running. *International Journal of Sports Nutrition*, 7, 174–184.

Nieman, D. C., Henson, D. A., Dumke, C. L., Lind, R. H., Shooter, L. R., & Gross, S. J. (in press). Relationship between salivary IgA secretion and upper respiratory tract infection following a 160-km race. *Journal of Sports Medicine and Physical Fitness*.

Nieman, D. C., Henson, D. A., Fagoaga, O. R., Utter, A. C., Vinci, D. M., Davis, J. M. *et al.* (2002a). Change in salivary IgA following a competitive marathon race. *International Journal of Sports Medicine*, 23, 69–75.

Nieman, D. C., Henson, D. A., Garner, E. B., Butterworth, D. E., Warren, B. J., Utter, A. *et al.* (1997c). Carbohydrate affects natural killer cell redistribution but not activity after running. *Medicine and Science in Sports and Exercise*, 29, 1318–1324.

Nieman, D. C., Henson, D. A., Gusewitch, G., Warren, B. J., Dotson, R. C., Butterworth, D. E. *et al.* (1993). Physical activity and immune function in elderly women. *Medicine and Science in Sports and Exercise*, 25, 823–831.

Nieman, D. C., Henson, D. A., McAnulty, S. R., McAnulty, L. S., Morrow, J. D., Ahmed, A. *et al.* (2004). Vitamin E and immunity after the Kona Triathlon World Championship. *Medicine and Science in Sports and Exercise*, 36, 1328–1335.

Nieman, D. C., Henson, D. A., McAnulty, S. R., McAnulty, L., Swick, N. S., Utter, A. C. et al. (2002b). Influence of vitamin C supplementation on oxidative and immune changes following an ultramarathon. *Journal of Applied Physiology*, 92, 1970–1977.

Nieman, D. C., Henson, D. A., Smith, L. L., Utter, A. C., Vinci, D. M., Davis, J. M. et al. (2001). Cytokine changes after a marathon race. *Journal of Applied Physiology*, 91, 109–114.

Nieman, D. C., Johanssen, L. M., & Lee, J. W. (1989). Infectious episodes in runners before and after a roadrace. *Journal of Sports Medicine and Physical Fitness*, 29, 289–296.

Nieman, D. C., Johanssen, L. M., Lee, J. W., Cermak, J., & Arabatzis, K. (1990a). Infectious episodes in runners before and after the Los Angeles Marathon. *Journal of Sports Medicine and Physical Fitness*, 30, 316–328.

Nieman, D. C., & Nehlsen-Cannarella, S. L. (1994). The immune response to exercise. *Seminars in Hematology*, 31, 166–179.

Nieman, D. C., Nehlsen-Cannarella, S. L., Fagoaga, O. R., Henson, D. A., Shannon, M., Davis, J. M. et al. (1999). Immune response to two hours of rowing in female elite rowers. *International Journal of Sports Medicine*, 20, 476–481.

Nieman, D. C., Nehlsen-Cannarella, S. L., Fagoaga, O. R., Henson, D. A., Shannon, M., Hjertman, J. M. E. et al. (2000a). Immune function in female elite rowers and non-athletes. *British Journal of Sports Medicine*, 34, 181–187.

Nieman, D. C., Nehlsen-Cannarella, S. L., Henson, D. A., Butterworth, D. E., Fagoaga, O. R., & Utter, A. (1998a). Immune response to exercise training and/or energy restriction in obese women. *Medicine and Science in Sports and Exercise*, 30, 679–686.

Nieman, D. C., Nehlsen-Cannarella, S. L., Henson, D. A., Butterworth, D. E., Fagoaga, O. R., & Utter, A. (1998b). Influence of carbohydrate ingestion and mode on the granulocyte and monocyte response to heavy exertion in triathletes. *Journal of Applied Physiology*, 84, 1252–1259.

Nieman, D. C., Nehlsen-Cannarella, S. L., Markoff, P. A., Balk-Lamberton, A. J., Yang, H., Chritton, D. B. W. et al. (1990b). The effects of moderate exercise training on natural killer cells and acute upper respiratory tract infections. *International Journal of Sports Medicine*, 11, 467–473.

Nieman, D. C., & Pedersen, B. K. (2000). *Nutrition and exercise immunology*. Boca Raton, FL: CRC Press.

Nieman, D. C., Peters, E. M., Henson, D. A., Nevines, E., & Thompson, M. M. (2000b). Influence of vitamin C supplementation on cytokine changes following an ultramarathon. *Journal of Interferon and Cytokine Research*, 20, 1029–1035.

Nieman, D. C., Simandle, S., Henson, D. A., Warren, B. J., Suttles, J., Davis, J. M. et al. (1995c). Lymphocyte proliferation response to 2.5 hours of running. *International Journal of Sports Medicine*, 16, 406–410.

Pedersen, B. K., & Bruunsgaard, H. (1995). How physical exercise influences the establishment of infections. *Sports Medicine*, 19, 393–400.

Peters, E. M. (1990). Altitude fails to increase susceptibility of ultramarathon runners to post-race upper respiratory tract infections. *South African Journal of Sports Medicine*, 5, 4–8.

Peters, E. M., & Bateman, E. D. (1983). Respiratory tract infections: An epidemiological survey. *South African Medical Journal*, 64, 582–584.

Peters, E. M., Goetzsche, J. M., Grobbelaar, B., & Noakes, T. D. (1993). Vitamin C supplementation reduces the incidence of postrace symptoms of upper-respiratory-tract infection in ultramarathon runners. *American Journal of Clinical Nutrition, 57,* 170–174.

Peters E. M., Goetzsche, J. M., Joseph, L. E., & Noakes, T. D. (1996). Vitamin C as effective as combinations of anti-oxidant nutrients in reducing symptoms of upper respiratory tract infection in ultramarathon runners. *South African Journal of Sports Medicine, 11,* 23–27.

Peters-Futre, E. M. (1997). Vitamin C, neutrophil function, and upper respiratory tract infection risk in distance runners: The missing link. *Exercise Immunology Reviews, 3,* 32–52.

Petersen, A. M., & Pedersen, B. K. (2005). The anti-inflammatory effect of exercise. *Journal of Applied Physiology, 98,* 1154–1162.

Petersen, E. W., Ostrowski, K., Ibfelt, T., Richelle, M., Offord, E., Halkjaer-Kristensen, J. et al. (2002). Effect of vitamin supplementation on cytokine response and on muscle damage after strenuous exercise. *American Journal of Physiology, 280,* C1570–C1575.

Plat, J., & Mensink, R. P. (2005). Food components and immune function. *Current Opinions in Lipidology, 16,* 31–37.

Pyne, D. B., Baker, M. S., Fricker, P. A., McDonald, W. A., & Nelson, W. J. (1995). Effects of an intensive 12-wk training program by elite swimmers on neutrophil oxidative activity. *Medicine and Science in Sports and Exercise, 27,* 536–542.

Rangan, G. K., Wang, Y., Tay, Y. C., & Harris, D. C. (1999). Inhibition of NFkappaB activation with antioxidants is correlated with reduced cytokine transcription in PTC. *American Journal of Physiology, 277,* F770–F789.

Rebelo, A. N., Candeias, J. R., Fraga, M. M., Duarte, J. A., Soares J. M., Magalhaes, C. et al. (1998). The impact of football training on the immune system. *Journal of Sports Medicine and Physical Fitness, 38,* 258–261.

Rohde, T., MacLean, D. A., & Pedersen, B. K. (1998). Effect of glutamine supplementation on changes in the immune system induced by repeated exercise. *Medicine and Science in Sports and Exercise, 30,* 856–862.

Rohde, T., Ullum, H., Rasmussen, J. P., Kristensen, J. H., Newsholme, E., & Pedersen, B. K. (1995). Effects of glutamine on the immune system: Influence of muscular exercise and HIV infection. *Journal of Applied Physiology, 79,* 146–150.

Ross, J. A., & Kasum, C. M. (2002). Dietary flavonoids: Bioavailability, metabolic effects, and safety. *Annual Reviews of Nutrition, 22,* 19–34.

Shephard, R. J., Kavanagh, T., Mertens, D. J., Qureshi, S., & Clark, M. (1995). Personal health benefits of Masters athletics competition. *British Journal of Sports Medicine, 29,* 35–40.

Shinkai, S., Kurokawa, Y., Hino, S., Hirose, M., Torii, J., Watanabe, S. et al. (1993). Triathlon competition induced a transient immunosuppressive change in the peripheral blood of athletes. *Journal of Sports Medicine and Physical Fitness, 33,* 70–78.

Singh, A., Papanicolaou, D. A., Lawrence, L. L., Howell, E. A., Chrousos, G. P., & Deuster, P. A. (1999). Neuroendocrine responses to running in women after zinc and vitamin E supplementation. *Medicine and Science in Sports and Exercise, 31,* 536–542.

Smith, J. A., & Pyne, D. B. (1997). Exercise, training, and neutrophil function. *Exercise Immunology Reviews, 3,* 96–117.

Strasner, A., Barlow, C. E., Kampert, J. B., & Dunn, A. L. (2001). Impact of physical activity on URTI symptoms in Project PRIME participants. *Medicine and Science in Sports and Exercise, 33* (suppl.), S304.

Urso, M. L., & Clarkson, P. M. (2003). Oxidative stress, exercise, and antioxidant supplementation. *Toxicology, 189,* 41–54.

Wiseman, H. (1999). The bioavailability of non-nutrient plant factors: Dietary flavonoids and phyto-estrogens. *Proceedings of the Nutrition Society, 58,* 139–146.

10 The brain and fatigue: New opportunities for nutritional interventions?

ROMAIN MEEUSEN, PHIL WATSON AND JIRI DVORAK

It is clear that the cause of fatigue is complex, influenced by events occurring in both the periphery and the central nervous system. Work conducted over the last 20 years has focused on the role of brain serotonin and catecholamines in the development of fatigue, and the possibility that manipulation of neuro-transmitter precursors may delay the onset of fatigue. While there is some evidence that branched-chain amino acid and tyrosine ingestion can influence perceived exertion and some measures of mental performance, the results of several apparently well-controlled laboratory studies have not demonstrated a positive effect on exercise capacity or performance under temperate conditions. As football is highly reliant upon the successful execution of motor skills and tactics, the possibility that amino acid ingestion may help to attenuate a loss in cognitive function during the later stages of a game would be desirable, even in the absence of no apparent benefit to physical performance. There are several reports of enhanced performance of high-intensity intermittent exercise with carbohydrate ingestion, but at present it is difficult to separate the peripheral effects from any potential impact on the central nervous system. The possibility that changes in central neurotransmission play a role in the aetiology of fatigue when exercise is performed in high ambient temperatures has recently been examined, although the significance of this in relation to the pattern of activity associated with football has yet to be determined.

Keywords: Branched-chain amino acids, carbohydrate, dopamine, neuro-transmission, serotonin, tyrosine

Introduction

Progressive fatigue that occurs during high-intensity intermittent exercise, characteristic of many team sports including football, has been typically ascribed to the depletion of muscle glycogen, reductions in circulating blood glucose, hyperthermia, and the progressive loss of body fluids (Mohr, Krustrup, & Bangsbo, 2005). These factors are thought to result in a reduction in distances covered, and the number and intensity of sprints undertaken by players, towards the end of the second half of play (Mohr, Krustrup, & Bangsbo, 2003). Although the idea that the central nervous system (CNS) is involved in feelings of tiredness, lethargy, and mood disturbances is not new, evidence has accumulated over the past 20 years to support a significant role of the brain in the aetiology of fatigue during strenuous exercise. It is now acknowledged that the cause of fatigue is a complex phenomenon influenced by both events occurring in the periphery and the CNS (Meeusen & De Meirleir, 1995; Nybo & Secher, 2004).

At the highest level, footballers have been reported to cover distances in excess of 10 km during competitive matches (Bangsbo, Norregaard, & Thorsoe, 1991). This activity typically consists of periods of walking and low- to moderate-intensity running, interspersed with explosive bursts of activity including sprinting, jumping, changes in speed and direction, and tackling. In many skill-based sports, participants have simultaneously to undertake mechanical work, often with a great physical demand, coupled with the precise performance of decisional and/or perceptual tasks. Football matches include periods of high-intensity activity, and successful football performance depends upon many factors, including technical, tactical, physical, physiological, and mental skills. Increased fatigue has commonly been observed after exercise and, although detrimental effects on mood or mental performance are typically small (Collardeau, Brisswalter, Vercruyssen, Audiffren, & Goubault, 2001), in sports such as football even minor decrements in mental performance can significantly influence the outcome of a game.

In this review, we discuss possible neurobiological mechanisms of fatigue and examine whether nutritional and pharmacological interventions to alter central neurotransmission are capable of influencing the development of fatigue during exercise.

The "central fatigue hypothesis"

The "central fatigue hypothesis" is based on the assumption that during prolonged exercise the synthesis and metabolism of central monoamines, in particular serotonin, dopamine, and noradrenaline, are influenced. It was first suggested by Newsholme, Ackworth and Blomstrand (1987) that prolonged exercise results in an increase in brain serotonergic activity that may augment lethargy, cause an altered sensation of effort, perhaps a differing tolerance of pain/discomfort, and a loss of drive and motivation, thus limiting physical and mental performance.

The rate of serotonin synthesis is largely dependent upon the peripheral availability of the essential amino acid tryptophan. An increase in the delivery of trypyophan to the CNS will increase serotonergic activity because the rate-limiting enzyme, tryptophan hydroxylase, is not saturated under physiological conditions. Furthermore, free tryptophan and the branched-chained amino acids share the same carrier in order to pass across the blood–brain barrier, meaning that the plasma concentration ratio of free trypyophan to branched-chain amino acids is thought to be an important determinant of serotonin synthesis.

The underlying mechanisms behind the central fatigue hypothesis as proposed by Newsholme *et al.* (1987) can be divided into two interrelated parts:

1. Under resting conditions, most tryptophan, the precursor of serotonin, circulates in the blood loosely bound to albumin, a transporter shared with free fatty acids (FFA). The shift in substrate mobilization that occurs as exercise progresses causes an increase in plasma FFA concentration. This displaces tryptophan from binding sites on albumin, leading to a marked increase in free tryptophan. Free tryptophan is then readily available for transport across the blood–brain barrier.
2. Plasma branched-chain amino acid concentrations either fall or are unchanged during prolonged exercise. Since free tryptophan and branched-chain amino acids share a common transporter across the blood–brain barrier, a reduction in competing large neutral amino acids (LNAA) would increase the uptake of tryptophan into the CNS. The resulting elevation in tryptophan delivery results in an increased central synthesis of serotonin.

Is there experimental evidence for central fatigue?

Since neurotransmitters, including serotonin, dopamine, and noradrenaline, have been implicated in the aetiology of a wide variety of psychiatric and mood disorders (e.g. depression, anxiety disorders, Parkinson's disease), a vast number of drugs have been developed to directly manipulate central neurotransmission. Through an understanding of the action of these pharmacological agents, it has been possible to examine the role of the CNS in the fatigue process. However, at present there appears to be no published reports of the effects of pharmacological manipulation of central neurotransmission on performance during high-intensity intermittent activity.

Bailey and co-workers were among the first to examine the effects of pharmacological manipulation of brain serotonin concentrations through the administration of specific serotonin agonists and antagonists to rodents (Bailey, Davis, & Ahlborn, 1992, 1993). This early work provided good evidence for a role of serotonin in the development of fatigue, with a dose-dependent reduction in exercise capacity reported when central serotonin activity was augmented by the acute administration of a general serotonin agonist (Bailey *et al.*, 1992). Brain serotonin and dopamine content progressively increased during exercise, but at the point of exhaustion a marked fall in tissue dopamine content was apparent. Furthermore, exercise capacity was enhanced by a serotonin antagonist (LY-53857), although this was apparent only when the highest dose was administered (Bailey *et al.*, 1993).

Selective serotonin reuptake inhibitors (SSRIs)

The SSRIs are a class of drugs that selectively inhibit the reuptake of serotonin into the pre-synaptic nerve terminal, thus increasing the extracellular concentration of serotonin present at the post-synaptic receptors. These agents have been widely administered in the treatment of various psychiatric disorders, in particular depression, and were the first to be employed in the study of central fatigue. To date, three studies have investigated the effects of an acute dose of paroxetine (Paxil, Seroxat), with two reporting a reduction in exercise time to exhaustion (Struder *et al.*, 1998; Wilson & Maughan, 1992). A number of subsequent studies have examined the effects of pharmacological agents acting on central serotonergic neurotransmission during prolonged exercise, with largely negative results, making it difficult at this stage to make a firm decision regarding the importance of serotonin in the fatigue process (Meeusen, Piacentini, Van den Eynde, Magnus, & De Meirleir, 2001; Meeusen, Roeykens, Magnus, Keizer, & De Meirleir, 1997; Pannier, Bouckaert, & Lefebvre, 1995; Strachan, Leiper, & Maughan, 2004).

The neuromuscular and performance effects of acute and long-term exposure to fluoxetine have also been examined (Parise, Bosman, Boecker, Barry, & Tarnopolsky, 2001). Serotonin was demonstrated to alter an individual's sensation of pain; this study differs from many others in this area by investigating whether manipulation of serotonergic neurotransmission could alter the response to high-intensity and resistance exercise. Following periods of acute and chronic (2 weeks) administration, Parise *et al.* concluded that SSRIs do not influence measures of strength or high-intensity exercise performance, including maximum voluntary contractions, voluntary activation percentage, repeated Wingate and high-intensity exercise tests to volitional exhaustion in young adult men.

Catecholaminergic drugs

Because of the complexity of brain functioning and the contradictory results of studies that have tried to manipulate only serotonergic activity, it is unlikely that one single neurotransmitter is responsible for a centrally mediated component of fatigue. In fact, alterations in catecholamines, as well as other excitatory and inhibitory neurotransmitters (glutamate, GABA, and acetylcholine), have been implicated as possible mediators of central fatigue during exercise (Meeusen & De Meirleir, 1995). These neurotransmitters are known to play a role in arousal, mood, motivation, vigilance, anxiety, and reward mechanisms, and could therefore, if adversely affected, impair performance. It is therefore necessary to explore the different transmitter systems and their effect on the neuroendocrine response to endurance exercise.

The neurotransmitters dopamine and noradrenaline have also been linked to the "central" component of fatigue, due to their well-known role in motivation and motor behaviour (Davis & Bailey, 1997; Meeusen & De Meirleir, 1995), and are therefore thought to have an enhancing effect on performance. Dopamine and noradrenaline are synthesized through a shared metabolic pathway, with the amino acid tyrosine acting as the precursor. Tyrosine is found in protein-rich dietary sources, including chicken and milk, but unlike tryptophan it is a non-essential LNAA that can also be synthesized from phenylalanine in the liver. Cerebral uptake of tyrosine is subject to competitive transport across the blood–brain barrier by the LNAA-carrier system, which is shared with tryptophan and the other LNAAs as discussed above.

Early pharmacological manipulation of central neurotransmission to improve exercise performance focused largely on the effects of amphetamines, which have a long history of abuse in sport. Amphetamine is a close analogue of dopamine and noradrenaline, and is thought to act directly on catecholaminergic neurones to produce a marked elevation in extracellular dopamine concentrations. This response is believed to be mediated through the stimulation of dopamine release from storage vesicles, inhibition of dopamine reuptake, and the inhibition of dopamine metabolism by monoamineoxidase. Amphetamines may also limit the synthesis of serotonin through a reduction in tryptophan hydroxylase activity and a direct interaction between dopamine release and serotonergic neurotransmission. Studies have demonstrated a clear performance benefit following the administration of amphetamine to both rodents (Gerald, 1978) and humans (Borg, Edstrom, Linderholm, & Marklund, 1972; Chandler & Blair, 1980). The ergogenic action of amphetamine is thought to be mediated through the maintenance of dopamine release late in exercise.

The importance of dopamine in the development of fatigue has been shown in animal studies (Heyes, Garnett, & Coates, 1985; Kalinski, Dluzen, & Stadulis, 2001). It would appear that at the point of fatigue extracellular dopamine concentrations are low, possibly due to the interaction with brain serotonin (Bailey *et al.*, 1992), or a depletion of central catecholamines (Davis & Bailey, 1997). In a series of studies, we supplemented athletes with (1) venlafaxine, a combined serotonin/noradrenaline reuptake inhibitor (SNRI; Piacentini, Meeusen, Buyse, De Schutter, & De Meirleir, 2002a), (2) reboxetine, a noradrenaline reuptake inhibitor (NARI; Piacentini *et al.*, 2002b), and (3) Buproprion, a combined noradrenaline/dopamine reuptake inhibitor (Piacentini, Meeusen, Buyse, De Schutter, & De Meirleir, 2004). Athletes performed two cycle time-trials requiring the completion of a predetermined amount of work as quickly as possible (~90 min), in a double-blind randomized crossover design. None of the agents above mentioned had a significant influence (either negative or positive) on exercise performance. Each drug clearly altered central neurotransmission, since different neuroendocrine effects were observed depending on the type of reuptake inhibitor administered.

Central fatigue and nutritional interventions

Much of the attraction of the hypothesis described by Newsholme and co-workers (1987) was the potential for nutritional manipulation of neurotransmitter precursors to delay the onset of central fatigue, potentially enhancing performance. In recent years, a number of studies have attempted to attenuate the increase in central serotonin levels and maintain/increase catecholaminergic neurotransmission through dietary supplementation with specific nutrients, including branched-chain amino acids, tyrosine, and carbohydrate.

Amino acid supplementation

As free tryptophan competes with branched-chain amino acids (BCAA) for transport across the blood–brain barrier into the CNS, reducing the plasma concentration ratio of free tryptophan to BCAA through the provision of exogenous BCAA has been suggested as a practice to attenuate the development of central fatigue. The first research to test the efficacy of BCAA supplementation in attenuating serotonin-mediated fatigue was a field study of the physical and mental performance of male volunteers competing in either a marathon or a 30 km cross-country race (Blomstrand, Hassmen, Ekblom, & Newsholme, 1991a). The results of this study suggested that both physical (race time) and mental (colour and word tests) performance were enhanced in the participants who received BCAA before exercise. However, enhanced performance was witnessed only in participants completing the marathon in times slower than 3 h 5 min, with the lack of a response in the faster runners being attributed to an increased resistance to the feelings associated with central and peripheral fatigue. The reliability of these results has been subsequently questioned, due to a number of methodological problems largely relating to the field-based nature of the study (Davis & Bailey, 1997).

While there is some additional evidence of BCAA ingestion influencing ratings of perceived exertion (RPE; Blomstrand, Hassmen, Ek, Ekblom, & Newsholme, 1997) and mental performance (Blomstrand, Hassmen, & Newsholme, 1991b; Hassmen, Blomstrand, Ekblom, & Newsholme, 1994), the results of several apparently well-controlled laboratory studies have not demonstrated a positive effect on exercise capacity or performance. No ergogenic benefit has been reported during prolonged fixed-intensity exercise to exhaustion (Blomstrand, Andersson, Hassmen, Ekblom, & Newsholme, 1995; Blomstrand *et al.*, 1997; Galiano *et al.*, 1991; Struder *et al.*, 1998; van Hall, Raaymakers, Saris, & Wagenmakers, 1995), prolonged time-trial (TT) performance (Hassmen *et al.*, 1994; Madsen, Kiens, & Christensen, 1996), or incremental exercise (Varnier *et al.*, 1994). Davis, Welsh, De Volve and Alderson (1999) investigated the effects of BCAA ingestion on the performance of a test specific to the intermittent, high-intensity activity involved in football. The effects of a sugar-free placebo, a carbohydrate solution (CHO), and a carbohydrate solution with added BCAA (CHO + BCAA) on exercise time to exhaustion were examined. Compared with the placebo trial, participants were able to run significantly longer when the CHO and CHO + BCAA solutions were ingested, but the addition of BCAA resulted in no further benefit. The possible influence of carbohydrate ingestion on the development of central fatigue is discussed below, but it is possible that the co-ingestion of BCAA together with carbohydrate may have masked any performance effect.

One possible explanation for a failure to observe an ergogenic effect in many BCAA studies, despite a good rationale for their use, is an increase in ammonia production (Davis & Bailey, 1997). During prolonged intense exercise, the plasma concentration of ammonia increases, with this increase amplified by BCAA ingestion. Since ammonia can readily cross the blood–brain barrier, it may enter the CNS where excessive accumulation may have a profound effect on cerebral function. Evidence suggests that hyperammonaemia has a marked effect of cerebral blood flow, energy metabolism, astrocyte function, synaptic transmission, and the regulation of various neurotransmitter systems (Felipo & Butterworth, 2002). Therefore, it has been considered that exercise-induced hyperammonaemia could also be a mediator of CNS fatigue during prolonged exercise (Davis & Bailey, 1997). Recently, Nybo, Dalsgaard, Steensberg, Moller and Secher (2005) reported that during prolonged exercise the cerebral uptake and accumulation of ammonia may provoke fatigue, through a disturbance to neurotransmitter metabolism. Marked increases in circulating ammonia concentrations have been reported during top-flight football matches (Mohr *et al.*, 2005), thus an accumulation of serum ammonia may contribute to the development of fatigue through disruptions in peripheral and cerebral metabolism.

The flip-side of the serotonin-fatigue hypothesis is the idea that increased catecholaminergic neurotransmission will favour feelings of arousal, motivation, and reward, consequently enhancing exercise performance. In a similar manner to serotonin, central dopamine and noradrenaline synthesis is reliant on the delivery of the non-essential amino acid tyrosine, but the rate of synthesis appears also to be limited by the activity of the catecholaminergic neurons (Davis & Bailey, 1997). Despite a good rationale for its use, evidence of an ergogenic benefit of tyrosine supplementation during prolonged exercise is limited. Work by Struder and colleagues (1998) failed to observe any change in the capacity to perform prolonged exercise following the ingestion of tyrosine immediately before (10 g) and during exercise (10 g). It has been suggested that the high dose of tyrosine administered in this study may have resulted in an inhibition of dopamine synthesis, but a recent report administering half the dose employed by Struder *et al.* (1998) also found no effect on time-trial performance (Chinevere, Sawyer, Creer, Conlee, & Parcell, 2002). Additionally, oral ingestion of tyrosine by humans had no measurable effect on endurance, muscle strength, or anaerobic power (Sutton, Coll, & Deuster, 2005).

While evidence for an effect of tyrosine on physical performance is limited, stress-related decrements in mood and task performance are reported to be reduced by tyrosine supplementation during sustained military operations exceeding 12 h, involving severe sleep deprivation and fatigue (Owasoyo, Neri, & Lamberth, 1992). There are also several reports indicating that tyrosine ingestion improves stress-induced cognitive and behavioural deficits, in particular working memory, tracking, and stress-sensitive attentional focus tasks (Banderet & Lieberman, 1989; Deijen, Wientjes, Vullinghs, Cloin, & Langefeld, 1999; Dollins, Krock, Storm, Wurtman, & Lieberman, 1995; Neri *et al.*, 1995;

Shurtleff, Thomas, Schrot, Kowalski, & Harford, 1994; Sutton *et al.*, 2005). As football is highly dependent on the successful execution of fine and gross motor skills, the possibility that tyrosine ingestion may attenuate a loss in cognitive function that occurs during the later stages of a game would be desirable, despite no apparent benefit to physical performance. It is yet to be seen whether these results can be reproduced in a football-specific protocol.

Carbohydrate supplementation

Analysis of the activity patterns and muscle biopsy data taken from football players suggest that there is a large reliance on carbohydrate utilization, and ingestion of exogenous carbohydrate before and during matches has been reported to enhance performance during the latter stages of a game (Kirkendall, 1993). The peripheral effects of carbohydrate ingestion will be discussed elsewhere in this issue, but it is clear that the provision of exogenous carbohydrate during exercise can also have a profound effect on the CNS.

Carbohydrate feeding suppresses lipolysis, consequently lowering the circulating concentration of plasma free fatty acids. Recognizing this, Davis *et al.* (1992) suggested carbohydrate ingestion as a means of reducing cerebral tryptophan uptake. A five- to seven-fold increase in the plasma concentration ratio of free tryptophan to BCAA was reported under placebo conditions. Supplementation with a 6% or 12% carbohydrate solution attenuated the increase in plasma free fatty acids and free tryptophan, reducing the plasma concentration ratio of free tryptophan to BCAA in a dose-dependent manner. Exercise capacity in the carbohydrate trials was increased compared with placebo, suggesting carbohydrate ingestion as an effective means of delaying the onset of central fatigue; however, it is difficult to separate the contribution of central factors from the widely reported benefits of carbohydrate at attenuating peripheral fatigue.

Several studies have directly examined the effect of carbohydrate supplementation on the development of fatigue during team sport-based activity (Davis *et al.*, 1999; Nicholas, Williams, Lakomy, Phillips, & Nowitz, 1995; Welsh, Davis, Burke, & Williams, 2002; Winnick *et al.*, 2005). It is clear that carbohydrate ingestion can have a profound effect on measures of physical fatigue during this type of exercise, with marked improvements in time to volitional exhaustion, maintenance of sprint performance, and vertical jump height. Recent work has also focused on the effects of carbohydrate supplementation on measures of CNS fatigue, assessed largely through the performance of skills-based tasks and psychological inventories. Ingestion of carbohydrate before and during exercise has been reported to attenuate decrements in performance of whole-body motor skills tasks (Welsh *et al.*, 2002; Winnick *et al.*, 2005).

The beneficial effect of carbohydrate supplementation during prolonged exercise could also relate to increased (or maintained) substrate delivery for the brain, with a number of studies indicating that hypoglycaemia affects brain function and cognitive performance. Exercise-induced hypoglycaemia has been reported to reduce brain glucose uptake and overall cerebral metabolic rate

(Nybo, Moller, Pedersen, Nielsen, & Secher, 2003), which is associated with a marked reduction in voluntary activation during sustained muscular contractions (Nybo, 2003). The reduction in CNS activation is abolished when euglycaemia was maintained. Ingestion of carbohydrate has also been reported to minimize the negative effect of prolonged exercise on cognitive function, with an improvement in the performance of complex cognitive tasks observed following running (Collardeau *et al.*, 2001). The results of animal studies suggest that glucose plays an important role in the regulation of central neurotransmission and alterations in extracellular glucose concentrations have been demonstrated to influence serotonin release and reuptake during exercise and recovery (Bequet, Gomez-Merino, Berthelot, & Guezennec, 2002). In addition to changes in circulating blood glucose, the possibility that the depletion of brain glycogen may be important to the development of fatigue during strenuous exercise has recently been explored (Dalsgaard, Ide, Cai, Quistorff, & Secher, 2002).

What other factors might be responsible for "central fatigue"?

Fatigue – and "central fatigue" in particular – is a complex and multifaceted phenomenon. There are several other possible cerebral factors that might limit exercise performance, all of which influence signal transduction, since the brain cells communicate through chemical substances. Not all of these relationships have been explored in detail, and the complexity of brain neurochemical interactions makes it difficult to construct a single or simple statement that covers the "central fatigue" phenomenon. Other neurotransmitters such as acetylcholine, GABA, and glutamate have been suggested to be involved to a lesser extent in the development of central fatigue (Abdelmalki, Merino, Bonneau, Bigard, & Guezennec, 1997; Conlay, Sabounjian, & Wurtman, 1992) and as such will not be discussed in this review. Attention has also been given to the influence of ammonia on cerebral levels of glutamate, glutamine, and GABA (Davis & Bailey, 1997; Nybo *et al.*, 2005).

In recent years, the role of central adenosine has been investigated, through its association with caffeine (Davis *et al.*, 2003). The ergogenic effect of caffeine was originally thought to be mediated through an increase in fat oxidation rate, thus sparing muscle glycogen (Costill, Dalsky, & Fink, 1978). Subsequent work has largely failed to provide convincing support for this mechanism, leading to the suggestion that the effects of caffeine supplementation are centrally mediated. Caffeine is a potent adenosine antagonist that readily crosses the blood–brain barrier, producing a marked reduction in central adenosine neurotransmission. Adenosine inhibits the release of many excitatory neurotransmitters, including dopamine and noradrenaline, consequently reducing arousal and spontaneous behavioural activity. The central effects of caffeine have recently been demonstrated by Davis and colleagues (2003), with a marked increase in exercise capacity observed following an infusion of caffeine into the brain of rodents. The influence of caffeine ingestion on both physical and mental performance is discussed by Hespel, Maughan and Greenhaff (2006).

One area of the CNS that has received little attention in relation to exercise is the blood–brain barrier, and the possibility that changes in its integrity may be involved in the fatigue process. The relative impermeability of the blood–brain barrier helps to maintain a stable environment for the brain by regulating exchange between the CNS and the extra-cerebral environment. While the blood–brain barrier is largely resistant to changes in permeability, there are circumstances in which the function of the blood–brain barrier may be either acutely or chronically compromised, with changes potentially resulting in a disturbance of a wide range of homeostatic mechanisms. There is some evidence that prolonged exercise may lead to increased blood–brain barrier permeability in both rodents (Sharma, Westman, Navarro, Dey, & Nyberg, 1996) and humans (Watson, Shirreffs, & Maughan, 2005b). A recent human study reported an increase in circulating serum S100β, a proposed peripheral marker of blood–brain barrier permeability, following prolonged exercise in a warm environment. This response was not apparent following exercise in temperate conditions (Watson *et al.*, 2005b). A similar increase in serum S100β has been reported following football drills involving the repeated heading of a football (Mussack, Dvorak, Graf-Baumann, & Jochum, 2003; Stalnacke, Tegner, & Sojka, 2004), although the authors of these studies perhaps incorrectly interpreted this change as an indication of neuronal damage. Serum S100β is now being employed as an index of brain trauma in individuals who suffer head injuries during sports. Changes in the permeability of the blood–brain barrier to this protein may give misleading results in exercising individuals, particularly under conditions that lead to significant heat stress. At present, the functional consequences of changes in blood–brain barrier permeability during exercise and whether nutritional supplementation can alter this response are not clear.

Other cerebral metabolic, thermodynamic, circulatory, and humoral responses could all lead to a disturbance of cerebral homeostasis and eventually central fatigue. To date there is evidence that because of the extreme disturbance of homeostasis that occurs during prolonged exercise, peripheral and central regulatory mechanisms will be stressed. However, for the moment it is not possible to determine the exact regulation and the importance of each factor.

Hyperthermia, fatigue, and central neurotransmission

The capacity to perform prolonged exercise is clearly impaired in high ambient temperatures (Galloway & Maughan, 1997; Parkin, Carey, Zhao, & Febbraio, 1999). While exercise capacity is thought to be primarily limited by thermoregulatory and fluid balance factors (Hargreaves & Febbraio, 1998), it has been suggested that the CNS may become important in the development of fatigue when body temperature is significantly elevated (Nielsen, 1992). During prolonged exercise in the heat, exhaustion in trained individuals appears to coincide with the attainment of an internal body temperature of around 40.0°C (Gonzalez-Alonso et al., 1999; Nielsen et al., 1993). Hyperthermia has been proposed to accelerate the development of central fatigue during exercise, resulting in a reduction in maximal muscle activation (Nybo & Nielsen, 2001a), altered EEG brain activity (Nielsen, Hyldig, Bidstrup, Gonzalez-Alonso, & Christoffersen, 2001), and increased perceived exertion (Nybo & Nielsen, 2001b). It is likely that this serves as a protective mechanism limiting further heat production when body temperature reaches values that may be detrimental to the organism as a whole, but the neurobiological mechanisms for these responses are not clear at present.

The suggestion that serotonin-mediated fatigue is important during exercise in the heat is partially supported by the work of Mittleman and colleagues (1998). A 14% increase in time to exhaustion in warm ambient conditions (34.4°C) was reported following BCAA supplementation when compared to a polydextrose placebo, with no apparent difference in peripheral markers of fatigue between trials. The authors concluded that the supplementation regimen was successful in limiting the entry of tryptophan into the CNS, attenuating serotonin-mediated fatigue. It is important to note that core temperature at fatigue was significantly below values described as limiting (< 38°C). Two subsequent studies have examined the effects of BCAA supplementation on human performance and thermoregulation in the heat (Cheuvront et al., 2004; Watson, Shirreffs, & Maughan, 2004). Cheuvront et al. (2004) reported that BCAA, when combined with carbohydrate, did not alter time-trial performance, cognitive performance, mood, ratings of perceived exertion (RPE), thermal comfort, or rectal temperature in the heat when participants were hypohydrated. In this study, hypohydration was used to increase plasma osmolality and increase thermoregulatory and cardiovascular strain. Additionally, ingestion of BCAA solution before, and during, prolonged exercise in glycogen-depleted individuals did not influence exercise capacity, rectal and skin temperature, heart rate, RPE, or perceived thermal stress despite a four-fold reduction in the plasma concentration ratio of free tryptophan to BCAA (Watson et al., 2004).

To date, there has been limited investigation of the influence of pharmacological agents acting on the CNS on the response to prolonged exercise in a warm environment. A recent series of studies examined the effects of acute serotonin (5-HT) agonist (paroxetine) and 5-HT_{2C} receptor antagonist (pizotifen) administration (Strachan, Leiper, & Maughan, 2004, 2005). Neither treatment influenced exercise performance, but pizotifen did produce a marked elevation in core temperature at rest and during exercise, suggesting a role for the 5-HT_{2C} receptor in the regulation of core temperature.

As dopamine and noradrenaline have been implicated in arousal, motivation, reinforcement and reward, the control of motor behaviour and mechanisms of addiction, we recently explored the possible interaction between high ambient temperature and possible underlying neurotransmitter drive during exercise using a dual dopamine/noradrenaline reuptake inhibitor (Watson et al.,

2005a). Participants ingested either a placebo or bupropion (Zyban) before exercise in temperate (18°C) or warm (30°C) conditions. Two important findings arose from this study. First, the participants completed a pre-loaded time-trial 9% faster when bupropion was taken before exercise in a warm environment than a placebo. This ergogenic effect was not apparent at 18°C. Second, seven of the nine participants in the heat attained core temperatures equal to, or greater than, 40°C in the bupropion trial, compared to only two participants in the placebo trial.

It is possible that this drug may dampen or override inhibitory signals arising from the CNS to cease exercise due to hyperthermia, and enable an individual to continue to maintain a high power output. It is important to note, however, that this response appeared to occur with the same perception of effort and thermal stress reported during the placebo trial, and may potentially increase the risk of developing heat illness. As evidence for a role of serotonin during exercise in the heat is limited (Cheuvront *et al.*, 2004; Strachan *et al.*, 2004; Watson *et al.*, 2004), these data suggest that catecholaminergic neurotransmission may act as an important neurobiological mediator of fatigue under conditions of heat stress.

It appears that when exercise is performed in high ambient temperatures, the development of central fatigue appears to be accelerated, leading to a loss of drive to continue. This may explain why individuals tend to cease exercise long before muscle glycogen stores reach levels thought to be limiting (Parkin *et al.*, 1999). Until recently, few studies had focused directly on the relationship between brain neurotransmission, thermoregulation, and exercise performance/exercise capacity in a warm environment. Therefore, further research, including both pharmacological and nutritional manipulation, are necessary to elucidate the role of specific neurotransmitter functions during exercise in the heat. Additionally, the significance of this in relation to the pattern of activity associated with football has yet to be determined.

Conclusions

The cause of fatigue is complex, influenced by both events occurring in the periphery and the CNS. The "central fatigue hypothesis" is based on the assumption that the synthesis and metabolism of central monoamines are influenced during prolonged exercise, consequently affecting subjective sensations of lethargy and tiredness, causing an altered sensation of effort, perhaps a differing tolerance of pain/discomfort, and a loss of drive and motivation to continue exercise. Since its conception, Newsholme's original hypothesis has been developed to include the possibility that other neurotransmitters and neuromodulators, in particular the catecholamines, dopamine, and noradrenaline, are also involved in the development of fatigue. Much of the attraction of neurotransmitter-mediated fatigue was the potential for nutritional manipulation of neurotransmitter precursors to delay the onset of central fatigue, potentially enhancing performance.

When exercise is performed in temperate conditions, it seems that manipulation of brain neuro-transmission through amino acid supplementation or pharmacological means has little effect (either negatively or positively) on physical performance. While there is some evidence that branched-chain amino acid and tyrosine ingestion can influence perceived exertion and various measures of mental performance (e.g. memory, tracking, cognitive function), the results of several apparently well-controlled laboratory studies have not demonstrated a positive effect on exercise capacity or performance. As football is highly dependent on the successful execution of motor skills and tactics, the possibility that amino acid ingestion may attenuate the loss in cognitive function that occurs during the later stages of a game would be desirable, despite no apparent benefit to physical performance.

It is clear that carbohydrate ingestion can have a profound effect on measures of physical fatigue during high-intensity intermittent activity, with marked improvements in time to volitional exhaustion, maintenance of sprint performance, and vertical jump height. The beneficial effect of carbohydrate supplementation during prolonged exercise may also relate to increased (or maintained) substrate delivery for the brain. Several studies have indicated that hypoglycaemia affects brain function and cognitive performance. There are indications that carbohydrate intake during exercise minimizes the negative effect of central fatigue induced by prolonged exercise on cognitive function.

Although these largely inconsistent findings make it difficult to reach a firm conclusion regarding the role of central neurotransmission in the fatigue process, it is premature to discount its importance in the light of studies investigating amphetamines and other CNS stimulants. Additionally, evidence for a central component of fatigue during prolonged exercise in a warm environment appears to be convincing, with hyperthermia demonstrated to reduce maximal muscle activation, alter brain activity, and increase perceived exertion. To date there has been limited investigation of the influence of nutritional or pharmacological manipulation of central neurotransmission on the response to exercise in a warm environment, and further research in this area is warranted.

Fatigue – and "central fatigue" in particular – is a complex and multifaceted phenomenon. There are several other possible cerebral factors that might limit exercise performance, all of which influence signal transduction, since the brain cells communicate through chemical substances. Not all of these relationships have been explored in detail, and the complexity of brain neurochemical interactions will probably make it very difficult to construct a single or simple statement that covers the phenomenon we call "central fatigue".

References

Abdelmalki, A., Merino, D., Bonneau, D., Bigard, A. X., & Guezennec, C. Y. (1997). Administration of a GABAB agonist baclofen before running to exhaustion in the rat: Effects on performance and on some indicators of fatigue. *International Journal of Sports Medicine*, 18, 75–78.

Bailey, S. P., Davis, J. M., & Ahlborn, E. N. (1992). Effect of increased brain serotonergic activity on endurance performance in the rat. *Acta Physiologica Scandinavica, 145,* 75–76.

Bailey, S. P., Davis, J. M., & Ahlborn, E. N. (1993). Serotonergic agonists and antagonists affect endurance performance in the rat. *International Journal of Sports Medicine, 14,* 330–333.

Banderet, L. E., & Lieberman, H. R. (1989). Treatment with tyrosine, a neurotransmitter precursor, reduces environmental stress in humans. *Brain Research Bulletin, 22,* 759–762.

Bangsbo, J., Norregaard, L., & Thorsoe, F. (1991). Activity profile of competition soccer. *Canadian Journal of Sports Sciences, 16,* 110–116.

Bequet, F., Gomez-Merino, D., Berthelot, M., & Guezennec, C. Y. (2002). Evidence that brain glucose availability influences exercise-enhanced extracellular 5-HT level in hippocampus: A microdialysis study in exercising rats. *Acta Physiologica Scandinavica, 176,* 65–69.

Blomstrand, E., Andersson, S., Hassmen, P., Ekblom, B., & Newsholme, E. A. (1995). Effect of branched-chain amino acid and carbohydrate supplementation on the exercise-induced change in plasma and muscle concentration of amino acids in human subjects. *Acta Physiologica Scandinavica, 153,* 87–96.

Blomstrand, E., Hassmen, P., Ek, S., Ekblom, B., & Newsholme, E. A. (1997). Influence of ingesting a solution of branched-chain amino acids on perceived exertion during exercise. *Acta Physiologica Scandinavica, 159,* 41–49.

Blomstrand, E., Hassmen, P., Ekblom, B., & Newsholme, E. A. (1991a). Administration of branched-chain amino acids during sustained exercise – effects on performance and on plasma concentration of some amino acids. *European Journal of Applied Physiology, 63,* 83–88.

Blomstrand, E., Hassmen, P., & Newsholme, E. A. (1991b). Effect of branched-chain amino acid supplementation on mental performance. *Acta Physiologica Scandinavica, 143,* 225–226.

Borg, G., Edstrom, C. G., Linderholm, H., & Marklund, G. (1972). Changes in physical performance induced by amphetamine and amobarbital. *Psychopharmacologia, 26,* 10–18.

Chandler, J. V., & Blair, S. N. (1980). The effect of amphetamines on selected physiological components related to athletic success. *Medicine and Science in Sports and Exercise, 12,* 65–69.

Cheuvront, S. N., Carter, R., III, Kolka, M. A., Lieberman, H. R., Kellogg, M. D., & Sawka, M. N. (2004). Branched-chain amino acid supplementation and human performance when hypohydrated in the heat. *Journal of Applied Physiology, 97,* 1275–1282.

Chinevere, T. D., Sawyer, R. D., Creer, A. R., Conlee, R. K., & Parcell, A. C. (2002). Effects of L-tyrosine and carbohydrate ingestion on endurance exercise performance. *Journal of Applied Physiology, 93,* 1590–1597.

Collardeau, M., Brisswalter, J., Vercruyssen, F., Audiffren, M., & Goubault, C. (2001). Single and choice reaction time during prolonged exercise in trained subjects: Influence of carbohydrate availability. *European Journal of Applied Physiology, 86,* 150–156.

Conlay, L. A., Sabounjian, L. A., & Wurtman, R. J. (1992). Exercise and neuromodulators: Choline and acetylcholine in marathon runners. *International Journal of Sports Medicine, 13* (suppl. 1), S141–S142.

Costill, D. L., Dalsky, G. P., & Fink, W. J. (1978). Effects of caffeine ingestion on metabolism and exercise performance. *Medicine and Science in Sports and Exercise*, *10*, 155–158.

Dalsgaard, M. K., Ide, K., Cai, Y., Quistorff, B., & Secher, N. H. (2002). The intent to exercise influences the cerebral O(2)/carbohydrate uptake ratio in humans. *Journal of Physiology*, *540*, 681–689.

Davis, J. M., & Bailey, S. P. (1997). Possible mechanisms of central nervous system fatigue during exercise. *Medicine and Science in Sports and Exercise*, *29*, 45–57.

Davis, J. M., Bailey, S. P., Woods, J. A., Galiano, F. J., Hamilton, M. T., & Bartoli, W. P. (1992). Effects of carbohydrate feedings on plasma free tryptophan and branched-chain amino acids during prolonged cycling. *European Journal of Applied Physiology*, *65*, 513–519.

Davis, J. M., Welsh, R. S., De Volve, K. L., & Alderson, N. A. (1999). Effects of branched-chain amino acids and carbohydrate on fatigue during intermittent, high-intensity running. *International Journal of Sports Medicine*, *20*, 309–314.

Davis, J. M., Zhao, Z., Stock, H. S., Mehl, K. A., Buggy, J., & Hand, G. A. (2003). Central nervous system effects of caffeine and adenosine on fatigue. *American Journal of Physiology*, *284*, R399–R404.

Deijen, J. B., Wientjes, C. J., Vullinghs, H. F., Cloin, P. A., & Langefeld, J. J. (1999). Tyrosine improves cognitive performance and reduces blood pressure in cadets after one week of a combat training course. *Brain Research Bulletin*, *48*, 203–209.

Dollins, A. B., Krock, L. P., Storm, W. F., Wurtman, R. J., & Lieberman, H. R. (1995). L-Tyrosine ameliorates some effects of lower body negative pressure stress. *Physiological Behaviour*, *57*, 223–230.

Felipo, V., & Butterworth, R. F. (2002). Neurobiology of ammonia. *Progressive Neurobiology*, *67*, 259–279.

Galiano, F. J., Davis, J. M., Bailey, S. P., Woods, J. A., Hamilton, M. T., & Bartoli, W. P. (1991). Physiological, endocrine and performance effects of adding branched-chain amino acids to a 6% carbohydrate electrolyte beverage during prolonged cycling. *Medicine and Science in Sports and Exercise*, *23*, S14.

Galloway, S. D., & Maughan, R. J. (1997). Effects of ambient temperature on the capacity to perform prolonged cycle exercise in man. *Medicine and Science in Sports and Exercise*, *29*, 1240–1249.

Gerald, M. C. (1978). Effects of (+)-amphetamine on the treadmill endurance performance of rats. *Neuropharmacology*, *17*, 703–704.

Gonzalez-Alonso, J., Teller, C., Andersen, S. L., Jensen, F. B., Hyldig, T., & Nielsen, B. (1999). Influence of body temperature on the development of fatigue during prolonged exercise in the heat. *Journal of Applied Physiology*, *86*, 1032–1039.

Hargreaves, M., & Febbraio, M. (1998). Limits to exercise performance in the heat. *International Journal of Sports Medicine*, *19* (suppl. 2), S115–S116.

Hassmen, P., Blomstrand, E., Ekblom, B., & Newsholme, E. A. (1994). Branched-chain amino acid supplementation during 30-km competitive run: Mood and cognitive performance. *Nutrition*, *10*, 405–410.

Hespel, P., Maughan, R. J., & Greenhaff, P. L. (2006). Dietary supplements for football. *Journal of Sports Sciences*, *24*, 749–761.

Heyes, M. P., Garnett, E. S., & Coates, G. (1985). Central dopaminergic activity influences rats' ability to exercise. *Life Sciences*, *36*, 671–677.

Kalinski, M. I., Dluzen, D. E., & Stadulis, R. (2001). Methamphetamine produces subsequent reductions in running time to exhaustion in mice. *Brain Research, 921,* 160–164.

Kirkendall, D. T. (1993). Effects of nutrition on performance in soccer. *Medicine and Science in Sports and Exercise, 25,* 1370–1374.

Madsen, K., MacLean, D. A., Kiens, B., & Christensen, D. (1996). Effects of glucose, glucose plus branched-chain amino acids, or placebo on bike performance over 100 km. *Journal of Applied Physiology, 81,* 2644–2650.

Meeusen, R., & De Meirleir, K. (1995). Exercise and brain neurotransmission. *Sports Medicine, 20,* 160–188.

Meeusen, R., Piacentini, M. F., Van den Eynde, S., Magnus, L., & De Meirleir, K. (2001). Exercise performance is not influenced by a 5-HT reuptake inhibitor. *International Journal of Sports Medicine, 22,* 329–336.

Meeusen, R., Roeykens, J., Magnus, L., Keizer, H., & De Meirleir, K. (1997). Endurance performance in humans: The effect of a dopamine precursor or a specific serotonin (5-HT2A/2C) antagonist. *International Journal of Sports Medicine, 18,* 571–577.

Mittleman, K. D., Ricci, M. R., & Bailey, S. P. (1998). Branched-chain amino acids prolong exercise during heat stress in men and women. *Medicine and Science in Sports and Exercise, 30,* 83–91.

Mohr, M., Krustrup, P., & Bangsbo, J. (2003). Match performance of high-standard soccer players with special reference to development of fatigue. *Journal of Sports Sciences, 21,* 519–528.

Mohr, A., Krustrup, P., & Bangsbo, J. (2005). Fatigue in soccer: A brief review. *Journal of Sports Sciences, 23,* 593–599.

Mussack, T., Dvorak, J., Graf-Baumann, T., & Jochum, M. (2003). Serum S-100β protein levels in young amateur soccer players after controlled heading and normal exercise. *European Journal of Medical Research, 8,* 457–464.

Neri, D. F., Wiegmann, D., Stanny, R. R., Shappell, S. A., McCardie, A., & McKay, D. L. (1995). The effects of tyrosine on cognitive performance during extended wakefulness. *Aviation, Space and Environmental Medicine, 66,* 313–319.

Newsholme, E. A., Ackworth, I., & Blomstrand, E. (1987). Amino acids, brain neurotransmitters and a function link between muscle and brain that is important in sustained exercise. In G. Benzi (Ed.), *Advances in myochemistry* (pp. 127–133). London: John Libbey Eurotext.

Nicholas, C. W., Williams, C., Lakomy, H. K., Phillips, G., & Nowitz, A. (1995). Influence of ingesting a carbohydrate-electrolyte solution on endurance capacity during intermittent, high-intensity shuttle running. *Journal of Sports Sciences, 13,* 283–290.

Nielsen, B. (1992). Heat stress causes fatigue! Exercise performance during acute and repeated exposures to hot, dry environments. In P. Marconnet, P. V. Komi, B. Saltin, & O. M. Sejersted (Eds.), *Muscle fatigue mechanisms in exercise and training* (Vol. 34, pp. 207–217). Basel: Karger.

Nielsen, B., Hales, J. R., Strange, S., Christensen, N. J., Warberg, J., & Saltin, B. (1993). Human circulatory and thermoregulatory adaptations with heat acclimation and exercise in a hot, dry environment. *Journal of Physiology, 460,* 467–485.

Nielsen, B., Hyldig, T., Bidstrup, F., Gonzalez-Alonso, J., & Christoffersen, G. R. (2001). Brain activity and fatigue during prolonged exercise in the heat. *Pflugers Archive, 442,* 41–48.

Nybo, L. (2003). CNS fatigue and prolonged exercise: Effect of glucose supplementation. *Medicine and Science in Sports and Exercise, 35,* 589–594.

Nybo, L., Dalsgaard, M. K., Steensberg, A., Moller, K., & Secher, N. H. (2005). Cerebral ammonia uptake and accumulation during prolonged exercise in humans. *Journal of Physiology*, 563, 285–290.

Nybo, L., Moller, K., Pedersen, B. K., Nielsen, B., & Secher, N. H. (2003). Association between fatigue and failure to preserve cerebral energy turnover during prolonged exercise. *Acta Physiologica Scandinavica*, 179, 67–74.

Nybo, L., & Nielsen, B. (2001a). Hyperthermia and central fatigue during prolonged exercise in humans. *Journal of Applied Physiology*, 91, 1055–1060.

Nybo, L., & Nielsen, B. (2001b). Perceived exertion is associated with an altered brain activity during exercise with progressive hyperthermia. *Journal of Applied Physiology*, 91, 2017–2023.

Nybo, L., & Secher, N.H. (2004). Cerebral perturbations provoked by prolonged exercise. *Progressive Neurobiology*, 72, 223–261.

Owasoyo, J. O., Neri, D. F., & Lamberth, J. G. (1992). Tyrosine and its potential use as a countermeasure to performance decrement in military sustained operations. *Aviation, Space and Environmental Medicine*, 63, 364–369.

Pannier, J. L., Bouckaert, J. J., & Lefebvre, R. A. (1995). The antiserotonin agent pizotifen does not increase endurance performance in humans. *European Journal of Applied Physiology*, 72, 175–178.

Parise, G., Bosman, M. J., Boecker, D. R., Barry, M. J., & Tarnopolsky, M. A. (2001). Selective serotonin reuptake inhibitors: Their effect on high-intensity exercise performance. *Archives of Physical Medicine and Rehabilitation*, 82, 867–871.

Parkin, J. M., Carey, M. F., Zhao, S., & Febbraio, M. A. (1999). Effect of ambient temperature on human skeletal muscle metabolism during fatiguing submaximal exercise. *Journal of Applied Physiology*, 86, 902–908.

Piacentini, M. F., Meeusen, R., Buyse, L., De Schutter, G., & De Meirleir, K. (2002a). No effect of a selective serotonergic/noradrenergic reuptake inhibitor on endurance performance. *European Journal of Sports Science*, 2, 1–10.

Piacentini, M. F., Meeusen, R., Buyse, L., De Schutter, G., & De Meirleir, K. (2004). Hormonal responses during prolonged exercise are influenced by a selective DA/NA reuptake inhibitor. *British Journal of Sports Medicine*, 38, 129–133.

Piacentini, M. F., Meeusen, R., Buyse, L., De Schutter, G., Kempenaers, F., Van Nijvel, J. et al. (2002b). No effect of a noradrenergic reuptake inhibitor on performance in trained cyclists. *Medicine and Science in Sports and Exercise*, 34, 1189–1193.

Sharma, H. S., Westman, J., Navarro, J. C., Dey, P. K., & Nyberg, F. (1996). Probable involvement of serotonin in the increased permeability of the blood–brain barrier by forced swimming: An experimental study using Evans blue and 131I-sodium tracers in the rat. *Behavioural Brain Research*, 72, 189–196.

Shurtleff, D., Thomas, J. R., Schrot, J., Kowalski, K., & Harford, R. (1994). Tyrosine reverses a cold-induced working memory deficit in humans. *Pharmacology, Biochemistry and Behaviour*, 47, 935–941.

Stalnacke, B. M., Tegner, Y., & Sojka, P. (2004). Playing soccer increases serum concentrations of the biochemical markers of brain damage S-100β and neuron-specific enolase in elite players: A pilot study. *Brain Injury*, 18, 899–909.

Strachan, A., Leiper, J., & Maughan, R. (2004). The failure of acute paroxetine administration to influence human exercise capacity, RPE or hormone responses during prolonged exercise in a warm environment. *Experimental Physiology*, 89, 657–664.

Strachan, A. T., Leiper, J. B., & Maughan, R. J. (2005). Serotonin2C receptor blockade and thermoregulation during exercise in the heat. *Medicine and Science in Sports and Exercise, 37,* 389–394.

Struder, H. K., Hollmann, W., Platen, P., Donike, M., Gotzmann, A., & Weber, K. (1998). Influence of paroxetine, branched-chain amino acids and tyrosine on neuro-endocrine system responses and fatigue in humans. *Hormone and Metabolic Research, 30,* 188–194.

Sutton, E., Coll, R., & Deuster, P. (2005). Ingestion of tyrosine: Effects on endurance, muscle strength, and anaerobic performance. *International Journal of Sports Nutrition and Exercise Metabolism, 15,* 173–185.

van Hall, G., Raaymakers, J. S., Saris, W. H., & Wagenmakers, A. J. (1995). Ingestion of branched-chain amino acids and tryptophan during sustained exercise in man: Failure to affect performance. *Journal of Physiology, 486,* 789–794.

Varnier, M., Sarto, P., Martines, D., Lora, L., Carmignoto, F., Leese, G. P. *et al.* (1994). Effect of infusing branched-chain amino acid during incremental exercise with reduced muscle glycogen content. *European Journal of Applied Physiology, 69,* 26–31.

Watson, P., Hasegawa, H., Roelands, B., Piacentini, M. F., Looverie, R., & Meeusen, R. (2005a). Acute dopamine/noradrenaline reuptake inhibition enhances human exercise performance in warm, but not temperate conditions. *Journal of Physiology, 565,* 873–883.

Watson, P., Shirreffs, S. M., & Maughan, R. J. (2004). The effect of acute branched-chain amino acid supplementation on prolonged exercise capacity in a warm environment. *European Journal of Applied Physiology, 93,* 306–314.

Watson, P., Shirreffs, S. M., & Maughan, R. J. (2005b). Blood–brain barrier integrity may be threatened by exercise in a warm environment. *American Journal of Physiology, 288,* R1689–1694.

Welsh, R. S., Davis, J. M., Burke, J. R., & Williams, H. G. (2002). Carbohydrates and physical/mental performance during intermittent exercise to fatigue. *Medicine and Science in Sports and Exercise, 34,* 723–731.

Wilson, W. M., & Maughan, R. J. (1992). Evidence for a possible role of 5-hydroxy-tryptamine in the genesis of fatigue in man: Administration of paroxetine, a 5-HT re-uptake inhibitor, reduces the capacity to perform prolonged exercise. *Experimental Physiology, 77,* 921–924.

Winnick, J. J., Davis, J. M., Welsh, R. S., Carmichael, M. D., Murphy, E. A., & Blackmon, J. A. (2005). Carbohydrate feedings during team sport exercise preserve physical and CNS function. *Medicine and Science in Sports and Exercise, 37,* 306–315.

11 Special populations: The female player and the youth player

CHRISTINE A. ROSENBLOOM, ANNE B. LOUCKS
AND BJORN EKBLOM

Females and youth are frequently described as "special" populations in football literature, but together these two populations outnumber male players. What makes females "special" is that they tend to eat less when training and competing than their male counterparts, leading to lower intakes of energy, carbohydrate, and some nutrients. Youth football players are special in regard to energy and nutrient requirements to promote growth and development, as well as to fuel sport. There is limited research on the dietary habits of these two populations, but the available literature suggests that many female and youth players need to increase carbohydrate intake, increase fluid intake, and develop dietary habits to sustain the demands of training and competition.

Keywords: Female athletes, young athletes, energy intakes

Introduction

Although exact numbers are not available it is safe to assume that, when combined, women and youth football players outnumber male players. Yet, there is insufficient research on the nutritional needs of these two groups of athletes. Most information on energy demands, training and conditioning strategies, and dietary habits is extrapolated from the research on male footballers. The purpose of this article is to review what is known about the nutrition needs and dietary habits of women and youth football players and to identify what is not known to encourage research of these two populations to gain a more comprehensive picture of these footballers.

Female players

FIFA estimates that in the year 2010, there will be more women playing football than men (Davies, 2005). Women have come a long way since the days when the Football Association of England (FA) banned women from playing on Football League grounds in 1921, stating that "the game of football is quite unsuitable for females and ought not to be encouraged" (The Football Association, 2002). Data from the Football 2000 Worldwide survey (www.FIFA.com) indicated that women in 132 countries played football. In 2002, the FA reported there were 131,000 registered female players and about 1.4 million females played football at various levels of competition in England (The Football Association, 2005). In the USA, it is estimated that 5.5 million women over the age of 7 years play football (NSGA, 2004a). Understanding the usual dietary patterns and nutritional intakes of females could help coaches, trainers, and sports dietitians to develop nutritional strategies to fuel performance and prevent fatigue over the course of a long competitive season.

Energy demands of football

Bangsbo (1994) reported that male players cover an average distance of 11 km during a match coupled with other energy-expending activities, including tackling, turning, and accelerating. Use of distance covered in a match as a way to assess energy expenditure underestimates the true cost of energy used in football (Reilly, 1997). Brewer (1994) reviewed nutritional aspects of female soccer players and reported that a female player covers less distance in a match than a male, but the relative intensity of activity is maintained around 70% of maximal oxygen uptake ($\dot{V}O_{2max}$), which is similar to that of males. Using data reported by Ekblom and Aginger, Brewer (1994) estimated an energy expenditure of about 1100 kcal for a 60 kg football player during a match. Fogelholm *et al.* (1995) estimated total energy expenditure to be $2218 \, kcal \cdot day^{-1}$ from measurements of resting energy expenditure and analyses of 7 day activity records of 12 female footballers. Because chronic undernutrition suppresses resting energy expenditure (Loucks, 2004), however, such calculations of total energy expenditure will underestimate the amount of dietary energy required to restore the healthy functioning of all physiological systems in undernourished individuals.

Energy and nutrient intakes

Information about the dietary intakes of female footballers is very limited. Two recent studies, conducted in the USA, assessed dietary intakes of female players from the U-21 national soccer team (Mullinix, Jonnalagadda, Rosenbloom, Thompson, & Kicklighter, 2003) and those competing in the National Collegiate Athletic Association (NCAA) Division I (Clark, Reed, Crouse, & Armstrong, 2003). The average energy, macronutrient, and micronutrient intakes in both groups of female athletes are shown in Table 1. The athletes in the U-21 national team (mean age 19.2 years) averaged $2015 \, kcal \cdot day^{-1}$, whereas the NCAA players averaged $2290 \, kcal \cdot day^{-1}$. Both groups of researchers found the women consumed less energy than would be predicted from estimated energy expenditure equations, and that most athletes consumed energy more suited to individuals with low activity levels. Clark *et al.* (2003) assessed energy intake pre- and post-season and found significantly lower intakes of energy and all macronutrients post-season. Both studies had small numbers of participants, but if energy expenditure during practice or a soccer match is about 1100 kcal, these women consumed much lower energy intakes than their actual

Table 1. Energy, macronutrient, and micronutrient intakes in female footballers
(mean ± s)

Nutrient	U-21 players[a] (n = 11)	NCAA players[b] (n = 13)	NCAA players[c] (n = 13)
Energy (kcal)	2015 ± 19	2290 ± 310	1865 ± 530
Carbohydrate (g)	282 ± 118	320 ± 70	263 ± 71
Protein (g)	79 ± 33	86.5 ± 18.7	58.8 ± 16.0
Fat (g)	67 ± 28	75.2 ± 13.3	65.9 ± 28.7
Fibre (g)	17.7 ± 5.2	14.5 ± 4.9	13.3 ± 5.7
Vitamin A (RE)	917 ± 505	894 ± 276	847 ± 425
Vitamin E (mg)	8.3 ± 8.8	7.2 ± 3.7	3.3 ± 3.3
Vitamin D (μg)	2.6 ± 2.4	2.4 ± 1.7	2.5 ± 2.6
Vitamin C (mg)	128 ± 110	100 ± 64	46 ± 32
Thiamin (mg)	1.6 ± 0.9	1.5 ± 0.6	1.0 ± 0.4
Niacin (mg)	21.5 ± 11.9	24.5 ± 8.5	15.2 ± 6.3
Riboflavin (mg)	1.7 ± 1.0	1.8 ± 0.7	1.2 ± 0.7
Folate (μg)	338 ± 213	271 ± 130	186 ± 113
Vitamin B6 (mg)	1.9 ± 1.2	1.8 ± 0.6	1.1 ± 0.6
Vitamin B12 (μg)	3.0 ± 2.8	4.5 ± 1.9	2.1 ± 1.7
Calcium (mg)	887 ± 510	931 ± 223	695 ± 289
Iron (mg)	16 ± 7.8	17.3 ± 4.7	12.2 ± 5.2
Magnesium (mg)	223 ± 103	178 ± 43	127 ± 71
Zinc (mg)	9.5 ± 6.1	10.4 ± 4.6	5.1 ± 2.5
Sodium (mg)	3780 ± 1679	Not reported	Not reported
Potassium (mg)	2312 ± 1049	Not reported	Not reported

[a] Mullinix et al. (2003: pre-season intakes), [b] Clark et al. (2003: pre-season intakes), [c] Clark et al. (2003: post-season intakes).

needs. Clark et al. (2003) also assessed body composition and reported a stable body weight in the football players from pre- to post-season, suggesting their energy needs were appropriate for the energy demands of the sport. Hinton, Sanford, Davidson, Yakushko and Beck (2004) reported nutrient intakes and dietary behaviours in 142 female collegiate athletes in the USA, including 20 footballers. Body composition was not assessed, but approximately 70% of the female footballers expressed a desire to lose weight and were intentionally restricting energy intake.

Under-reporting of energy intake is common when collecting dietary information by recall methods, and stability of body weight may not be the best predictor of energy balance. Researchers have repeatedly observed endocrine signs of energy deficiency in both amenorrhoeic and eumenorrhoeic female athletes (Loucks, 2004). Research directed at accurate assessment of energy intake, energy expenditure, body composition, and hormone status would help to answer the question of energy needs in female footballers.

Absolute carbohydrate intake in these two groups of female footballers was lower than the recommendations in the Joint Position Statement of the American Dietetic Association, the Dietitians of Canada, and the American

College of Sports Medicine (2000). Females were reported to consume an average of 4.7 g carbohydrate $\cdot$ kg^{-1} $\cdot$ day^{-1} (Mullinix *et al.*, 2003), and 5.2 g carbohydrate $\cdot$ kg^{-1} $\cdot$ day^{-1} in the pre-season and 4.3 g carbohydrate $\cdot$ kg^{-1} $\cdot$ day^{-1} in the post-season (Clark *et al.*, 2003). These values are below the recommendations of 7–8 g carbohydrate $\cdot$ kg^{-1} $\cdot$ day^{-1} for athletes participating in heavy training and competition. Mean carbohydrate intake failed to approach values of dietary carbohydrate sufficient to maintain glycogen levels. When carbohydrate intake is expressed as a percentage of total energy intake, these women were eating approximately 52% of energy intake as carbohydrate, but their absolute intake of carbohydrate was not optimal.

In a comprehensive review of carbohydrate needs for athletes, Burke, Cox, Cummings and Desbrow (2001) concluded that female athletes, especially endurance athletes, are less likely than their male counterparts to achieve the recommendations for carbohydrate intake. The most likely reason for a less than desirable energy intake was to achieve or maintain a lower body weight and/or percentage body fat. In a study on eating patterns of elite athletes, Burke *et al.* (2003) suggested that female athletes may ingest less energy and carbohydrate than males because women may have less rigorous training and may under-report food intake on dietary food records compared with men.

Energy and macronutrients needs – are there differences between the sexes?

It is clear that energy and macronutrient intakes of male athletes are generally greater than those of female athletes, but energy and macronutrient needs may be different in females. Loucks (2004) reported that energy intake is a special concern for females because of reproductive disorders associated with an energy intake that is too low to support high energy demands in sport. When energy and carbohydrate intakes are normalized by body weight, female athletes consume far less than men – about 30% less (Burke *et al.*, 2001; Loucks, 2004). Insufficient energy and carbohydrate intake can compromise hormonal patterns, leading to alterations in growth, impaired performance, and decreased bone mineralization. Loucks (2004) argued that because many female athletes strive for a low body weight and percentage body fat, and they find it difficult to consume sufficient energy, a focus on manipulating carbohydrate, protein, and fat intake might be a more useful, albeit challenging, strategy.

Kirkendall (2000) summarized the physiological aspects of football and concluded that there are three trends that are seen in football players: (1) pregame concentrations of glycogen are lower in footballers than in other athletes; (2) significant glycogen depletion occurs in the first 45 min (first half) of play; and (3) at the end of the game, glycogen is totally depleted. While these trends are not specific for female athletes, the limited research suggests that female athletes ingest less energy and less carbohydrate than males, so a logical conclusion is that female players may have lower pre-game and half-time glycogen than male players. Low glycogen stores can lead to sub-optimal performance during the match.

Burke, Keins and Ivy (2004) presented practical suggestions for improving carbohydrate intake in athletes, although the recommendations are not gender-specific. Revised guidelines for carbohydrate intake include:

- Immediately after exercise (0–4 h): 1.0–$1.2\,\mathrm{g\cdot kg^{-1}\cdot h^{-1}}$ consumed at frequent intervals.
- Daily intake for recovery from training of low-intensity and moderate duration: 5–$7\,\mathrm{g\cdot kg^{-1}\cdot h^{-1}}$.
- Daily intake for recovery from endurance training of moderate to heavy duration: 7–$12\,\mathrm{g\cdot kg^{-1}\cdot h^{-1}}$.

Providing food choices to a football team, based on their training and competition schedule, is a useful tool to help athletes meet carbohydrate needs. This is especially important in the USA, where carbohydrate is often viewed as the fattening enemy.

Recent research on carbohydrate storage and utilization of both endogenous and exogenous sources has shed new light on the frequent observation that women store and utilize less glycogen than men. Although increasing the carbohydrate content of the diet to 65% increased glycogen stores only in men, the absolute carbohydrate intake of the women was substantially lower because their total energy intake was lower, even when normalized to body size (Tarnopolsky, Atkinson, Phillips, & MacDougall, 1995). When normalized, absolute as well as relative carbohydrate intakes of the women were matched to those of men in a subsequent experiment; the gender difference in glycogen storage had disappeared (Tarnopolsky *et al.*, 2001a).

Gender differences in substrate utilization during exercise also disappeared when the dietary intake of women, normalized to body size, was matched to that of men for 8 days (Roepstorff *et al.*, 2002). Similarly, M'Kaouar, Peronnet, Massicotte and Lavoie (2004) recently demonstrated that men and women utilized carbohydrate at similar levels when fed glucose during prolonged activity. Glucose ingestion during prolonged exercise increases carbohydrate oxidation with improvements in performance (Baile, Zacher, & Mittleman, 2000). Thus, the frequent observation that women store and utilize less glycogen than men may be a result of their lower carbohydrate intake.

Riddell *et al.* (2003) studied healthy females ($n = 7$) and males ($n = 7$) completing two 90 min cycle ergometer tests at 60% $\dot{V}O_{2peak}$. Exercise bouts were separated by one week. The participants were given an 8% carbohydrate drink or a placebo beverage. The researchers found that in the final 60 min of the 90 min exercise bout, women utilized more of the ingested carbohydrate than males. Exogenous carbohydrate may spare more endogenous carbohydrate in females than in males in endurance events. These data are preliminary and small numbers of participants were studied, but gender differences in utilization of fuels should be investigated.

Another concern for active women is the effect of the menstrual cycle on exercise. Campbell, Angus and Febbraio (2001) observed that women have better exercise performance (i.e. greater time to exhaustion in cycle ergometer tests) in the follicular phase than in the luteal phase of the menstrual cycle when exercising in the fasted state. When researchers fed the women glucose during the exercise trials there was no difference in exercise performance between the menstrual cycle phases. The results of this study give women another reason to consume adequate carbohydrate when training and competing.

Protein

Many athletes, as well as sedentary individuals, consume protein in excess of their biological requirement, and this holds true for men and women alike. It is generally recommended that endurance athletes and those involved in "stop and go" sports like football should consume 1.2–$1.4\,g\cdot kg^{-1}\cdot day^{-1}$, with no advantage to consuming amounts in excess of $2.0\,g\cdot kg^{-1}\cdot day^{-1}$ (Tipton & Wolfe, 2004). Little is known about gender differences in protein metabolism in athletes, perhaps because athletes usually have adequate protein intakes. Female athletes in the two dietary intake studies reviewed for this paper showed that females consumed protein in adequate amounts in the pre-season [$1.3\,g\cdot kg^{-1}\cdot day^{-1}$ (Mullinix *et al.*, 2003) and $1.4\,g\cdot kg^{-1}\cdot day^{-1}$ (Clark *et al.*, 2003)]. However, these data are reported as averages and most likely there are some athletes consuming less than the recommended amount of protein in their diets. Athletes in the post-season consumed significantly less protein compared to the preseason ($0.95\,g\cdot kg^{-1}\cdot day^{-1}$) (Clark *et al.*, 2003). However, protein recommendations are established when energy intakes are adequate. If inadequate energy intake is consumed, protein needs will be higher. Lemon (1994) suggests that soccer players should consume about 1.4–$1.7\,g$ protein$\cdot kg^{-1}\cdot day^{-1}$, slightly more than the amounts recommended by Tipton and Wolfe (2004).

A recent focus of research has been on the timing of protein intake to support muscle anabolism. Providing essential amino acids before and after exercise has been shown to stimulate protein synthesis (Tipton & Wolfe, 2004). This dietary strategy is usually employed by strength and power athletes. Dietary protein recommendations are usually made for endurance athletes (1.2–$1.4\,g\cdot kg^{-1}\cdot day^{-1}$) and strength athletes (1.2–$1.7\,g\cdot kg^{-1}\cdot day^{-1}$), but footballers undertake both types of training. Presenting protein recommendations for both types of training would be useful and practical for footballers.

Fluids

Fluid losses in female footballers are not well documented. A summary of sweat losses in male players, published by Maughan and Leiper (1994), revealed that athletes can lose 1.0–2.5 litres in matches held in temperate climates and as much as 3.5 litres in the heat. In 2005, the FIFA Medical Committee added a provision that "players are entitled to take liquid refreshment during a stoppage in the match but only on the touch line". In many parts of the world (Central and South America, Mexico, southern USA), football is often played in hot conditions and on a field of play that offers no shade or relief from the heat. Fluid intake is especially challenging in football (whether in hot or cool climates), as there are no time-outs and at many levels of the sport matches are scheduled in short time frames with little time for recovery (Kirkendall, 2004). Coyle (2004) reviewed the fluid needs of athletes during exercise and summarized the recommendations, although no research is available to assess gender differences. For both health and performance, Coyle (2004) recommends:

- Fluid intake that matches sweating rate and, when exercising in hot environmental conditions, dehydration of 1% of body weight should be the limit of fluid loss.
- During exercise lasting more than an hour (football match), ingesting 30–60 g carbohydrate $\cdot$ h^{-1} can delay fatigue.

Burke and Hawley (1997) reported fluid balance of a women's football team during international competition in a hot climate. The women's mean sweat losses were approximately 0.8 litres $\cdot$ h^{-1} during training and 1.5 litres $\cdot$ h^{-1} during a match. The rate of fluid replacement was the same during training and competition at about 0.4 litres $\cdot$ h^{-1}.

Shirreffs *et al.* (2004) reviewed pre- and post-exercise hydration and concluded that athletes who fail to hydrate after exercise can compromise the subsequent exercise bout. This is especially relevant in football when training and competition frequently occur on consecutive days. Rehydrating with electrolyte-containing beverages is preferred, as volume losses as well as sodium and chloride need to be replaced (Shirreffs *et al.*, 2004). Shirreffs conducted a number of on-field tests to assess sweat sodium and hydration practices, and about 30 of the athletes were women (Burke, 2005). Shirreffs noted that many females gained weight over the training sessions. Females may be more conscious of hydration than males. Mullinix *et al.* (2003) found that women responded appropriately to questions on the importance of hydration (100% knew that fluids should be replaced before, during, and after exercise), but were not as knowledgeable about the most appropriate fluids to consume (only 11% agreed with the statement that "PowerAde and other sports drinks are better than water at replacing fluids").

Micronutrients

Micronutrient intakes of female soccer players (Table 1) were adequate for all nutrients except vitamin D, vitamin E, folate, calcium, magnesium, phosphorus, and zinc, which were less than 100% of the dietary reference intakes (DRIs). The DRIs are established for healthy individuals and intense physical activity may increase the need for several vitamins and minerals. However, most authors conclude that supplementation of micronutrients does not improve performance (Akabas and Dolins, 2005; Fogelholm, 1994), but athletes with suboptimal nutrient status may see a further decline in nutrient stores with heavy exercise (Manore, 2000). In a recent review of micronutrient requirements in athletic women, Akabas and Dolins (2005) concluded that "despite an upsurge in interest in physical activity, for most vitamins and minerals, current research is not conclusive enough to provide specific micronutrient recommendations to physically active women. It is clear that they need to get at least the RDA [recommended daily allowance] for micronutrients, and that many women fail to do so for several vitamins and minerals".

Two micronutrients of concern in exercising females are iron and calcium. The impact of iron deficiency anaemia on performance is well documented. In a review on haemoglobin and iron deficiency, Ekblom (1997) states that iron supplementation in anaemic athletes can increase aerobic power and improve performance. It is less clear if athletes with iron deficiency without anaemia (usually defined as low serum ferritin with normal haemoglobin) benefit from treatment with iron supplementation. Ekblom (1997) concludes that no studies show positive effects on performance when iron is supplemented in non-anaemic athletes. In two recent studies, Brutsaert *et al.* (2003) and Brownlie, Utermohlen, Hinton, Giordano and Haas (2002) studied women with iron deficiency supplemented with iron for 6 weeks. Brutsaert *et al.* (2003) had their participants perform knee contraction and extension exercises and Brownlie *et al.* (2004) had their participants work on cycle ergometers. Both researchers found women in the iron supplementation group improved exercise tolerance compared with the placebo group. Because these studies are not soccer-specific and knee contraction exercises maybe irrelevant to endurance, more research is needed on females and iron status. Athletes who manifest with iron deficiency should be monitored to make sure the deficiency does not develop into anaemia. Athletes who are vegetarian or eat little haem-iron-containing foods should be monitored for iron status. Ekblom (1997) speculated that a high-carbohydrate diet may result in a less than desirable iron intake.

Fallon (2004) screened 174 elite female athletes, 33 of them footballers, for haematological variables. Fifty-eight percent of the football players had abnormalities in their haematological profile, suggesting that elite female footballers should be routinely screened for iron deficiency with or without anaemia.

Encouraging female footballers to include haem-iron-containing foods, as well as pairing non-haem-iron-containing foods with vitamin C-containing foods, is a good strategy. In addition, many women can benefit from a vitamin–mineral preparation that contains the DRI for iron.

Football is not a sport associated with extreme leanness or thinness, but many females feel social pressure to maintain a desirable body weight and percentage body fat, which could lead to insufficient energy intake to fuel sport. The presence of menstrual irregularities is well documented in distance runners and ballet dancers (DeSouza *et al.*, 1998), but the prevalence is unclear in female footballers. Mullinix *et al.* (2003) and Clark *et al.* (2003) reported that their participants did not have amenorrhoea. However, in a higher energy demand sport, like football, females could have insufficient energy intake to support activity, leading to hormonal imbalances without obvious symptoms (Loucks, 2004). DeSouza *et al.* (1998) studied 46 women aged 18–36 years with normal menses and no history of eating disorders. Women were classified as sedentary or recreational runners (running at least 2 h a week or 16 km per week in the past year) and hormonal data were collected for three consecutive menstrual cycles. The recreational runners ran, on average, 32 km per week. The incidence of abnormal menstrual function in the runners was 79%, with defects noted in menstrual cycle inconsistencies from month to month. The runners presented with luteal phase deficiency and anovulation, whereas none of the sedentary group had abnormalities.

The question arises if female footballers have unrecognized menstrual irregularities that could affect their bone mineral status. Soderman, Bergstrom, Lorentzon and Alfredson (2000) measured bone mineral density (BMD) in teenage female footballers (age 16 years) who had been playing football for an average of 8 years and age-matched inactive girls. The footballers reached menarche, on average, at age 13.0 years, similar to the age of 12.8 year for the sedentary girls. The athletes had greater bone mass in the hip and lumbar spine than the sedentary girls. The authors noted that the increase in BMD is evident in early adolescence and becomes more pronounced in late adolescence as more time is spent in football practice and competition (Soderman *et al.*, 2000).

Pettersson, Nordstrom, Alfredson, Henriksson-Larsen and Lorentzon (2000) compared BMD in female footballers and competitive rope-skippers. Both groups of young women (average age about 17.5 years) trained about 6 h · week^{-1}. The athletes were compared with age-matched sedentary controls and all had regular menses at the time of the study. Both groups of athletes had higher BMD than the controls in the sites that were most affected by weight-bearing exercise (lumbar spine, femur, tibia).

It can be concluded that female footballers have superior BMD than inactive females, indicating that hormonal status in these women is sufficient to promote bone health. However, because some athletic women strive for thinness, monitoring menstrual status in this population is warranted.

Dietary supplements

Mullinix *et al.* (2003) reported that 55% of the US Under-21 female players took nutrient supplements occasionally, 33% took supplements daily, and 11% did not take any supplements. The most popular supplements were multivitamin/mineral preparations, vitamin C, calcium, iron, and zinc. Clark *et al.* (2003) reported that female collegiate footballers took multivitamin/mineral supplements and iron, but did not report the percentage of athletes using supplements.

Although creatine use was not reported by either group of female athletes in the studies reviewed for this paper, creatine supplementation has been investigated as a performance-enhancing supplement in both endurance and power athletes. Creatine is found in the diet in meat and fish with less than $1 \, g \cdot day^{-1}$ ingested from animal foods (Hespel, Maughan, & Greenhaff, 2006). Creatine supplementation is popular in strength and power sports relying on the anaerobic energy system. Creatine is also used by athletes to enhance training response (Volek & Kraemer, 1996). Creatine supplementation does not benefit endurance athletes. Balsom, Harridge, Soderlund, Sjodin and Ekblom (1993) studied 18 trained men in a double-blind design and gave them creatine monohydrate or placebo for 6 days prior to the endurance exercise trials. There were no significant differences in performance between groups, but the creatine-supplemented group gained weight after supplementation.

Larson-Meyer *et al.* (2000) studied creatine supplementation in female collegiate soccer players to assess changes in body composition and muscle strength. Fourteen members of the team were recruited to participate in the study in the off-season. Seven players were given a loading dose of creatine monohydrate ($0.24 \, g \cdot kg$ body $mass^{-1}$ or about $15 \, g$) in a sports drink for 5 days, and $5 \, g$ of creatine in a sports drink for a maintenance dose. Seven players served as controls and the sports drink without creatine was used as placebo. The participants completed strength workouts at baseline and every 2 weeks for a total of 13 weeks. Soccer practice was started 2 weeks after supplementation with creatine and consisted of soccer-specific drills. At the end of 13 weeks, both groups increased body mass with no significant difference between creatine supplementation and placebo. The creatine-supplemented group showed a greater improvement in bench press and squat and the effects were most pronounced after 5 weeks of supplementation. Despite the limitations of the study (small number of participants, not all participants completed all strength measures, and the placebo did not contain protein), the authors suggested that creatine supplementation in female soccer players could have some advantages. Players may improve maximal strength, which could help them shield the ball and maintain possession. The authors also noted that creatine supplementation did cause additional weight gain beyond usual weight gain from weight training. Many female athletes avoid creatine use because the main side-effect is weight gain.

Special considerations

There are no reports of the number of female footballers who practise vegetarianism, but vegetarian athletes face unique challenges to proper nutrition (Barr & Rideout, 2004). Vegetarians usually consume sufficient protein, but may be at risk for iron deficiency. It has been reported that vegetarians have a lower mean muscle creatine concentration than meat eaters (Delanghe *et al.*, 1989) and it has been suggested that vegetarian athletes might benefit from creatine supplementation. Vegetarianism can be a healthy eating practice if nutrient-dense foods are selected and special attention is paid to consumption of vitamin B12, calcium, zinc, iron, and magnesium. However, some women choose vegetarian diets for weight control and this practice may conceal a disordered eating pattern.

Youth players

Type in the words "youth soccer" in the search engine "Google" and 4,690,000 pages appear. FIFA reported that in 2000, almost 18 million youth played football worldwide (www.FIFA.com). The American Youth Soccer Organization (youth aged 4–12 years) identifies 50,000 teams with more than 650,000 participants (AYSO, 2005). The National Sporting Goods Association reports a 6.2% increase in the number of 7- to 11-year-olds participating in soccer since 1994 (NSGA, 2004b). The Football Association reports that girls' football is "booming" in England. Figures for May 2002 revealed that 85% of girls aged 7–15 years played football and 65% of that age group played football at least once a week, a figure of 1.4 million girls (The Football Association, 2003).

Youth players have unique physical demands for growth and development that make nutrition more important than just as a fuel for sport. In addition, there is wide variation in physical growth and maturation of young athletes at the same chronological age. Rules governing youth football are different from adult rules, and vary by age group. The purposes of the rules for youth are to make matches fun (e.g. smaller fields), make matches safer (e.g. no slide tackling), and more evenly matched (e.g. small sided) (Bar-Or & Unnithan, 1994; www.usyouthsoccer.org). For example, children under 6 play four 8 min quarters with a 2 min break between quarters and a 5 min half-time. Each player plays a minimum of 50% of total playing time. Children under 10 play two 25 min halves with a 5 min break at half-time. Many youth leagues allow unlimited substitutions during matches (www.usyouthsoccer.com).

Rowland (2000) reviewed what is known about the effects of exercise on the young athlete and concluded that both growth and functional changes that occur in children make it difficult to assess the effects of exercise on growth and development. It is clear that thermoregulatory responses of children are different from those of adults: children expend more energy per kilogram to perform work than adults and children sweat less during activity (Rowland, 2000), making thermoregulation more challenging.

Energy and nutrient intakes

Few studies have addressed the energy and nutrient intakes of youth football players (for a comprehensive review of general nutritional considerations in young, competitive athletes, see Petrie, Stover, & Horswill, 2004). Iglesias-Gutierrez *et al.* (2005) and Ruiz *et al.* (2005) recently published studies of nutritional intake in male youth players. Table 2 summarizes the mean energy and macronutrient intakes of young (14–16 years) players participating at high

Table 2. Daily mean energy and macronutrient intakes of adolescent footballers

	Spanish adolescents (14–16 years) [a] (n = 32)	Arenas FC players (14 years) [b] (n = 18)	Arenas FC players (15 years) [b] (n = 20)	Arenas FC players (16 years) [b] (n = 19)	Arenas FC players (21 years) [b] (n = 25)
Energy (kcal $\cdot$ day^{-1})	3003	3456	3418	3478	3030
Energy (kcal $\cdot$ kg^{-1})	46.5	54.6	51.5	48.4	41.4
Protein (g $\cdot$ day^{-1})	123	128.5	141.9	150.2	132.8
Protein (g $\cdot$ kg^{-1})	1.9	2.0	2.1	2.0	1.8
Carbohydrate (g $\cdot$ day^{-1})	364	422	391	392	334
Carbohydrate (g $\cdot$ kg^{-1})	5.6	6.7	5.9	5.3	4.6
Fat (g $\cdot$ day^{-1})	127	139	142	154	128
Fat (g $\cdot$ kg^{-1})	1.95	2.2	2.15	2.15	1.8

[a] Iglesias-Gutierrez et al. (2005), [b] Ruiz et al. (2005).

levels of the sport. Ruiz *et al.* (2005) compared young players in different age groups (14-, 15-, and 16-year-olds) and collected dietary data using weighed food records. Iglesias-Gutierrez *et al.* (2005) reported mean data obtained from the youths' home environment. Both groups of researchers reported mean data but noted a wide range in individual nutrient intakes and heterogeneity of anthropometric measures.

Iglesias-Gutierrez *et al.* (2005) estimated mean energy expenditure at 2983 kcal · day^{-1} and an energy intake of 3003 kcal · day^{-1}. Carbohydrate intake was 45% of energy intake or 5.6 g · kg^{-1} on average; this is less than the recommendations for highly active athletes. Protein intake averaged 1.9 g · kg^{-1}. Micronutrient intakes were below the DRIs for folate, vitamin E, calcium, magnesium, and zinc. Biochemical and haematological values were measured and 48% of these young athletes had iron deficiency without anaemia, as assessed by low ferritin levels, despite a diet adequate in iron (143% of DRI).

Ruiz *et al.* (2005) compared energy and nutrient intake among players of different ages (14-, 15-, 16-, and 20-year-olds). Younger athletes had higher energy intakes, consumed more monounsaturated fatty acids, and were more likely to eat breakfast than the 20-year-old players, but energy and carbohydrate intakes did not meet recommendations for any age group. The researchers also collected information on consumption of meals and snacks and noted a trend for the older athletes to skip meals, especially breakfast, which could contribute to the decline in energy and nutrient intakes seen in this age group. The authors concluded that younger players live in a more controlled food environment (eating at school or home) than the older players. A nutrition education programme, starting with younger players, may help promote healthy dietary habits as players get older.

None of the boys in the above two studies (Iglesias-Gutierrez *et al.*, 2005; Ruiz *et al.*, 2005) consumed adequate carbohydrate to support energy expenditure in training or competition. Fat intake was adequate in both relative and absolute amounts. Boys use more fat (~70% more) and less carbohydrate (~23% less) than men during activity performed at about the same intensity (Timmons, Bar-Or, & Riddell, 2003). Recent findings that the lower carbohydrate storage and utilization of women appears to be due to their lower carbohydrate intake (M'Kaouar *et al.*, 2004; Roepstorff *et al.*, 2002; Tarnopolsky *et al.*, 2001a) support the suggestion that increasing carbohydrate intake during activity of high intensity lasting longer than 60 min may also improve the performance and spare endogenous stores for growth and development of boys (Timmons *et al.*, 2003).

Athletes who engage in regular sports activities need slightly higher protein than sedentary people (Institute of Medicine, 2002). Boisseau, LeCreff, Loyens and Poortmans (2002) compared youth football players (age 15 years) with sedentary age-matched non-athletes. Seven-day food diaries were collected and protein status was assessed by nitrogen balance techniques. Both the athletes and the sedentary adolescents needed a protein intake of 1.6 g · kg^{-1} · day^{-1} to obtain a positive nitrogen balance. This study is the first to address protein needs of youth football players. However, researchers have questioned the benefit of using nitrogen balance as an assessment tool to recommend higher protein intake in athletes (Millward, 2004). Further research is warranted to assess protein needs in young athletes.

Fluids

Few studies have assessed the hydration status of young athletes. Active children do not adapt to conditions of high heat and humidity as effectively as adults, and the adaptation of adolescents has been described as somewhere between that of children and adults (American Academy of Pediatrics, 2000). The US Soccer Federation issued guidelines to prevent heat illness in young football players in 2002 and these are summarized in Table 3.

Rico-Sanz et al. (1996) assessed the effect of increased fluid intake on temperature regulation in eight elite youth footballers and found that those who hyperhydrated improved the ability to regulate body temperature during a 90 min match played in hot, humid conditions. There was no effect on soccer performance.

Dietary supplements

Young athletes are increasingly using dietary supplements that are touted as performance enhancing. The reasons cited for use of dietary supplements in youth include the following:

- Athletes reach a plateau in training and the use of a performance-enhancing supplement may allow him or her to break through the plateau.

Table 3. US Soccer Federation (2002) youth soccer heat stress guidelines

Before activity
- Players should be well hydrated
  - Check urine colour for hydration status

During activity
- Drink early
- Consume 5–9 ounces (5 ounces for a player weighing less than 90 pounds, 9 ounces for a player weighing more than 90 pounds) every 20 min while active
- Sports drinks are preferred to water

After activity
- Drink every 20 min for one hour after activity, regardless of thirst

Fluids to avoid during practice or a game
- Fruit juice
- Carbonated beverages
- Caffeinated beverages
- Energy drinks

- Peer pressure from coaches, parents, and team-mates to use supplements.
- The cultural norm in some sports is to use supplements.
- Knowledge that competitors use supplements.
- Dietary supplements are readily available for purchase and are advertised as "safe and natural" ways to improve physical and mental performance.
- Trickle down effect from elite adult athletes using supplements to young athletes who want to emulate a sports hero.
- No drug testing in many youth sports (DesJardins, 2002; Metzl, 2002; Metzl, Small, Levene, & Gershel, 2001).

While not popular in all countries, the prevalence of creatine use in adolescent athletes is reported to be 7–30% in the USA, with athletes as young as 12 years using creatine (DesJardins, 2002). The American College of Sports Medicine (2000) does not advise creatine use in those under the age of 18 years, but it is clear that some young athletes use this dietary supplement.

Ostojic (2004) studied creatine use in young football players. He randomly assigned 20 young soccer players (mean age 16.6 years) to creatine monohydrate (at $10 g \times 3$ doses per day) or placebo and measured soccer-specific skills at baseline and after 7 days of creatine or placebo ingestion. Significant improvements were noted in a dribbling test, a power test, and vertical jump between pre- and post-creatine ingestion and between the creatine group and placebo group. The authors concluded that acute creatine ingestion may improve performance in soccer-related tasks, but cautioned that creatine use is not recommended for those under 18 years. The dose of creatine given in this study ($30 g \cdot day^{-1}$) is higher than the usual doses of creatine recommended to athletes and the placebo was a cellulose pill. Tarnopolsky *et al.* (2001b) believed that comparing a creatine supplemented experimental group with a control group receiving a non-protein-containing placebo is not a good experimental design. They showed that when energy and protein are equivalent (i.e. creatine versus a carbohydrate and a nitrogen-containing placebo), strength and mass are similar (Tarnopolsky *et al.*, 2001b).

Special considerations

Elite youth players frequently play several matches within a short time frame, which can have consequences for the immune system. Malm, Ekblom and Ekblom (2004) studied elite football players (16 to 19 years) who played two consecutive games separated by 20 h. Blood measures of cells of the immune system were taken before the first match, immediately after the second match, and at 6, 24, 48, and 72 h after the second match. Players with greater aerobic capacity demonstrated smaller changes in some measures of immunity, but at least 72 h was needed to reach normal levels of cells of the immune system after two competitive matches.

Summary and recommendations

Little is known about the nutrient intake or nutritional status of female and young footballers. From the few studies reviewed, it is clear that some female and young players do not get adequate carbohydrate to fuel the demands of training and competition. Micronutrients of concern in both females and young athletes include folate, vitamin E, calcium, magnesium, and zinc. Biochemical assessment reveals concern for iron deficiency without anaemia, although it is unlikely that this haematological abnormality affects performance. However, if left undetected and untreated, iron deficiency anaemia could be the result.

Female athletes appear to have good knowledge about hydration in general, but may need more guidance in choosing the most appropriate beverage during exercise and for recovery. Young athletes may have better nutrient intakes and food behaviours than older athletes because they have a more controlled dietary environment.

Recommendations for female players

- Provide carbohydrate recommendations in absolute terms ($g \cdot kg^{-1}$) versus relative terms (percent of energy) and provide levels of carbohydrate consumption for pre-season, in-season, and post-season.
- Monitor post-season intake to ensure adequate intake of nutrients so athletes report for pre-season training with adequate nutrient stores.
- Educate athletes on hydration and the preferred beverages for rehydration.
- Monitor iron status in females and recommend consumption of an iron-rich diet with adequate energy for those with iron deficiency without anaemia.
- Explore new methodologies to obtain dietary data. Food diaries are difficult to obtain and under-reporting is common. One methodology worthy of exploration is the use of the cell phone camera to take pictures of meals and snacks consumed, which can then be analysed and timely feedback provided. One US company (www.myfoodphone.com) is using this technology as a dieting tool but it could be adapted for use as a research tool for athletes.

Recommendations for young players

- Provide nutrition education to athletes at an early age with the goal of improving nutritional status and nutrient intakes as the players get older.
- Monitor young players for iron deficiency without anaemia.
- Provide carbohydrate to athletes during training and competition.
- Assess protein needs of young athletes to determine the most appropriate dietary protein guidelines.

References

Akabas, S. R., & Dolins K. R. (2005). Micronutrient requirements of physically active women: What can we learn from iron? *American Journal of Clinical Nutrition, 81,* 1246S–1251S.

American Academy of Pediatrics (2000). Climatic heat stress and the exercising child and adolescent. *Pediatrics, 106,* 158–159.

American College of Sports Medicine (2000). The physiological and health effects of oral creatine supplementation. *Medicine and Science in Sports and Exercise, 32,* 706–717.

American Dietetic Association, Dietitians of Canada, and the American College of Sports Medicine (2000). Position statement: Nutrition and athletic performance. *Journal of the American Dietetic Association, 100,* 1543–1556.

American Youth Soccer Organization (2005). *American youth soccer* (available at: http://soccer.org; accessed 6 July 2005).

Bailey, S. P., Zacher, C. M., & Mittleman, K. D. (2000). Effect of menstrual cycle phase on carbohydrate supplementation during prolonged exercise to fatigue. *Journal of Applied Physiology, 88,* 690–697.

Balsom, P. D., Harridge, S. D. R., Soderlund, K., Sjodin, B., & Ekblom, B. (1993). Creatine supplementation *per se* does not enhance endurance exercise performance. *Acta Physiologica Scandinavica, 149,* 521–523.

Bangsbo, J. (1994). Energy demands in competitive soccer. *Journal of Sports Sciences, 12,* S5–S12.

Bar-Or, O., & Unnithan, V. B. (1994). Nutritional requirements of young soccer players. *Journal of Sports Sciences, 12,* S39–S42.

Barr, S., & Rideout, C. A. (2004). Nutritional considerations for vegetarian athletes. *Nutrition, 20,* 696–703.

Boisseau, N., LeCreff, C., Loyens, M., & Poortmans, J. R. (2002). Protein intake and nitrogen balance in male non-active adolescents and soccer players. *European Journal of Applied Physiology, 88,* 288–293.

Brewer, J. (1994). Nutritional aspects of women's soccer. *Journal of Sports Sciences, 12,* S35–S38.

Brownlie, T., Utermohlen, V., Hinton, P. S., Giordano, C., & Haas, J. D. (2002). Marginal iron deficiency without anemia impairs aerobic adaptation among previously untrained women. *American Journal of Clinical Nutrition, 78,* 702–710.

Brutsaert, T. D., Hernandez-Cordero, S., Rivera, J., Viola, T., Hughes, G., & Haas J. D. (2003). Iron supplementation improves progressive fatigue resistance during dynamic knee extensor exercise in iron-depleted, nonanemic women. *American Journal of Clinical Nutrition, 77,* 441–448.

Burke, L. M. (2005). Fluid balance testing for elite team athletes: An interview with Dr. Susan Shirreffs. *International Journal of Sport Nutrition and Exercise Metabolism, 15,* 323–327.

Burke, L. M., Cox, G. R., Cummings, N. K., & Desbrow, B. (2001). Guidelines for daily carbohydrate intake. Do athletes achieve them? *Sports Medicine, 31,* 267–299.

Burke, L. M., & Hawley, J. A. (1997). Fluid balance in team sports. *Sports Medicine, 24,* 38–53.

Burke, L. M., Keins, B., & Ivy, J. L. (2004). Carbohydrates and fat for training and recovery. *Journal of Sports Sciences, 22,* 15–30.

Burke, L. M., Slater, G., Broad, E. M., Haukka, J., Modulon, S., & Hopkins, W. G. (2003). Eating patterns and meal frequency of elite Australian athletes. *International Journal of Sport Nutrition and Exercise Metabolism, 13*, 521–538.

Campbell, S. E., Angus, D. J., & Febbraio, M. A. (2001). Glucose kinetics and exercise performance during phases of the menstrual cycle: Effect of glucose ingestion. *American Journal of Physiology: Endocrinology and Metabolism, 281*, E817–E825.

Clark, M., Reed, D. B., Crouse, S. F., & Armstrong, R. B. (2003). Pre- and post-season dietary intake, body composition and performance indices of NCAA Division I female soccer players. *International Journal of Sport Nutrition and Exercise Metabolism, 13*, 303–319.

Coyle, E. F. (2004). Fluid and fuel intake during exercise. *Journal of Sports Sciences, 22*, 39–55.

Davies, H. (2005). The fan. *The New Statesman*, 4 April.

Delanghe, J., DeSlypere, J. P., Dehuyzere, M., Robbrecht, J., Wieme, R., & Vermeulen, A. (1989). Normal reference values for creatine, creatinine, and carnitine are lower in vegetarians. *Clinical Chemistry, 35*, 1802–1803.

DesJardins, M. (2002). Supplement use in the adolescent athlete. *Current Sports Medicine Reports, 1*, 369–373.

DeSouza, M. J., Miller, B. E., Loucks, A. B., Luciano, A. A., Pescatello, L. S., Campbell, C. G. *et al.* (1998). High frequency of luteal phase deficiency and anovulation in recreational women runners: Blunted elevation in follicle-stimulating hormone observed during luteal-follicular transition. *Journal of Clinical Endocrinology and Metabolism, 83*, 4220–4232.

Ekblom, B. (1997). Micronutrients: Effects of variation in [Hb] and iron deficiency on physical performance. In A. P. Simopoulos & K. N. Pavlou (Eds.), *Nutrition and fitness: Metabolic and behavioral aspects in health and disease* (pp. 122–130). Basel: Karger.

Fallon, K. E. (2004). Utility of haematological and iron-related screening in elite athletes. *Clinical Journal of Sports Medicine, 14*, 145–152.

FIFA (2005). *FIFA laws of the game 2005/2006* (available at http://dps.twiihosting.net/USSF/doc; accessed 10 August 2005).

Fogelholm, M. (1994). Vitamins, minerals and supplementation in soccer. *Journal of Sports Sciences, 12*, S23–S27.

Fogelholm, M., Kukkonen-Harjula, T. K., Taipale, S. A., Sievanen, H. T., Oja, P., & Vuori, I. M. (1995). Resting metabolic rate and energy intake in female gymnasts, figure skaters, and soccer players. *International Journal of Sports Medicine, 16*, 551–556.

Hespel, P., Maughan, R. J., & Greenhaff, P. L. (2006). Dietary supplements for soccer. *Journal of Sports Sciences, 24*, 749–761.

Hinton, P. S., Sanford, T. C., Davidson, M. M., Yakushko, O. F., & Beck, N. C. (2004). Nutrient intakes and dietary behaviors of male and female collegiate athletes. *International Journal of Sport Nutrition and Exercise Metabolism, 14*, 389–405.

Iglesias-Gutierrez, E., Garcia-Roves, P. M., Rodriguez, C., Braga, S., Garcia-Zapico, P., & Patterson, A. M. (2005). Food habits and nutritional status assessment of adolescent soccer players: A necessary and accurate approach. *Canadian Journal of Applied Physiology, 30*, 18–32.

Institute of Medicine (2002). *Dietary reference intakes for energy, carbohydrates, fiber, fat, protein, and amino acids (macronutrients)*. Washington, DC: National Academy Press (available at: http://www.nap.edu/books; accessed 26 July 2005).

Kirkendall, D. T. (2000). Physiology of soccer. In W. E. Garrett & D. T. Kirkendall (Eds.), *Exercise and sport science* (pp. 875–884). Philadelphia, PA: Lippincott Williams & Wilkins.

Kirkendall, D. T. (2004). Creatine, carbs, and fluids: How important in soccer nutrition? *Sports Science Exchange, 17*, 1–6.

Larson-Meyer, D. E., Hunter, G. R., Trowbridge, C. A., Turk, J. C., Ernest, J. M., Torman, S. L. *et al.* (2000). The effect of creatine supplementation on muscle strength and body composition during off-season training in female soccer players. *Journal of Strength and Conditioning Research, 14*, 434–442.

Lemon, P. W. R. (1994). Protein requirements of soccer. *Journal of Sports Sciences, 12*, S17–S22.

Loucks, A. B. (2004). Energy balance and body composition in sports and exercise. *Journal of Sports Sciences, 22*, 1–14.

Malm, C., Ekblom, O., & Ekblom, B. (2004). Immune system alteration in response to two consecutive soccer games. *Acta Physiologica Scandinavica, 180*, 143–155.

Manore, M. M. (2000). Effect of physical activity on thiamine, riboflavin, and vitamin B-6 requirements. *American Journal of Clinical Nutrition, 72*, 598S–606S.

Maughan, R. J., & Leiper, J. B. (1994). Fluid replacement requirements in soccer. *Journal of Sports Sciences, 12*, S29–S34.

Metzl, J. D. (2002). Performance-enhancing drug use in the young athlete. *Pediatric Annals, 31*, 27–32.

Metzl, J. D., Small, E., Levine, S. R., & Gershel, J. C. (2001). Creatine use among young athletes. *Pediatrics, 108*, 421–425.

Millward, D. J. (2004). Protein and amino acid requirements of athletes. *Journal of Sports Sciences, 22*, 143–145.

M'Kaouar, H., Peronnet, F., Massicotte, D., & Lavoie, C. (2004). Gender difference in metabolic response to prolonged exercise with [^{13}C] glucose ingestion. *European Journal of Applied Physiology, 92*, 462–469.

Mullinix, M. C., Jonnalagadda, S. S., Rosenbloom, C. A., Thompson, W. R., & Kicklighter, J. A. (2003). Dietary intake of female U.S. soccer players. *Nutrition Research, 23*, 585–593.

National Sporting Goods Association (2004a). *Women's participation – ranked by total female participation* (available at: www.nsga.org; accessed 10 July 2005).

National Sporting Goods Association (2004b). *Youth participation in selected sports with comparisons to 1994* (available at: www.nsga.org; accessed 10 July 2005).

Ostojic, S. J. (2004). Creatine supplementation in young soccer players. *International Journal of Sport Nutrition and Exercise Metabolism, 14*, 95–103.

Pettersson, U., Nordstrom, P., Alfredson, H., Henriksson-Larsen, K., & Lorentzon, R. (2000). Effect of high impact activity on bone mass and size in adolescent females: A comparative study between two different types of sports. *Calcified Tissue International, 67*, 207–214.

Petrie, H. J., Stover, E. A., & Horswill, C. A. (2004). Nutritional concerns for the child and adolescent competitor. *Nutrition, 20*, 620–631.

Reilly, T. (1997). Energetics of high-intensity exercise (soccer) with particular reference to fatigue. *Journal of Sports Sciences, 15*, 257–263.

Rico-Sanz, J., Frontera, W. R., Rivera, M. A., Rivera-Brown, A., Mole, P. A., & Meredith, C. N. (1996). Effects of hyperhydration on total body water, temperature regulation and performance of elite young soccer players in a warm climate. *International Journal of Sports Medicine, 17*, 85–91.

Riddell, M. C., Partington, S. L., Stupka, N., Armstrong, D., Rennie, C., & Tarno-polsky, M. A. (2003). Substrate utilization during exercise performed with and without glucose ingestion in female and male endurance-trained athletes. *International Journal of Sport Nutrition and Exercise Metabolism*, 13, 407–421.

Roepstorff, C., Steffensen, C. H., Madsen, M., Stallknecht, B., Kanstrup, I., Richter, E. A. *et al.* (2002). Gender differences in substrate utilization during submaximal exercise in endurance-trained subjects. *American Journal of Physiology: Endocrinology and Metabolism*, 282, E435–E447.

Rowland, T. W. (2000). Exercise and the child athlete. In W. E. Garrett & D. T. Kirkendall (Eds.), *Exercise and sport science* (pp. 339–349). Philadelphia, PA: Lippincott Williams & Wilkins.

Ruiz, F., Irazusta, A., Gil, S., Irazusta, J., Casis, L., & Gil, J. (2005). Nutritional intake in soccer players of different ages. *Journal of Sports Sciences*, 23, 235–242.

Shirreffs, S. M., Armstrong, L. E., & Cheuvoront, S. N. (2004). Fluid and electrolyte needs for training, competition, preparation and recovery. *Journal of Sports Sciences*, 22, 57–63.

Soderman, K., Bergstrom, E., Lorentzon, R., & Alfredson, H. (2000). Bone mass and muscle strength in young female soccer players. *Calcified Tissue International*, 67, 297–303.

Tarnopolsky, M. A., Atkinson, S. A., Phillips, S. M., & MacDougall, J. D. (1995). Carbohydrate loading and metabolism during exercise in men and women. *Journal of Applied Physiology*, 78, 1360–1388.

Tarnopolsky, M. A., Parise, G., Yardley, N. J., Ballantyne, C. S., Olatunji, S., & Phillips, S. M. (2001b). Creatine-dextrose and protein-dextrose induce similar strength gains during training. *Medicine and Science in Sports and Exercise*, 33, 2040–2052.

Tarnopolsky, M. A., Zwada, C., Richmond, L. B., Carter, S., Shearer, J., Graham, T. *et al.* (2001a). Gender differences in carbohydrate loading are related to energy intake. *Journal of Applied Physiology*, 91, 225–230.

The Football Association (2002). *A brief history: Women's football* (available at: http://www.thefa.com/Womens/EnglandSenior/History; accessed 3 August 2002).

The Football Association (2003). *Participation figures* (available at: http://wwwthefa.com/Womens/Reference-FAQ/Posting/2003/11/Participation+Figures.htm; accessed 1 August 2005).

The Football Association (2005). *Studying the game* (available at: http://www.thefa.com/Womens/EnglandSenior/NewsAndFeatures; accessed 1 August 2005).

Timmons, B. W., Bar-Or, O., & Riddell, M. C. (2003). Oxidation rate of exogenous carbohydrate during exercise is higher in boys than men. *Journal of Applied Physiology*, 94, 278–284.

Tipton, K. D., & Wolfe, R. R. (2004). Protein and amino acids for athletes. *Journal of Sports Sciences*, 22, 65–79.

US Soccer Federation (2002). *Youth soccer heat stress guidelines* (available at: www.ussoccer.com; accessed 3 July 2005).

Volek, J. S., & Kraemer, W. J. (1996). Creatine supplementation: Its effect on human muscular performance and body composition. *Journal of Strength and Conditioning Research*, 10, 200–210.

12 Special populations: The referee and assistant referee

THOMAS REILLY AND WARREN GREGSON

The referee has responsibility for control of players' behaviour during competitive football and implementing the rules of the game. To do this, the referee and the two assistant referees are obliged to keep up with play. Referees cover 10,000 m on average during a game, mean heart rate is about 160–165 beats $\cdot$ min^{-1} and oxygen uptake is close to 80% of maximum ($\dot{V}O_{2max}$). Assistant referees cover approximately 7500 m, mean heart rate is about 140 beats $\cdot$ min^{-1} and the corresponding oxygen uptake is 65% $\dot{V}O_{2max}$. Both groups display evidence of fatigue towards the end of the game, a phenomenon that has not been thoroughly examined for nutritional interventions. The estimated energy expenditure of referees during a game exceeds 5600 kJ. Both referees and assistant referees execute unorthodox patterns of movement during match-play that increase energy expenditure over normal locomotion. As high standards of fitness and decision making are expected of professional referees, there are nutritional consequences associated with the training regimes they adopt. The effects of nutritional interventions on cognitive performance during the later stages of a game are in need of further investigation.

Keywords: Assistant referees, energy expenditure, fatigue, fitness, mental performance

Introduction

The referee is charged with responsibility for implementing the rules of the game and guaranteeing that players abide by its regulations. These requirements mean that the referee is obliged to keep up with play to be in a good position to notice infringements. In addition to this requirement for mobility about the pitch, the referee must also maintain mental concentration and make split-second decisions about competitive incidents. In many circumstances, he or she has recourse to consult one of the two assistant referees (linesmen).

Most research on nutritional requirements in football has been directed towards the players, with the referee being relatively neglected until recently. The omission reflects the fact that the players form the centre of attention of spectators until refereeing decisions are considered controversial. In a review by Eissmann (1994), it was stated that the physical and psychological demands on referees increased enormously in the 1980s. The claim was based on the health checks and fitness tests imposed by FIFA on referees qualifying for the international list rather than any observations of physiological responses to officiating of match-play. National associations have tended to follow the examples of FIFA and the ruling confederations in implementing these assessments.

Advice on nutritional provision for referees tends to be general rather than specific. The US Soccer Association currently provides guidelines to referees for allowing hydration of players during a game but there is no mention of rules regarding rehydration for referees. Eissmann (1994) recognized that the referee has to "prepare before a game in the same way as a player, i.e. with proper nutrition", but no further direction was given. With the advent of professional referees at the elite level of competition by the turn of the century, a more scientific approach towards the task of officiating is now feasible.

To place the energetic demands of refereeing in a nutritional context, the activities of referees during match-play are reviewed. The physiological demands imposed by these activities are then considered. The training programmes undertaken to meet these demands and the fitness standards set as targets by the ruling bodies are also addressed. These areas are all relevant to any inferences about specific nutritional counselling of referees.

Activities of referees during match-play

The work rate of referees during matches may be determined by motion analysis using procedures that have been adopted for monitoring players (Bangsbo, 1994; Drust, Reilly, & Rienzi, 1998; Reilly & Thomas, 1976). The overall distance covered yields an indirect indication of the energy expenditure (Reilly & Thomas, 1979) but can be broken down according to exercise intensity. In general, a distinction is made between low-intensity activities such as walking and jogging and high-intensity activity such as striding or cruising (with effort but submaximal) and sprinting. Periods of inactivity when the referee is stationary and bouts of unorthodox movements such as backing or shuffling sideways may also be recorded.

Observations on referees in the English, Danish, Italian, and Tasmanian leagues indicate that referees cover between 9 and 13 km in a game. The highest individual values recorded were 13.1 km in the Italian League (D'Ottavio & Castagna, 2001) and 11.1 km in the Danish League (Krustrup & Bangsbo, 2001). The Danish referees were found to spend significantly more time standing and less time engaged in high-speed running and sprinting in the second half compared with the first half. Similarly, Catterall, Reilly, Atkinson and Coldwells (1993) reported a significant reduction in the distance covered by English referees during the second half. The Serie A referees studied by Castagna, Abt and D'Ottavio (2004) covered less distance running backwards and sideways in the second half compared with the first half; no differences were observed in the other movement categories. In footballers, a decline in performance in the second half has been linked to a run down of muscle glycogen stores (Saltin, 1973). This cause of fatigue has not been confirmed in referees and it may be linked to the fall in tempo of the game associated with the drop in work rate of the players. Krustrup and Bangsbo (2001) reported that referees were further away from infringements in the second half than in the first, suggesting that the fall in work rate manifests as true fatigue. The referee has to follow movements of the ball rather than those of players and so must be prepared for direct methods of attacking play towards the end of the game. The distance covered at high intensity decreased in the second half compared with the first so that any shift towards a strategy of long passes for distance would increase the load on the referee while sparing the players.

Most of the activity of referees is conducted at a low intensity, comprising walking and jogging (see Figure 1). The time spent inactive by the Danish referees amounted to 21.8% of the total time and constituted on average a 7–8 s period standing still once every 35 s (Krustrup & Bangsbo, 2001). The corresponding figure for Italian referees was 16.9% of the total time played (D'Ottavio & Castagna, 2001). The total number of activities recorded was 1268, representing a change in activity every 4.3 s on average. There were few significant differences in activities between the referees classed as top class and those described as high standard. The data from the studies cited in Table 1

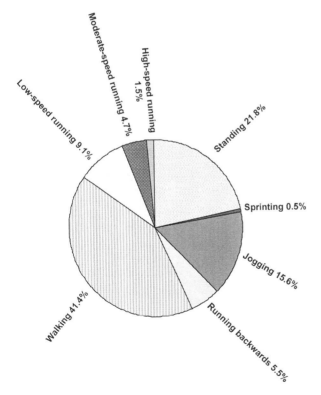

Figure 1. The percent of total time occupied by different categories of activity in top-class Danish referees. The diagram was drawn using the data of Krustrup and Bangsbo (2001).

Table 1. Distance covered by referees during football matches (mean ± *s*)

Competition	*n*	Age	Distance covered (m)	Reference
Japan Soccer League	10	–	10 168 ± 756	Asami *et al.* (1988)
International matches	7	–	9736 ± 1077	Asami *et al.* (1988)
English Premier League and First Division	14	–	9438 ± 707	Catterall *et al.* (1993)
Tasmanian State League	10	38.1 ± 3.8	9408 ± 838	Johnston and McNaughton (1994)
Italian Serie A	18	37.5 ± 2.1	11 376 ± 1604	D'Ottavio and Castagna (2001)
	13	37.0 ± 3.0	12 956 ± 548	Castagna *et al.* (2004)
Danish Superliga and First Division	27	38.0 (29–47)	10 070 ± 130	Krustrup and Bangsbo (2001)
European Cup matches	13	38.0 ± 3.0	11 218 ± 1056	Castagna *et al.* (2004)

imply that energy contribution is mainly from aerobic sources but there are episodes of appreciable anaerobic efforts during a match. Altogether, referees sprint for about 10–12% of the total distance (Catterall *et al.*, 1993; Friedman & Klein, 1988). Operating on a time-base and combining high-intensity running and sprinting, Krustrup and Bangsbo (2001) found that on average the referees performed 161 of these runs with a mean duration of 2.3 s during a game.

It would appear that the work rate of referees expressed as total distance covered approximates and overlaps with that of professional players (see Reilly, 1997). A difference is that the referee is not called upon to make angled runs, accelerate and decelerate as abruptly as players or engage with agility and power in game-related actions. All these activities are energetically costly. The Danish referees covered 850 m moving backwards, the distance being greater in the first than in the second half (Krustrup & Bangsbo, 2001). The distance reported for reverse running for English referees was much greater, amounting to an average of 1722 m, while for the Australian referees the value was 1521 m. This unorthodox mode of motion adds to the energy expenditure (Reilly & Bowen, 1984) and is necessitated by moving backwards at free kicks and goal kicks to keep an eye on the ball and anticipate the location of the next possession.

Physiological responses to match-play

The monitoring of heart rate has been adopted as a means of indicating the physiological strain during match-play. It has been used also in conjunction with regression equations determining the relationship between heart rate and oxygen uptake ($\dot{V}O_2$) derived from laboratory assessments to estimate energy expenditure. Despite the irregular fluctuations in exercise intensity during match-play, the mean heart rate during a game can provide a reasonable estimate of the energy expended (Bangsbo, 1994; Reilly, 1997).

Catterall *et al.* (1993) reported resting heart rates of 100 beats·min^{-1} in English referees in the dressing room before going on to the pitch. Allowing for emotional tachycardia, the main cause was the light exercise undertaken as a warm-up. A similar value (98 beats·min^{-1}) was reported for the Australian referees studied by Johnston and McNaughton (1994) after a similar light warm-up. Since these studies were published, the warm-up of referees has become more structured but still entails a low outlay of energy and is less intensive than that undertaken by players.

The mean heart rate of referees has shown a remarkable agreement between studies, within a range 162–165 beats·min^{-1} (see Table 2). There were no significant differences between halves even when work rates declined towards the end of the game. This consistency in heart rate throughout the game accompanied by a fall in work rate has been attributed to the cardiovascular drift that occurs with prolonged exercise (Catterall *et al.*, 1993). The mean heart rates suggest a similar relative cardiovascular strain on referees as on players, allowing for the greater age of the referees. The relative strain may be decreased at the

Table 2. Heart rate of referees during matches (mean ± *s*)

Competition	n	Hear rate (beats · min$^{-1)}$	Reference
English Premier League and First Division	14	165 ± 8	Catterall *et al.* (1993)
Tasmanian State League	10	163	Johnston and McNaughton (1994)
Italian Serie A	18	163 ± 5	D'Ottavio and Castagna (2001)
Danish Superliga and First Division	27	162 (137–179)	Krustrup and Bangsbo (2001)
UEFA 2000 Finals	17	155 ± 16	Helsen and Bultynck (2004)

lower divisions, Weston, Helsen, Bird, Nevill and Castagna (2005) reporting a higher mean heart rate and perception of exertion in the Premier League than in the Football League in England.

The variation in heart rate during competition may prove as insightful as the mean value. The high variability in the referees' responses in the European Nations Championship (Helsen & Bultynck, 2004) in France mid-summer may explain why mean values were lower than those observed in the professional national leagues. In studies of Danish referees, Krustrup and Bangsbo (2001) noted that heart rate was within the range 150–170 beats · min^{-1} for 56% of the time and above 170 beats · min^{-1} for 27% of total time. Heart rate exceeded 90% of maximum for more than 25 min. The highest heart rate observed was 196 beats · min^{-1}, while Catterall *et al.* (1993) reported a peak value of 200 beats · min^{-1} in English referees. Such values reflect the periodic bouts of anaerobic exercise superimposed on the predominantly aerobic activity. For those referees who had been studied twice, intra-individual variation in mean heart rate was 4 beats · min^{-1} (range 2–7 beats · min^{-1}) with a coefficient of variation of 2% (Krustrup & Bangsbo, 2001).

The cardiovascular strain does not seem to be accentuated at international championship finals. Helsen and Bultynck (2004) monitored 17 top-class referees at the 2000 UEFA Championship, recording heart rates throughout matches (see Figure 2). The mean value was 155 (*s* = 16) beats · min^{-1} and was higher at the beginning of the first half than after the resumption following the half-time interval. It is in the first 15 min that tackles with a high risk of injury are most frequently executed (Rahnama, Reilly, & Lees, 2002), which may have an impact on the referee's behaviour. The risk rises again in the last 15 min, the period in which both players and referee are most likely to experience fatigue. The authors, Helsen and Bultynck (2004), concluded that their results supported the adoption of specialized intensive and intermittent training sessions by referees.

Krustrup and Bangsbo (2001) used the relationship between heart rate and oxygen uptake to estimate the oxygen consumption during a game. Oxygen uptake was calculated to be 3.03 litres · min^{-1}, which corresponded to 81%

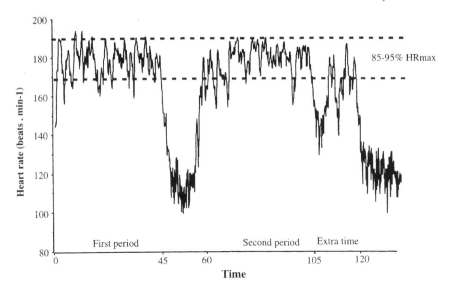

Figure 2. Graphical output of heart rate recordings, showing heart rate versus time for the referee during the final of the 2000 European Championship between France and Italy (from Helsen & Bultynck, 2004 Physical and perceptual-cognitive demands of top-class refereeing in association football, *Journal of Sports Sciences, 22*, 179–189).

(73–88%) of maximum ($\dot{V}O_{2max}$). This value is in agreement with estimates of relative metabolic loading on players (Bangsbo, 1994). Assuming the transformations employed by Reilly and Thomas (1979), this value would amount to 5616 kJ over 90 min.

Mean blood lactate concentration has been recorded as 4.8 and 5.1 mmol·l⁻¹ at the end of the first and second halves (Krustrup & Bangsbo, 2001). Values tend to reflect the activities before sampling, a significant correlation being observed between blood lactate concentration and mean heart rate in the 5 min before sampling the blood. The intra-individual variability was high with a coefficient of variation of 31%. These data are broadly in line with observations on players (Bangsbo, 1994).

Exercise at an intensity of 75–85% $\dot{V}O_{2max}$ over 90 min has consequences for thermoregulation, especially when matches are played in hot conditions. Da Silva and Fernandez (2003) focused on changes in hydration status of referees in Brazil during the autumn months. Mean temperature over six games was 20.3°C and relative humidity averaged 76.8%. Nude body mass was determined before and after matches and values were used together with water intake at half-time and urinary volume to estimate total body water loss. The referees lost 1.22 ($s = 0.10$) kg during the match, amounting to 1.55% of their pre-match body weight. Total water lost averaged 1.6 ($s = 0.13$) litres, corresponding to a sweat rate exceeding 1 litre·h⁻¹ and representing 2.05% ($s = 0.18$%) of body weight determined before the start of the game. These changes are close to the dehydration of 2% body weight thought to induce negative changes in exercise performance (Barr, 1999). The significant reduction in plasma volume of 5% was linearly related to total body water loss. The volitional intake of water during the half-time interval represented only 24% of the total water lost during the game. The question remains as to whether a more aggressive approach towards rehydration and attention to the content of fluid provided for referees would enhance their performance, particularly during the later stages of the game and when environmental temperatures are likely to induce heat stress.

Fitness and health-related assessments

The fitness targets for referees have been based on performance criteria rather than physiological measures. Standards to achieve accreditation at national and international level have been raised successively to improve fitness. Unless referees maintain their level of performance in these tests, their accreditation is withdrawn.

At the time of Eissmann's (1994) review, Cooper's 12 min run test was used for endurance. The minimum distance allowed was 2700 m for males and 2000 m for females. The test was performed 15 min after completing a series of four sprints alternating between 50 m and 200 m with 15 min allowed between sprints. The maximum time permitted for 50 m was 7.5 and 9.0 s, and for the 200 m 32 and 42 s, for males and females respectively. A 4×10 m shuttle run was added in 1994 with an upper limit of 11.5 s.

The mean distance covered in the 12 min run by 10 top-class Danish referees was 2905 m (range 2720–3200 m) (Krustrup & Bangsbo, 2001). Their mean $\dot{V}O_{2max}$ was 46.3 ml · kg^{-1} · min^{-1}, while mean performance in the Yo-Yo recovery test of Bangsbo (1995) was 1308 m (range 1040–1960 m). The distance covered when performing high-intensity running was more highly correlated with performance in this Yo-Yo test ($r = 0.75$, $n = 18$) than was $\dot{V}O_{2max}$ ($r = 0.54$) or performance in the 12 min run test ($r = 0.46$).

Rontoyannis, Stalikas, Sarros and Vlastaris (1998) reported data from medical and functional assessments of 188 referees in Greece aged 36.3 ($s = 4.5$) years. Performances in all the FIFA running tests were satisfactory, being 7.45 ($s = 0.3$) and 7.5 ($s = 0.3$) s for 50 m, 31.2 ($s = 1.7$) and 31.9 ($s = 1.6$) s for 200 m, and 10.25 ($s = 0.3$) s for 4×10 m shuttle run. Performance in the 12 min run test was 2719 ($s = 172$) m, but there was a systematic decline from Divisions A to D of the league. Despite the broadly satisfactory performances, a majority of referees displayed a predisposition to coronary heart disease based on one to four risk factors. The mean body mass index was 25.9 ($s = 2.1$) and percent body fat was estimated to be 16.7 ($s = 2.5$) %. These values are higher than those found in professional players. Over 40% of the referees smoked more than 20 cigarettes a day, and 27% had resting blood pressures above upper normal limits. For these referees, a restriction of safe

Table 3. Body composition data for Premier League referees and for Premier League players measured November 2004 (mean ± s)

	Referees (n = 6)	Players (n = 13)
Age (years)	37.5 ± 4.7	26.3 ± 5.0
Height (m)	1.82 ± 0.03	1.84 ± 0.05
Body mass (kg)	89.8 ± 4.8	84.7 ± 6.9
Body mass index	27.1 ± 5.3	25.0 ± 2.4
Body fat (%)	18.9 ± 3.7	13.0 ± 2.0
Bone mineral density (g · cm^{-2})	1.37 ± 0.34	1.46 ± 0.1

cigarette consumption to five-a-day was recommended and a decrease in energy intake was advised for the referees deemed to be overweight.

Assessment of body composition of referees provides insight into health-related status and indirectly yields information of nutritional relevance. The percent body fat values (mean 18.9%) of the sample of Premier League referees represent normal figures for their respective age but are much higher than values for players (see Table 3). The body mass index would place the referees within the overweight category but is likely explained by the higher than normal values for bone mineral density. While weight control may be a concern for some referees (the range for percent body fat was 14.0–22.7), the data demonstrate the limitations of the body mass index for both referees and footballers. The high bone mineral density for both groups suggests that the exercise stimulus for bone health and the dietary mineral content were adequate for both samples.

Training

A common feature in feedback to referees after fitness assessments is advice on training requirements. Generally, improvement of aerobic power is advocated and intermittent running is recommended to provide specificity for match activities. In an era of full-time professional referees, an optimization of training regimens would be expected. Compliance with guidelines for players on sports nutrition should be of benefit in the conduct of training as well as in matches, the referees being deemed athletes in their own right.

Castagna et al. (2004) attributed the difference of 1738 m between Serie A referees and international-match referees to the high-volume training conducted by the Italian officials. Krustrup and Bangsbo (2001) demonstrated how a systematic regimen of training can improve performance of match activities. The programme entailed three to four sessions per week of intermittent exercise over 12 weeks during a break in the competitive season. The first 4 weeks consisted of three long-duration interval sessions (4 × 4 min or 8 × 2 min), the second 4 weeks comprised three long-duration interval sessions and one short-duration session (16 × 1 min or 24 × 30 s), while the final weeks involved two short-duration and two long-duration interval sessions. There was a 2:1 ratio for exercise and rest. The programme improved performance in the Yo-Yo recovery test by 31 ($s = 7$) % and increased the amount of high-intensity running in a match by 23 ($s = 8$) %. This effect was evident in the number rather than in the distance of high-intensity runs, which remained at an average of 17 m.

Weston, Helsen, MacMahon and Kirkendall (2004) adopted a programme of high-intensity running in training sessions on both playing pitch and running track. Mean heart rate and intensity during these sessions were 86 ($s = 3$) % and 88.2 ($s = 2.4$) % maximal heart rate respectively. Over a period of 16 months, the performance of the referees on the Yo-Yo intermittent recovery test improved by 46.5% to a level deemed comparable with that of professional players.

It is clear that a regimen of physical training is required to enable professional referees to keep up with play at an elite level in contemporary football. The main emphasis may rightly be on aerobic training, but anaerobic elements, agility, and unorthodox movements should also be included. To cope with the repeated cycles of training and matches, referees must adopt nutritional strategies that resemble those used by players.

Assistant referees

Assistant referees would appear to have a physically less demanding task than that of the main match official. Their path is approximately 50 m along the verge of the sideline, from end-line to half-way line. Assistant referees tend to be drawn from accredited referees and so might be expected to have similar fitness levels even if activity is not as strenuous as that of the referee. Indeed, assistant referees in the top Danish league had mean $\dot{V}O_{2max}$ values of 45.9 (40.9–53.6) ml·kg^{-1}·min^{-1}, covered 2889 (2760–3175) m in the 12 min run, and were aged 40 (32–47) years (Krustrup, Mohr, & Bangsbo, 2002).

The movement patterns of 15 Danish Superliga assistant referees were monitored over 22 matches. The mean total distance covered was 7.28 ($s = 0.17$) km. This figure included 0.31 ($s = 0.04$) km of sprinting, 0.34 ($s = 0.03$) km of high-speed running, and 0.50 ($s = 0.03$) km of moderate-speed running. When these three categories were combined as high-intensity running, the total was significantly correlated with performance of repeated sprints. Sideways and backwards running accounted for 1.22 ($s = 0.15$) km or 16.8% of the total distance covered, while on 240 occasions the officials were standing for a mean duration of 10.9 s. Mean heart rate was 137 ($s = 3$) beats·min^{-1}, corresponding to 73% of individual maximal heart rate and 65% $\dot{V}O_{2max}$. Blood lactate concentration was 4.7 (1.6–11.0) mmol·l^{-1} at half-time and 4.8 (1.1–13.7) mmol·l^{-1} at the end of the game; blood glucose concentrations at these times were 5.1 ($s = 0.1$) and 4.4 ($s = 0.2$) mmol·l^{-1}. The officials spent more time standing, less time walking, and less time moving backwards and sideways in the second half than in the first. Sprinting performance in three 30 m runs was poorer after the game than it was pre-match, suggesting a fatigue effect. The peak distance to the offside line was greater in the second half than it was in the first half, reflecting the decreased ability of the officials to keep up with play. These observations indicate frequent short periods of inactivity during the game, a moderate aerobic energy production with episodes of high aerobic and anaerobic energy turnover.

Assistant referees ($n = 17$) at the 2000 European Championship finals were monitored by Helsen and Bultynck (2004). Mean heart rate was 144 ($s = 14$) beats · min^{-1} for the game as a whole and was higher at the beginning of the first half (0–15 min) than at the beginning of the second half (45–60 min). The mean value was 77 ($s = 7$) % of individual maximal heart rate and was lower than that for referees ($85 \pm 5\%$) at the same tournament.

In the Danish study (Krustrup *et al.*, 2002), the weight loss of the assistant referees during a game was 0.81 (0.49–1.56) kg or 1.0 (0.6–2.0) % of body mass. Mean fluid intake was 360 (200–500) ml and sweat loss was estimated to be 1.17 (0.83–1.81) litres, corresponding to 1.5 (1.0–2.3) % of body mass. These values are higher than observed for assistant referees in Brazil who consumed 250 ($s = 9$) ml of fluid, lost 0.63% of body mass and 1.05% of total body water (Da Silva & Fernandez, 2003). These figures amounted to less than half of the dehydration levels of the main official in Brazilian matches and may reflect the more conservative pace of the game in South America (Rienzi, Drust, Reilly, Carter, & Martin, 2000).

Cognitive function

Referees and assistant referees as well as players must make frequent game-related decisions during match-play. The intensity of exercise undertaken by the match officials during matches is frequently in the zone where cognitive function can be affected (Reilly & Smith, 1986). Although referees may experience increased difficulty in keeping up with play in the later stages of a game when carbohydrate reserves in active muscles are reduced, whether there is a concomitant change in the quality of decision making is unknown.

Helsen and Bultynck (2004) calculated that a top referee makes 137 observable decisions on average in a match, manifested as an intervention in play. They estimated also the frequency of invisible decisions and made allowance for the effective playing time to conclude that referees take three to four decisions each minute. The number of observed decisions is uniform throughout a match and in roughly two-thirds of cases is based on communication with the assistant referee. Choices are made against a background where noise from an excitable crowd and a home advantage can have an influence on the result.

There are numerous questions with respect to the influence of ergogenic aids and nutritional preparation on cognitive function. First, it is uncertain whether physiological fatigue necessitates a decline in mental performance related to the game. Nor is it known whether the executive function of the brain is aloof from the physiological strain and the performance deteriorations experienced by referees and assistant referees. It may be that deterioration in decision making occurs when cerebral metabolism is affected but existing laboratory-based assessments of cognitive function are not sensitive enough to detect the decline. While rehydration and energy provision can help to delay and offset muscular fatigue, their effects on "central factors" in match officials are not established.

Recommendations

Based on research already conducted, the following recommendations can be made:

1. Access to fluids should be equally available to match officials as to players during natural breaks in match-play.
2. Referees at the top level can adopt the nutritional guidelines used by players in preparing for and recovering from training and matches.
3. At lower standards of play, attention may need to be directed towards harmonizing nutritional and fitness measures in any instance of health-related concern.
4. At the international standard of refereeing, further research is needed to examine the variations in the physiological responses to match-play.

References

Asami, T., Togari, H., & Ohashi, J. (1988). Analysis of movement patterns of referees during soccer matches. In T. Reilly, A. Lees, K. Davids, & W. J. Murphy (Eds.), *Science and football* (pp. 341–345). London: E & FN Spon.

Bangsbo, J. (1994). The physiology of soccer with special reference to intense intermittent exercise. *Acta Physiologica Scandinavica, 151* (suppl. 619), 1–156.

Bangsbo, J. (1995). *Fitness training in football: A scientific approach.* Bagsvaerd, Denmark: HO+Storm.

Barr, S. I. (1999). Effects of dehydration on exercise performance. *Canadian Journal of Applied Physiology, 24,* 164–172.

Castagna, C., Abt, G., & D'Ottavio, S. (2004). Activity profile of international-level soccer referees during competitive matches. *Journal of Strength and Conditioning Research, 18,* 486–490.

Catterall, C., Reilly, T., Atkinson, G., & Coldwells, A. (1993). Analysis of the work rates and heart rates of association football referees. *British Journal of Sports Medicine, 27,* 193–196.

Da Silva, A. I., & Fernandez, R. (2003). Dehydration of football referees during a match. *British Journal of Sports Medicine, 37,* 502–506.

D'Ottavio, S., & Castagna, C. (2001). Physiological load imposed on elite soccer referees during actual match play. *Journal of Sports Medicine and Physical Fitness, 41,* 27–32.

Drust, B., Reilly, T., & Rienzi, E. (1998). Analysis of work rate in soccer. *Sports Exercise and Injury, 4,* 151–155.

Eissmann, H. J. (1994). The referee. In B. Ekblom (Ed.), *Football (soccer)* (pp. 100–101). Oxford: Blackwell Scientific.

Friedman, Z., & Klein, K. (1988). What are the physical activities of a soccer referee in the field. *Soccer Journal, 33* (4), 35–37.

Helsen, W., & Bultynck, J.B. (2004). Physical and perceptual-cognitive demands of top-class refereeing in association football. *Journal of Sports Sciences, 22,* 179–189.

Johnston, L., & McNaughton, L. (1994). The physiological requirements of soccer refereeing. *Australian Journal of Science and Medicine in Sport, 26* (3/4), 67–72.

Krustrup, P., & Bangsbo, J. (2001). Physiological demands of top-class soccer refereeing in relation to physical capacity: Effect of intense intermittent exercise training. *Journal of Sports Sciences, 19,* 881–891.

Krustrup, P., Mohr, M., & Bangsbo, J. (2002). Activity profile and physiological demands of top-class soccer assistant refereeing in relation to training status. *Journal of Sports Sciences, 20,* 861–871.

Rahnama, N., Reilly, T., & Lees, A. (2002). Injury risk associated with playing actions during competitive soccer. *British Journal of Sports Medicine, 36,* 354–359.

Reilly, T. (1997). Energetics of high intensity exercise (soccer): With particular reference to fatigue. *Journal of Sports Sciences, 5,* 257–263.

Reilly, T., & Bowen, T. (1984). Exertional costs of changes in directional modes of running. *Perceptual and Motor Skills, 58,* 149–150.

Reilly, T., & Smith, D. (1986). Effect of work intensity on performance in a psychomotor task during exercise. *Ergonomics, 29,* 601–606.

Reilly, T., & Thomas, V. (1976). A motion analysis of work-rate in different positional roles in professional football match-play. *Journal of Human Movement Studies, 2,* 87–97.

Reilly, T., & Thomas, V. (1979). Estimated daily energy expenditures of professional association footballers. *Ergonomics, 22,* 541–548.

Rienzi, E., Drust, B., Reilly, T., Carter, J. E. L., & Martin, A. (2000). Investigation of anthropometric and work-rate profiles of elite South American international soccer players. *Journal of Sports Medicine and Physical Fitness, 40,* 162–169.

Rontoyannis, G. P., Stalikas, A., Sarros, G., & Vlastaris, A. (1998). Medical, morphological and functional aspects of Greek football referees. *Journal of Sports Medicine and Physical Fitness, 38,* 208–214.

Saltin, B. (1973). Metabolic fundamentals in exercise. *Medicine and Science in Sports, 5,* 137–146.

Weston, M., Helsen, W., Bird, S., Nevill, A., & Castagna, C. (2005). The effect of match standard on objective and subjective demands on elite soccer players. *Journal of Sports Sciences, 23,* 189.

Weston, M., Helsen, W., MacMahon, C., & Kirkendall, D. (2004). The impact of specific high-intensity training sessions on football referees' fitness levels. *American Journal of Sports Medicine, 32* (suppl. 1), 54–615.

Index

Note: page numbers in *italics* refer to figures and tables.

An environmentally friendly book printed and bound in England by www.printondemand-worldwide.com

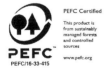

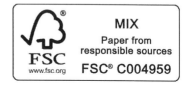

This book is made entirely of chain-of-custody materials; FSC materials for the cover and PEFC materials for the text pages.

#0086 - 300113 - C0 - 234/156/14 [16] - CB